Machine Learning and Data Analytics for Predicting, Managing, and Monitoring Disease

Manikant Roy
Lovely Professional University, India

Lovi Raj Gupta
Lovely Professional University, India

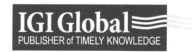

A volume in the Advances in Medical Technologies and Clinical Practice (AMTCP) Book Series

Published in the United States of America by
> IGI Global
> Medical Information Science Reference (an imprint of IGI Global)
> 701 E. Chocolate Avenue
> Hershey PA, USA 17033
> Tel: 717-533-8845
> Fax: 717-533-8661
> E-mail: cust@igi-global.com
> Web site: http://www.igi-global.com

Library of Congress Cataloging-in-Publication Data

Names: Roy, Manikant, 1989- editor. | Gupta, Lovi Raj, editor.
Title: Machine learning and data analytics for predicting, managing, and
  monitoring disease / Manikant Roy and Lovi Raj Gupta, editors.
Description: Hershey : Engineering Science Reference, [2022] | Includes
  bibliographical references and index. | Summary: "This book provides the
  recent various theoretical frameworks, empirical research and
  application of advanced analytics methods for disease detection,
  pandemic management, disease prediction etc. using the data analysis
  methods and their usages for taking timely decisions for prevention of
  such spread of pandemic and how people in government, society and
  administer can use these insights for overall management"-- Provided by
  publisher.
Identifiers: LCCN 2021027657 (print) | LCCN 2021027658 (ebook) | ISBN
  9781799871880 (hardcover) | ISBN 9781799871897 (paperback) | ISBN
  9781799871903 (ebook)
Subjects: LCSH: Epidemiology--Data processing. | Epidemics--Mathematical
  models. | Machine learning. | Artificial intelligence--Medical
  applications.
Classification: LCC RA652.2.M3 M33 2022 (print) | LCC RA652.2.M3 (ebook)
  | DDC 614.40285--dc23
LC record available at https://lccn.loc.gov/2021027657
LC ebook record available at https://lccn.loc.gov/2021027658

This book is published in the IGI Global book series Advances in Medical Technologies and Clinical Practice (AMTCP) (ISSN: 2327-9354; eISSN: 2327-9370)

British Cataloguing in Publication Data
A Cataloguing in Publication record for this book is available from the British Library.

For electronic access to this publication, please contact: eresources@igi-global.com.

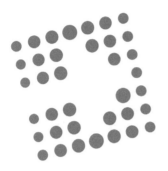

Advances in Medical Technologies and Clinical Practice (AMTCP) Book Series

Srikanta Patnaik
SOA University, India
Priti Das
S.C.B. Medical College, India

ISSN:2327-9354
EISSN:2327-9370

Mission

Medical technological innovation continues to provide avenues of research for faster and safer diagnosis and treatments for patients. Practitioners must stay up to date with these latest advancements to provide the best care for nursing and clinical practices.

The **Advances in Medical Technologies and Clinical Practice (AMTCP) Book Series** brings together the most recent research on the latest technology used in areas of nursing informatics, clinical technology, biomedicine, diagnostic technologies, and more. Researchers, students, and practitioners in this field will benefit from this fundamental coverage on the use of technology in clinical practices.

Coverage

- Clinical Studies
- Clinical Nutrition
- Medical Imaging
- E-Health
- Patient-Centered Care
- Clinical Data Mining
- Biomechanics
- Clinical High-Performance Computing
- Nutrition
- Neural Engineering

IGI Global is currently accepting manuscripts for publication within this series. To submit a proposal for a volume in this series, please contact our Acquisition Editors at Acquisitions@igi-global.com or visit: http://www.igi-global.com/publish/.

Titles in this Series

For a list of additional titles in this series, please visit:
http://www.igi-global.com/book-series/advances-medical-technologies-clinical-practice/73682.

Advancing the Investigation and Treatment of Sleep Disorders Using AI
M. Rajesh Kumar (Vellore Institute of Technology, Vellore, India) Ranjeet Kumar (Vellore Institute of Technology, Vellore, India) and D. Vaithiyanathan (National Institute of Technology, Vellor, India)
Medical Information Science Reference • © 2021 • 291pp • H/C (ISBN: 9781799880189) • US $345.00

Machine Learning in Cancer Research With Applications in Colon Cancer and Big Data Analysis
Zhongyu Lu (University of Huddersfield, UK) Qiang Xu (University of Huddersfield, UK) Murad Al-Rajab (University of Huddersfield, UK & Abu Dhabi University, UAE) and Lamogha Chiazor (University of Huddersfield, UK)
Medical Information Science Reference • © 2021 • 263pp • H/C (ISBN: 9781799873167) • US $345.00

Handbook of Research on Nano-Strategies for Combatting Antimicrobial Resistance and Cancer
Muthupandian Saravanan (Mekelle University, Ethiopia & Saveetha Dental College, Saveetha Institute of Medical and Technical Sciences (SIMATS), India) Venkatraman Gopinath (University of Malaya, Malaysia) and Karthik Deekonda (Monash University, Malaysia)
Medical Information Science Reference • © 2021 • 559pp • H/C (ISBN: 9781799850496) • US $375.00

Handbook of Research on Solving Modern Healthcare Challenges With Gamification
Ricardo Alexandre Peixoto de Queirós (uniMAD, Escola Superior de Media Artes e Design, Portugal) and António José Marques (LabRP, School of Health, Polytechnic of Porto, Portugal)
Medical Information Science Reference • © 2021 • 382pp • H/C (ISBN: 9781799874720) • US $425.00

Diagnostic Applications of Health Intelligence and Surveillance Systems
Divakar Yadav (National Institute of Technology, Hamirpur, India) Abhay Bansal (Amity University, India) Madhulika Bhatia (Amity University, India) Madhurima Hooda (Amity University, India) and Jorge Morato (Universidad Carlos III de Madrid, Spain)
Medical Information Science Reference • © 2021 • 332pp • H/C (ISBN: 9781799865278) • US $285.00

AI Innovation in Medical Imaging Diagnostics
Kalaivani Anbarasan (Department of Computer Science and Engineering, Saveetha School of Engineering, India & Saveetha Institute of Medical and Technical Sciences, Chennai, India)
Medical Information Science Reference • © 2021 • 248pp • H/C (ISBN: 9781799830924) • US $345.00

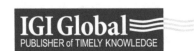

701 East Chocolate Avenue, Hershey, PA 17033, USA
Tel: 717-533-8845 x100 • Fax: 717-533-8661
E-Mail: cust@igi-global.com • www.igi-global.com

Editorial Advisory Board

Table of Contents

Detailed Table of Contents

Neurological disorders are diseases of the central and peripheral nervous system and most commonly affect middle- or old-age people. Accurate classification and early-stage prediction of such disorders are very crucial for prompt diagnosis and treatment. This chapter discusses a new framework that uses image processing techniques for detecting neurological disorders so that clinicians prevent irreversible changes that may occur in the brain. The newly proposed framework ensures reliable and accurate machine learning techniques using visual saliency algorithms to process brain magnetic resonance imaging (MRI). The authors also provide ample hints and dimensions for the researchers interested in using visual saliency features for disease prediction and detection.

The growth of COVID-19 (SARS-CoV-2) in India has been rampant. Despite having a relatively small value of R0, the spread of disease increases exponentially every consecutive day. This chapter aims to analyze and conduct a concise study for the southern state of Tamil Nadu in India and build non-linear predictive models that evaluate the transmission of coronavirus amongst locals. A logistic regression and SIR model are deployed to understand the potential spread of disease. Through descriptive analysis on theoretical segmented portions, districts in Tamil Nadu with a higher number of confirmed cases are identified. Computation of crude mortality rate, infection fatality rate, predictive models, illustrations, and their results are discussed analytically.

# Chapter 3

India, with a population of over 1.38 billion, is facing high number of daily COVID-19 confirmed cases. In this chapter, the authors have applied ARIMA model (auto-regressive integrated moving average) to predict daily confirmed COVID-19 cases in India. Detailed univariate time series analysis was conducted on daily confirmed data from 19.03.2020 to 28.07.2020, and the predictions from the model were satisfactory with root mean square error (RSME) of 7,103. Data for this study was obtained from various reliable sources, including the Ministry of Health and Family Welfare (MoHFW) and http://covid19india.org/. The model identified was ARIMA(1,1,1) based on time series decomposition, autocorrelation function (ACF), and partial autocorrelation function (PACF).

# Chapter 4

COVID-19 is a major pandemic disease exploited in this century in the whole world. COVID-19 was started om Wuhan, China in November 2019. The main reason for spreading this disease was that test kits were not available in huge amounts to diagnose the COVID-19, and no vaccine was available to cure this disease. Many researchers are trying to make a vaccine for the treatment of this disease. Prevention is better than cure. Therefore, prevention from this epidemic disease is diagnosis at early stages, and treatment should be given to the patient at an accurate time so that patient can escape death. Millions of people were infected by this disease, and most of them lost their lives after suffering from this disease. As we all know, this disease diagnosis test is complicated. Therefore, many smart apps like Siri, Cova App, Arogya Setu App, etc. and digital systems are used to detect and diagnose cases of infected people. These systems are embedded with artificial intelligence techniques. For diagnosis, the COVID-19 computer tomography is based on deep learning convolutional neural network.

# Chapter 5

Recognizing landmarks in images with machine learning is an excellent topic for research today. Landmark recognition is an important field in computer vision. In this field, we train the machine learning models to identify and recognize the closed distinctly distinguishable objects in a digital image. In general, if we consider a digital image to be a set of coordinates of different pixels, a landmark is said to be enclosed in that closed polygon formed by the pixels that may be considered as a distinct and distinguishable thing in one or the other sense. Landmark recognition is an important subject area of image classification since it is considered as one of the first steps towards reaching complete computer vision. The extremely broad definition of a landmark makes it eligible to be considered as one of the leading problems in image classification tasks. Since the task is considered to be a very broad one, the solutions to the task hold no easy procedures. This chapter explores landmark recognition using ensemble-based machine learning models.

Chapter 6

Sukanta Ghosh, Lovely Professional University, India
Amar Singh, Lovely Professional University, India

Facial expression recognition is an activity that is performed by every human in their day-to-day lives. Each one of us analyses the expressions of the individuals we interact with to understand how people interact and respond with us. The malicious intentions of a thief or a person to be interviewed can be recognized with the help of his facial features and gestures. Face recognition from picture or video is a well-known point in biometrics inquiry. Numerous open places, for the most part, have reconnaissance cameras, and these cameras have their noteworthy security incentives. It is generally recognized that face recognition has assumed a significant job in reconnaissance framework. The genuine favorable circumstances of face-based distinguishing proof over different biometrics are uniqueness. Since the human face is a unique item having a high level of inconstancy in its appearance, face location is a troublesome issue in computer vision. This chapter explores emotion detection using facial images.

Chapter 7

Megha Nain, Manipal University Jaipur, India
Shilpa Sharma, Manipal University Jaipur, India
Sandeep Chaurasia, Manipal University Jaipur, India

The pandemic corona virus disease (COVID-19) caused by the virus 'SARS-CoV-2' continues affecting the health and affluence of the worldwide population. The role of artificial intelligence in improving safety and health conditions has been studied in the chapter. The various fields of artificial intelligence such as machine learning, computer vision, deep learning, and natural language processing are contributing to almost every field ranging from healthcare, agriculture, automotive, astronomy, and many others. For overcoming a global outbreak such as COVID-19, conventional approaches are not feasible enough, and therefore the requirement for the more robust and automated techniques for making predictions in advance is essential. The vision of this chapter is to assess and survey the impact of artificial intelligence-based approaches in the management of pandemics and recommend procedures for the enhancement of the currently used techniques along with the imminent research areas in artificial intelligence for controlling pandemics.

Chapter 8

Anoop V. S., Rajagiri College of Social Sciences (Autonomous), Kochi, Kerala, India

Health informatics deals with applying informatics to medicine and healthcare that aims to store, process, and retrieve large amounts of healthcare data to enable optimal collaboration between different stakeholders. This has several applications in the healthcare domain from extracting information from medical documents such as case reports and prescriptions to analyzing data from sensors available in wearable devices. Recent advancements in information and communication technologies fueled the need of devising intelligent technologies for analyzing such data – not only in various forms but also in large quantities. This has posed many challenges and opportunities to use techniques such as text mining, natural language processing (NLP), and deep learning to unearth the latent themes from the vast array of textual data. This chapter proposes some prominent works in health informatics that use text mining and NLP and also discusses some active research areas in these dimensions. This chapter will be useful to understand the recent advancements and future research dimensions.

Sukanta Ghosh, School of Computer Applications, Lovely Professional University, India
Shubhanshu Arya, School of Computer Application, Lovely Professional University, India
Amar Singh, School of Computer Application, Lovely Professional University, India

Agricultural production is one of the main factors affecting a country's domestic market situation. Many problems are the reasons for estimating crop yields, which vary in different parts of the world. Overuse of chemical fertilizers, uneven distribution of rainfall, and uneven soil fertility lead to plant diseases. This forces us to focus on effective methods for detecting plant diseases. It is important to find an effective plant disease detection technique. Plants need to be monitored from the beginning of their life cycle to avoid such diseases. Observation is a kind of visual observation, which is time-consuming, costly, and requires a lot of experience. For speeding up this process, it is necessary to automate the disease detection system. A lot of researchers have developed plant leaf detection systems based on various technologies. In this chapter, the authors discuss the potential of methods for detecting plant leaf diseases. It includes various steps such as image acquisition, image segmentation, feature extraction, and classification.

Rahul Sharma, Lovely Professional University, India
Amar Singh, Lovely Professional University, India

Agriculture is one of the important sources of earning worldwide. With the rapid expansion of the human population and food security for all, the agriculture sector needs to be boosted to increase the yield. Agriculture is the prime source of livelihood in India for more than 50% of the total population. As per Indian agriculture and allied industries industry report, agriculture is one of the major contributors in gross value. Agricultural crops suffer heavy losses due to insect damage and plant diseases. Worldwide, out of the crop losses, major losses are caused by plant pests. In this chapter, various image pre-processing methods and the need of pre-preprocessing are discussed in detail. For image classification, TensorFlow deep neural network is presented. Deep learning model is used for automatic and early detection of paddy pests. Early detection of the pests will aid farmers in adopting necessary preventive measures. Multiple ways to reduce overfitting during model training are also suggested.

Gowhar Mohiuddin Dar, Lovely Professional University, India
Ashok Sharma, University of Jammu, India
Parveen Singh, Government SPMR College of Commerce, Jammu, India

The chapter explores the implications of deep learning in medical sciences, focusing on deep learning concerning natural language processing, computer vision, reinforcement learning, big data, and blockchain influence on some areas of medicine and construction of end-to-end systems with the help of these computational techniques. The deliberation of computer vision in the study is mainly concerned with medical imaging and further usage of natural language processing to spheres such as electronic wellbeing record data. Application of deep learning in genetic mapping and DNA sequencing termed as genomics and implications of reinforcement learning about surgeries assisted by robots are also overviewed.

Chapter 12

Developments in machine learning techniques for classification and regression exposed the access of detecting sophisticated patterns from various domain-penetrating data. In biomedical applications, enormous amounts of medical data are produced and collected to predict disease type and stage of the disease. Detection and prediction of diseases, such as diabetes, lung cancer, brain cancer, heart disease, and liver diseases, requires huge tests and that increases the size of patient medical data. Robust prediction of a patient's disease from the huge data set is an important agenda in in this chapter. The challenge of applying a machine learning method is to select the best algorithm within the disease prediction framework. This chapter opts for robust machine learning algorithms for various diseases by using case studies. This usually analyzes each dimension of disease, independently checking the identified value between the limits to monitor the condition of the disease.

Chapter 13

The global pandemic has led to an undeniable surge in using digital technologies due to the social distancing norms and nationwide lockdowns. Firms and organizations are conforming to the new culture of work and life. The use of internet services, digital devices, and cloud systems has seen surges in usage from 40% to 100%, compared to pre-lockdown levels. With the rapid growth of this technological use, people are exposing their digital assets, presence, and behavior out to the binary world where AI-driven data analysis algorithms, data-gathering systems, and spyware are continuously monitoring their behavior. These subconsciously exposed data are then carried forward for delivering customized ads and recommend features.

Chapter 14

COVID-19 is very dynamic in nature, and it is varying drastically with time, and this requires continuous monitoring of the situation for better resource management during the pandemic such as medical facilities and daily necessities. The situation needs to be evaluated on a regular interval by all the stakeholders such as all the government officials for making strategic decisions such as lockdown or lifting lockdown in a phase-wise manner. In order to manage pandemics such as COVID-19, the administration needs to know statistical information, trends, forecasting, and overall aggregated real-time information, and this can be achieved through a well-designed dashboard. A dashboard is used for efficient monitoring of continuously evolving situations, and it provides an overall picture in addition to historical information.

This chapter proposes a real-time dashboard design for COVID-19, and it will provide insight about different elements such as design and application of the dashboard in pandemic management.

    Mansha Sharma, Mithibai College, Mumbai University, India
    Ajay Kumar Sharma, Human Resource Development Centre, Lovely Professional University,
      India

Coronavirus has come up as the worst nightmare in the form of a pandemic for progressive sapiens in terms of health, wealth, prosperity, and social wellbeing. To date, coronavirus has mutated to seven different shapes evolving into various variants. The main deliberation of catching the disease is carelessness and negligence of the citizens, and in developing countries like India, population and illiteracy makes it even more difficult to control the disease. However, immunity can be the superhero in fighting against the virus that invades the host. Although a strong immunity is important to fight the disease, the symptoms show at a later stage by the body of a human with a stronger immunity and cases are getting critical in this case. After a long struggle, scientists have come up with vaccines that are 90% efficient and show some side effects. The world is expected to function only if 'herd immunity' is achieved, but it is expected that wearing masks would be the new normal.

Preface

Machine Learning, Data Analytics are no longer buzz word in media news. The Analytics ecosystem is now all-pervading. Be it entertainment, eCommerce, industry 4.0, you can find the application of Analytics. The entire cutting-edge technology is mature enough to provide real-time benefits.

This book presents the various method and techniques of Artificial Intelligence, Machine Learning for Diseases prediction, monitoring, diagnosis, etc. Students in undergraduate, graduate, faculty members, and those who want to use the cutting-edge technology application in their research will find the helpful book. They will also find many ideas for managing pandemic-like situations using a data-driven approach.

Chapter 1: This chapter discusses how neurological disorders diseases can be diagnosed by collecting MRI data and applying Machine Learning techniques to detect such conditions promptly and help the early treatment.

Chapter 2: Managing the pandemic situation is very difficult yet very important, applying a data-driven model to understand the spread of disease and how to control it. This chapter proposes SIR Model and Logistics regression for COVID 19 prediction.

Chapter 3: The data-driven approach in pandemic-like situations helps everyone, be it citizens, administrators, and Government officials, to be prepared for handling and managing the resources.

Chapter 4: This chapter explores the application of computer tomography & Artificial Intelligence for the detection of COVID -19. As we all know, this disease diagnosis test is complicated; hence applying cutting-edge technology can help in early and accurate detection.

Chapter 5: This chapter covers the deep learning-based model for landmark recognition in images and as its one of the critical areas in image processing & Computer Vision.

Chapter 6: This chapter provides deep learning for detecting emotion in an image by extracting facial expressions. It can be used in various places for security over traditional biometric authentication.

Chapter 7: This chapter explains how the artificial intelligence can be applied for safety measures and providing the preventive recommendations.

Chapter 8: The utilization of AI through (ML) and natural language processing (NLP) can bring a colossal measure of significant worth across the current medical services continuum to the conveyance of further developed results. This chapter presents health informatics as an important field of study.

Chapter 9: This chapter presents the Track down a compelling plant illness identification procedure. Plants should be checked from the start of their life cycle to keep away from such sicknesses. Perception is a sort of visual perception, which is tedious, expensive, and requires a ton of involvement. For accelerating this interaction, it is essential to robotize the illness discovery framework.

Chapter 10: This chapter is about a profound learning model for programmed and early paddy bugs. Early discovery of the bugs will help ranchers in receiving essential preventive measures. Various approaches to diminish overfitting during model preparation are likewise recommended.

Chapter 11: This chapter provides direction for use of profound learning in hereditary planning and DNA sequencing named genomics and Implications of support finding out about medical procedures helped by robots.

Chapter 12: This chapter is to monitoring disease; this usually analyzes each dimension of disease, independently checking the identified value between the limits to monitor the condition of the disease.

Chapter 13: This chapter highlights the importance of data privacy in today's era. Data Protection is an integral part of any analytical process.

Chapter 14: This chapter proposes a real-time dashboard design for Covid-19, and it will provide insight into different elements such as the design and application of the dashboard in pandemic management.

Chapter 15: This chapter provides a pragmatic view of the effect of Corona Virus in our life.

This entire book presents the state of art methods, techniques for managing the pandemic, detecting disease.

Acknowledgment

At the outset, I would like to express my sincere thanks to Professor (Dr.) Lovi Raj Gupta, Executive Dean, Faculty of Technology & Sciences, Lovely Professional University (LPU), Punjab, India, allowed me to work under his guidance and belief in me. We want to thank IGI Global for providing the opportunity to contribute through this edited book. I also take this opportunity to thank all the authors who contributed to the book's development and sharing their knowledge. We would also like to acknowledge all participants of the "Online Short-Term course on Pandemic Analytics using Machine Learning – 2020" held at Lovely Professional University Punjab, India, and all the members of at Academic Staff College, LPU, India.

I am deeply indebted to my mother Smt. Lal Roy for always inspiring me to explore the new horizon in life with unconditional support. Thanks to my wife Rita Roy & son Medhansh Kant Roy for giving me uninterrupted time to focus on my work. Special thanks to Santosh Kumar for everything.

Manikant Roy

Lovi Raj Gupta

Chapter 1
Prediction of Neurological Disorders Using Visual Saliency:
Current Trends and Future Directions

Sreelakshmi S.
Indian Institute of Information Technology and Management - Kerala (IIITM-K), Thiruvananthapuram, India

Anoop V. S.
Rajagiri College of Social Sciences (Autonomous), Kochi, India

ABSTRACT

Neurological disorders are diseases of the central and peripheral nervous system and most commonly affect middle- or old-age people. Accurate classification and early-stage prediction of such disorders are very crucial for prompt diagnosis and treatment. This chapter discusses a new framework that uses image processing techniques for detecting neurological disorders so that clinicians prevent irreversible changes that may occur in the brain. The newly proposed framework ensures reliable and accurate machine learning techniques using visual saliency algorithms to process brain magnetic resonance imaging (MRI). The authors also provide ample hints and dimensions for the researchers interested in using visual saliency features for disease prediction and detection.

INTRODUCTION

Neurological disorders are medically defined as disorders that affect the brain as well as the nerves found throughout the human body and the spinal cord. Structural, biochemical, or electrical abnormalities in the brain, spinal cord, or other nerves can result in a range of symptoms. Machine learning (ML) techniques have influenced all aspects of human life and neurology is no exception to this growing trend. Modern medical imaging techniques are powered by ML and several ML architectures are using this ability to analyze medical data in disease prevention, diagnosis, and patient monitoring. Visual saliency detection is a crucial application of medical image processing, and it made a considerable movement in the easy

DOI: 10.4018/978-1-7998-7188-0.ch001

and accurate diagnosis of the disease. The visual saliency algorithms predict eye fixations on a visual scene and it improves the accuracy of complex scene analysis. These algorithms have shown tremendous improvements over the classic models on disease prediction and perform close to the human observer. This chapter discusses the current trends in visual saliency-based approaches for predicting neurological disorders and throws light on the future directions on the same. A new framework for detecting and predicting a neurological disorder using visual saliency is also proposed in this chapter. This chapter will act as a guideline that provides ample hints and dimensions for the researchers and academicians interested in using visual saliency features to detect and predict neurological disorders.

BACKGROUND

Neurological Disorders

Neurological disorders are among the most common diseases of this age, and their global prevalence has increased over the past decades. Neurological disorders are brain and nervous system disorders including Alzheimer's, brain tumors, dementia, depression, epilepsy, memory loss, stroke, psychotic, and Parkinson's disease, to mention but a few. The exact reason for these may vary but can include genetic disorders, congenital abnormalities or disorders, infections, lifestyle or environmental health problems including malnutrition, and brain injury, spinal cord injury, or nerve injury. The World Health Organization (WHO) indicated that hundreds of millions of people worldwide are affected by neurological disorders (Bali & Garba, 2021). These disorders increase the mortality rate, disability rate, and have a significant effect on global economies. The WHO has provided the latest global health estimates that Alzheimer's, Stroke and heart neurological disorders are among the top 5 global causes of death and the top 5 global causes of disability-adjusted life years in 2020. An early and accurate diagnosis can reduce the progression of disorders, But unfortunately, no such strategies or devices are available for accurate early detection. But researchers are making an effort to find appropriate treatment for these disorders which can improve the quality of life for both the patients and their families.

Neurological disorders are the most challenging to diagnose, manage and monitor due to the complex nervous system. Diagnosis of neurological diseases and their treatments demand high precision, dedication, and experience. Nowadays, modern technology and systems allow neurologists to provide proper neurological care (Siuly & Zhang, 2016). Recently, varieties of advanced diagnosis technologies (figure.1) have been used to detect, manage and treat neurological diseases, such as Magnetic Resonance Imaging, Magnetoencephalography, Positron Emission Tomography, Computed Axial Tomography, Diffuse Optical Imaging, etc. to name a few.

Structural MRI (sMRI) and Functional MRI (fMRI) are the most commonly used imaging modalities for classifying neurological disorders. Magnetic Resonance Imaging (MRI) is a non-invasive imaging technique used to capture both the anatomical structures and the functional signatures of the brain. It is based on the principle of Nuclear Magnetic Resonance (NMR). It uses magnetic fields and radio waves to produce detailed images of the brain and other organs. Structural MRI qualitatively and quantitatively describes the size, shape, and integrity of the brain's y and white matter structures. It can also measure volumes of brain regions and sub-regions and identify any localized lesions. In contrast to Functional MRI which is used to map the physiological mechanisms of the brain over time, structural MRI is static and captures only anatomical information. Figure 2 shows the MRI sequence of normal brain and dis-

Figure 1. Neuroimaging modalities a) MRI b) fMRI c) CT d) DTI e) PET f) TMS

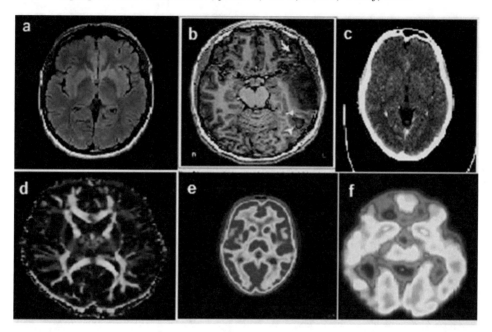

eased brain. The first row (a,b,c) contains the normal brain MRI images and the second row contains the corresponding d) Alzheimer's affected,e) tumorous, f) stroke affected MR images.

Visual Saliency

Visual saliency detection is an important application of medical image processing and it simulates the human visual system to perceive the scene. Recently it made a considerable movement in the easy and accurate diagnosis of several diseases. The visual saliency map highlights relevant visual patterns in an image, possibly associated with objects or specific concepts. The analysis of medical images allows the radiologist or clinical expert to focus the attention on image abnormalities or specific patterns that could suggest the presence of pathology (Daza & Rueda, 2016). In clinical practice, visual assessment and analysis is the most widely used method for brain atrophy evaluation. The radiologists focus attention on brain regions susceptible to change in specific dementia and then achieve structured reporting of these findings. The development of an automated approach for objective visual interpretation could potentially augment the visual skills of radiologists by extracting image features that may be relevant to the diagnostic. This also makes diagnosis easier for clinicians without the expertise to extract diagnostically useful information. The visual assessment strategies used by radiologists for neurological disorder diagnosis consist usually in restricting eye movements to some regions of interest in the image while scrolling through slices of a given MRI projection. This visual search is guided by the so-called "visual attention" which is the cognitive process of selectively attending to a Region of Interest (ROI) while filtering out irrelevant information. In a second step, the clinician identifies relationships between the perceived patterns and possible diagnosis.

The visual computational models have been used to characterize ROIs in natural images, but their investigation in medical images for computer aided-diagnosis has remained very limited. Modeling clinician

Figure 2. Normal vs. affected brain MRIs

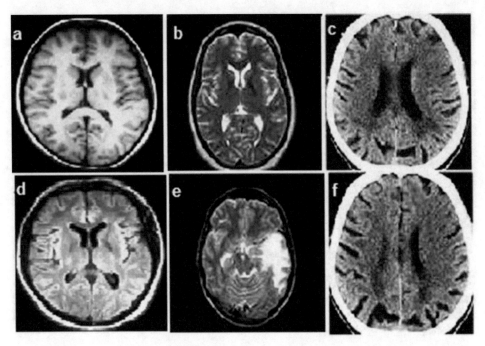

visual attention by reading medical images can automate pathology detection and diagnosis processes. In the context of medical images, the bottom-up influences correspond to image features whereas top-down influences correspond to the knowledge and expertise of radiologists. Saliency-based methods for

Figure 3. Brain MRIs vs the corresponding saliency maps a) Normal brain b) Tumorous brain c) Par-kinson's affected brain

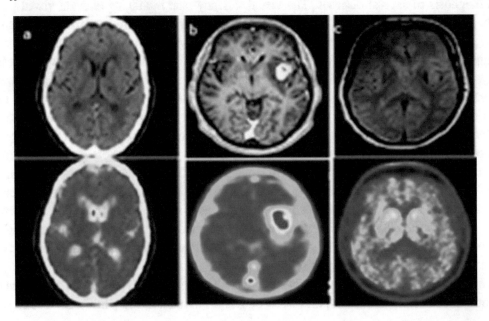

computer-aided diagnosis have attracted much attention for brain abnormality detection and suspicious regions identification(Ben-Ahmed et al., 2017). Figure 3 showcased the MRI images of a normal brain, Tumor affected brain, and Parkinson's diseased brain, and their visual saliency mapping respectively.

RELATED WORK

There are several approaches reported very recently in the medical image processing literature on visual saliency detection. Some of the very prominent approaches that are closely related to the idea discussed in this chapter are given in this section. Gadgil et al., (Gadgil et al., 2021) developed a semi-supervised method for multi-pathology segmentation using visual saliency that leverages the benefits of both available medical image classification models and expert pixel-level annotations. Han et al., (Han et al., 2021) proposed a new deep learning approach using saliency detection and aims to improve the utility of prosthetic vision for people blinded from retinal degenerative diseases. Serte et al., (Serte & Serener, 2021) introduced a new graph-based saliency region detection for early and advanced glaucoma classification. Sran et al., (Sran et al., 2020) proposed an efficient non-uniform compression algorithm based on visual saliency that emulates the human visual system. This hybrid technique has two phases, first, the automatic saliency-based Fuzzy C-Means clustering algorithm is designed for Region of Interest (ROI) detection and extraction, and the second phase, the encoding of ROI and the background are carried out using the SPIHT algorithm at a high and low bit rate respectively. Verma et al., (Verma et al., 2020) proposed a saliency-based model to detect Covid-19 positive cases from x-ray images. Kundu et al., (Kundu et al., 2020) proposed a least-square saliency transformation model for detecting multiple Gastrointestinal diseases from WCE (Wireless capsule endoscopy) videos. Wei et al., (Wei et al., 2020) proposed a deep convolutional neural network model specialized in atypical visual saliency for predicting autism spectrum disorders. Mehran et al., (Mehran & Saraf Esmaili, 2020) proposed a new method based on the graph-based visual saliency model, along with the watershed segmentation algorithm and region growing algorithm to detect optic disc area in retinal fundus images have been suggested to help diagnose eye diseases including glaucoma. Ferreira et al., (Ferreira et al., 2019) proposed a CNN-based system for cell image classification, which first identifies critical cells using a saliency prediction algorithm and later classifies the ROI. They provide evidence that classification systems driven by saliency methods trained on expert's attention data are a viable strategy in cell analysis.

Adeel et al., (Adeel et al., 2019) proposed an automated system based on a novel saliency approach for segmentation and recognition of grape leaf diseases. Pesce et al., (Pesce et al., 2019) introduced two novel neural network architectures for the detection of chest radiographs containing pulmonary lesions. Both architectures make use of a large number of weakly labeled images combined with a smaller number of manually annotated x-rays. The annotated lesions are used during training to deliver a type of visual attention feedback informing the networks about their lesion localization performance. Ali Borji et al., (Borji, 2018) conducted a detailed survey on the landscape of the field emphasizing new deep saliency models, benchmarks, and datasets. And proposed several avenues for future research. Banerjee et al., (Banerjee et al., 2018) presented a novel approach for the reliable, automated, and accurate 3D segmentation of brain tumors from multi-sequence magnetic resonance images using visual saliency. And the tumor volume, detected using visual saliency, is evaluated in three dimensions for small as well as large ROIs and/or VOIs.Mitra et al., (Mitra et al., 2017) developed a new algorithmic approach to the detection of saliency in a three-dimensional multi-channel MR image sequence for the glioblastoma multiforme.

Zou X et al., (Zou et al., 2016) introduced a learning-based visual saliency model method for detecting diagnostic diabetic macular edema (DME) regions of interest in the retinal image. The new visual saliency model using the Bayesian probability theory and machine learning techniques. The method presented the cognitive process of visual selection of relevant regions that arise during an ophthalmologist's image examination. Banerjee et al.,(Banerjee et al., 2016) designed a novel framework based on visual saliency used for the identification of tumor regions from MR images of the brain. This model is designed by taking cues from the concept of visual saliency in natural scenes and it improves the accuracy of automatic detection techniques. Mahapatra et al.,(Mahapatra et al., 2016) proposed a novel algorithmic approach that calculates saliency values for every image pixel at multiple scales to capture global and local image information. This approach also extracts the generalized image information in an unsupervised manner using convolutional neural networks. Rueda et al., (Rueda et al., 2013) proposed a new method to build up a saliency map for the classification of brain Magnetic Resonance (MR) images from healthy and diseased subjects. The saliency map extracts regions of relative change in three different dimensions: intensity, orientation, and edges. The proposed framework employs a segmentation approach with the classification phase so that better classification and prediction of neurological disorders will be possible. The proposed framework is explained in detail in the subsequent sections.

PREDICTION OF NEUROLOGICAL DISORDERS USING VISUAL SALIENCY

The concept of the proposed framework is based on visual saliency prediction, which is an important task in computer vision and image processing. Research on human vision can effectively solve application problems in computer vision. And scientists have become interested in its capability to find objects or regions representing a scene, which is generally referred to as saliency detection. Saliency detection is generally described as the automatic estimation of significant (salient) objects and regions of images without any prior assumption or knowledge. Saliency usually is described as the difference between a pixel and its surrounding neighborhood. In addition, saliency models (i.e., models of saliency detection) include visual models, purely computational models, and their combination. Purely computational models do not consider the visual characteristics of the human eye whereas others do. Generally, more attention is on visual models, which can be roughly classified into two categories: attention models (predicting fixation points) and salient region detection models (highlighting the whole salient object areas). The former uses the selective visual attention mechanism to dynamically sample the important visual content in the scene. These models acquire a series of visual fixation points which locate the salient objects. The latter detects and segments the whole object or region (Li et al., 2018).

Here, the authors introduced a novel framework for predicting neurological disorders using visual saliency techniques. The model progresses through different stages and finally, it will predict whether the given data is affected or not. The major advantage of this model is incorporating the segmentation algorithm in this framework. The block diagram of the proposed work is given in figure.4.

Diagnosis of neurological disorders can be made by imaging modalities MRI/CT/PET/DTI and by physical examination. This proposed work comprises image acquisition, preprocessing of the images, saliency map generation and segmentation of affected area which is highlighted by saliency map, and classification of data into affected or normal classes. The process starts by collecting the brain images and after that needs to preprocess the images. The image pre-processing is done to remove the unwanted labels present in the image and enhance brain regions. To remove the unnecessary details of the brain

Figure 4. Overall workflow of the proposed framework

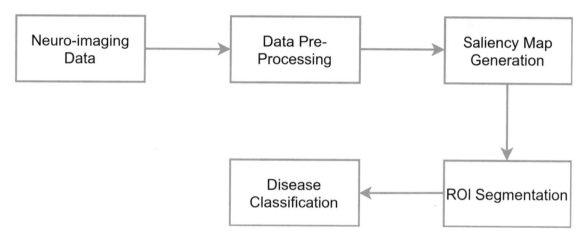

images that might cause the model to learn unneeded features. The authors suggest performing skull stripping for removing unwanted labels and other noises. And it also helps to remove the skull(cranium) and other non-brain areas from the input image. To enhance the edges of neuroimages, there are lots of image processing techniques available. Image enhancement is the method of improving the quality and information content of original data and it improves the accuracy of segmentation and classification. Histogram equalization, filtering, morphological operations are some of the major image enhancement techniques widely used in the brain image processing field.

The next stage of the proposed work is the generation of a visual saliency map. A saliency map is an image in which the brightness of a pixel represents how salient the pixel is i.e brightness of a pixel is directly proportional to its saliency. It is generally a grayscale image. Saliency maps are also called a heat map where hotness refers to those regions of the image which have a big impact on predicting the class which the object belongs to. The purpose of the saliency map is to find the regions which are prominent or noticeable at every location in the visual field and to guide the selection of attended locations, based on the spatial distribution of saliency. Each image has basic features like color, orientation, and intensity is extracted from the image. These processed images are used to create Gaussian pyramids to create features Maps. A saliency map is created by taking the mean of all the feature maps. Researchers can adapt any suitable method for generating a saliency map. The concept of visual saliency is employed to enable the algorithms to quickly focus on the ROI.

A crucial and important stage of the framework is the segmentation of the affected area/region of interest(ROI). Brain image segmentation is an essential task in many clinical applications because it influences the outcome of the entire analysis. This is because different processing steps rely on the accurate segmentation of anatomical regions. Image segmentation aims to divide an image into a set of semantically meaningful, homogeneous, and non-overlapping regions of similar attributes such as intensity, depth, color, or texture. The segmentation result is either an image of labels identifying each homogeneous region or a set of contours that describe the region boundaries.

The final stage of the proposed approach is the classification. Classifying an image according to its visual content is referred to as image classification. The process of classification is to sort all pixels in a digital image into several classes.

Figure 5. The workflow of the proposed framework on brain tumor detection

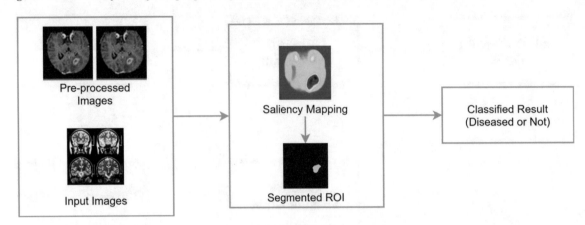

The Authors try to demonstrate the proposed framework on MRI images for brain tumor detection. The steps followed by the authors are given below;

1. Collecting neuroimaging data from an MRI scanner.
2. Performing preprocessing on the input data. Removing the skull and other non-brain regions is done with the help of FreeSurfer software. Performing other noise removal and edge enhancement using the median adaptive filtering technique.
3. Generating the saliency map of the preprocessed data using the pseudo-coloring strategy. The pseudo-coloring strategy for MR images efficiently generates the saliency map for highlighting the location of the tumor.
4. After computing the saliency, the authors performed the segmentation using watershed segmentation techniques. Watershed segmentation is an advanced region-based technique that utilizes image morphology.
5. In the end, the authors performed the classification and successfully classified the brain images into normal and affected classes. Logistic Regression, Naive Bayes, K-Nearest Neighbors, Decision Tree, Support Vector Machines, and artificial neural networks are the best classifiers used in machine learning algorithms.

Other saliency-based approaches first generate and compute saliency and then passes the same to the classifier. The major issue with these approaches is that the classifiers may not work well on noisy data and the wrongly identified regions while computing the saliency. The proposed approach incorporates a segmentation process before the classification phase that segments the ROI from the saliency. Thus this approach can better classify images into normal and affected classes and this will help identify neurological disorders. This will save a lot of time in analyzing medical data to find out potential neurological disorders. To verify and establish the usability of the proposed approach, the authors have applied the proposed framework for classifying Brain MRI images into tumourous and non-tumorous classes with real-life datasets. The end results are promising and the authors have identified significant improvements in the accuracy of the classification tasks. This will throw light on further research and discussions on using the proposed approach for medical image analysis and prediction of neurological disorders.

SOME POTENTIAL RESEARCH DIMENSIONS

Brain image analysis and disorder classification is a challenging and time-consuming task for clinicians. This is due to the very complex structure of the human brain and the nervous system. There were several approaches reported in the recent literature on classifying and predicting neurological disorders, that use different approaches, with varying degrees of success. The visual saliency-based approach was one among them that got significant attention among medical image processing researchers. Even though these approaches work well to some extent on identifying the disorders, there is much scope for further research to improve the accuracy. In this dimension, the authors list the following avenues for further research.

1. Using deep learning architecture for better segmentation and classification of neurological disorders using visual saliency.
2. Usage of pre-trained models such as U-Net and VGG-Net for better segmentation of medical images is a dimension worth exploring. The major advantage of these pre-trained models is that they will work with large datasets.
3. Semantic segmentation is an emerging segmentation technique that has many advantages over traditional segmentation algorithms. Incorporating semantic segmentation techniques with saliency computing would be an interesting research dimension.
4. Apart from Brain images, the proposed framework can be extended for the detection of abnormalities from the lung, heart, and other parts of the human body.

CONCLUSION

This chapter proposes a framework for the classification and prediction of neurological disorders using a visual saliency-based machine learning approach. Even though there is much medical image processing literature that discusses visual saliency-based approaches for the detection and prediction of neurological disorders, there is still room for improvements. While the majority of the approaches directly classify the outcome of the saliency computation using the machine learning approach, the proposed framework employs a segmentation phase before the classification. This approach better classifies the images and this may aid in better prediction of neurological disorders.

REFERENCES

Adeel, A., Khan, M. A., Sharif, M., Azam, F., Shah, J. H., Umer, T., & Wan, S. (2019). Diagnosis and recognition of grape leaf diseases: An automated system based on a novel saliency approach and canonical correlation analysis based multiple features fusion. *Sustainable Computing: Informatics and Systems*, *24*, 100349. doi:10.1016/j.suscom.2019.08.002

Bali, B., & Garba, E. J. (2021). Neuro-fuzzy Approach for Prediction of Neurological Disorders: A Systematic Review. *SN. Computer Science*, *2*(4), 307. doi:10.100742979-021-00710-9

Banerjee, S., Mitra, S., & Shankar, B. U. (2018). Automated 3D segmentation of brain tumor using visual saliency. *Information Sciences*, *424*, 337–353. doi:10.1016/j.ins.2017.10.011

Banerjee, S., Mitra, S., Shankar, B. U., & Hayashi, Y. (2016). A novel GBM saliency detection model using multi-channel MRI. *PLoS One, 11*(1), e0146388. doi:10.1371/journal.pone.0146388 PMID:26752735

Ben-Ahmed, O., Lecellier, F., Paccalin, M., & Fernandez-Maloigne, C. (2017). Multi-view visual saliency-based MRI classification for Alzheimer's disease diagnosis. In *2017 Seventh International Conference on Image Processing Theory, Tools and Applications (IPTA)* (pp. 1-6). IEEE. 10.1109/IPTA.2017.8310118

Borji, A. (2018). *Saliency prediction in the deep learning era: Successes, limitations, and future challenges.* arXiv preprint arXiv:1810.03716.

Daza, J. C., & Rueda, A. (2016, September). Classification of Alzheimer's disease in mri using visual saliency information. In *2016 IEEE 11th Colombian Computing Conference (CCC)* (pp. 1-7). IEEE. 10.1109/ColumbianCC.2016.7750796

Ferreira, D. S., Ramalho, G. L., Medeiros, F. N., Bianchi, A. G., Carneiro, C. M., & Ushizima, D. M. (2019, April). Saliency-Driven System With Deep Learning for Cell Image Classification. In *2019 IEEE 16th International Symposium on Biomedical Imaging (ISBI 2019)* (pp. 1284-1287). IEEE. 10.1109/ISBI.2019.8759398

Gadgil, S., Endo, M., Wen, E., Ng, A. Y., & Rajpurkar, P. (2021). *CheXseg: Combining Expert Annotations with DNN-generated Saliency Maps for X-ray Segmentation.* arXiv preprint arXiv:2102.10484.

Han, N., Srivastava, S., Xu, A., Klein, D., & Beyeler, M. (2021). *Deep Learning—Based Scene Simplification for Bionic Vision.* arXiv preprint arXiv:2102.00297.

Kundu, A. K., Fattah, S. A., & Wahid, K. A. (2020). Least square saliency transformation of capsule endoscopy images for PDF model based multiple gastrointestinal disease classification. *IEEE Access: Practical Innovations, Open Solutions, 8*, 58509–58521. doi:10.1109/ACCESS.2020.2982870

Li, N., Bi, H., Zhang, Z., & Kong, X. (2018). Performance Comparison of Saliency Detection. Advances in Multimedia. doi:10.1155/2018/9497083

Mahapatra, D., Roy, P. K., Sedai, S., & Garnavi, R. (2016). Retinal image quality classification using saliency maps and CNNs. In *International Workshop on Machine Learning in Medical Imaging* (pp. 172-179). Springer. 10.1007/978-3-319-47157-0_21

Mehran, M., & Saraf Esmaili, S. (2020). Optic Disc Detection in Retinal Fundus Images Based on Saliency Map. *Signal Processing and Renewable Energy, 4*(4), 65–80.

Mitra, S., Banerjee, S., & Hayashi, Y. (2017). Volumetric brain tumour detection from MRI using visual saliency. *PLoS One, 12*(11), e0187209. doi:10.1371/journal.pone.0187209 PMID:29095877

Pesce, E., Withey, S. J., Ypsilantis, P. P., Bakewell, R., Goh, V., & Montana, G. (2019). Learning to detect chest radiographs containing pulmonary lesions using visual attention networks. *Medical Image Analysis, 53*, 26–38. doi:10.1016/j.media.2018.12.007 PMID:30660946

Rueda, A., González, F., & Romero, E. (2013). Saliency-based characterization of group differences for magnetic resonance disease classification. *Dyna, 80*(178), 21–28.

Serte, S., & Serener, A. (2021). Graph-based saliency and ensembles of convolutional neural networks for glaucoma detection. *IET Image Processing*, *15*(3), 797–804. doi:10.1049/ipr2.12063

Siuly, S., & Zhang, Y. (2016). Medical Big Data: Neurological Diseases Diagnosis Through Medical Data Analysis. *Data Sci. Eng.*, *1*(2), 54–64. doi:10.100741019-016-0011-3

Sran, P. K., Gupta, S., & Singh, S. (2020). Segmentation based image compression of brain magnetic resonance images using visual saliency. *Biomedical Signal Processing and Control*, *62*, 102089. doi:10.1016/j.bspc.2020.102089

Verma, P., Negi, C. S., Pant, M., & Saxena, A. (2020). *Deep Saliency: A Deep Learning based Saliency Approach to detect Covid-19 through x-ray images*. Academic Press.

Wei, W., Liu, Z., Huang, L., Nebout, A., Le Meur, O., Zhang, T., ... Xu, L. (2020). Predicting atypical visual saliency for autism spectrum disorder via scale-adaptive inception module and discriminative region enhancement loss. *Neurocomputing*. Advance online publication. doi:10.1016/j.neucom.2020.06.125

Zou, X., Zhao, X., Yang, Y., & Li, N. (2016). Learning-Based Visual Saliency Model for Detecting Diabetic Macular Edema in Retinal Image. *Computational Intelligence and Neuroscience*, *2016*, 7496735. doi:10.1155/2016/7496735 PMID:26884750

Chapter 2
An Exploratory Analysis and Predictive SIR Model for the Early Onset of COVID–19 in Tamil Nadu, India

Chandan Tanvi Mandapati
Lovely Professional University, India

ABSTRACT

The growth of COVID-19 (SARS-CoV-2) in India has been rampant. Despite having a relatively small value of R_0, the spread of disease increases exponentially every consecutive day. This chapter aims to analyze and conduct a concise study for the southern state of Tamil Nadu in India and build non-linear predictive models that evaluate the transmission of coronavirus amongst locals. A logistic regression and SIR model are deployed to understand the potential spread of disease. Through descriptive analysis on theoretical segmented portions, districts in Tamil Nadu with a higher number of confirmed cases are identified. Computation of crude mortality rate, infection fatality rate, predictive models, illustrations, and their results are discussed analytically.

INTRODUCTION

The earliest cases of Covid-19 surfaced in January 2020, which posed to be a dire threat to India; exposure to an Influenza-like disease could prove to be fatal to a country inhabited by 1.3 billion. Predicting the probable transmission of an airborne pathogen (like SARS-CoV-2) is a laborious but necessary task in excessively populated countries, and failing to anticipate the contagion of diseases like Covid-19 could cause epidemic-control bodies, such as Epidemic Intelligence Service (EIS) of India, to harbour a handicap; in turn, leading to inadequacies and risking the lives of millions.

Epidemic models, for contagious and non-contagious diseases, have been employed to predict and analyse the spread of infections to curb the escalation of disease among humans since the dawn of mathematical epidemic models. An epidemic model that relies on documented data might not consider

DOI: 10.4018/978-1-7998-7188-0.ch002

plausible interactions an infected person has had. In cases of a newly-emerged disease (like Covid-19), data might be scarce and of smaller size; a dataset of such population is insufficient for a machine-learning algorithm to grasp patterns from. Parameters that incorporate transmissibility (i.e., rate at which the infection is spreading) are principal aspects for building an appropriate model which considers probable secondary transmitted cases. The primary goals of this paper are defined below.

1. Build a predictive model that works with deterministic parameters (factors that are estimable through mathematical, i.e., differential methods) for Tamil Nadu (from January 2020 to August 2020)
2. Analyse the spread of Covid-19 in Tamil Nadu
3. Obtain an estimate of the Crude Mortality Rate and Infection Fatality Rate.

For objective (a), a SIR (Susceptible-Infected-Recovered) model, built using Covid-19 data from Tamil Nadu (an Indian state whose confirmed reports were higher than the other states), exemplifies the use of a predictive model using differential processes. Non-linear mathematical epidemiological models are popularly utilized for diseased environments in various situations using simulations (such as Monte Carlo Simulation) for foresights on the spread of disease. The SIR model is a mathematical epidemic model that works with constants such as population, the number of confirmed, recovered cases (deceased are clubbed with recovered, as they no longer belong to the susceptible pool), and principal parameters – R_0 and gamma. It is a theoretical model in nature, and unlike most machine learning models, the SIR model doesn't rely on past data. Additionally, a logistic regression model is deployed between confirmed and recovered cases, where confirmed cases are the independent (predictor) variables and recovered cases are dependent (predicted) variables.

(b) To examine the outspread of disease in Tamil Nadu, the state has been segmented into four clusters and visualized through facet grid; the grids revealed that the majority of confirmed cases arose from the cluster of districts situated in the northern part of the state. The final objective calls for estimation of crude mortality rate and infection fatality rate till the mid of August 2020 in Tamil Nadu, which is computed through Python. This paper examines the contagion of Covid-19 through visual analysis and predictive modelling, which helps in understanding the spread of this disease, and could aid in the prevention of further contamination.

BACKGROUND

The Basic SIR Model

The SIR model (Kermack & McKendrick, 1927) predicts the rise/decline in diseased cases over a specified period, utilizing a function of constants and parameters. Differential equations are integral tools for implementing the model; they instigate changes in susceptible and diseased pools with respect to time over a specified period. The model presumes that at a given time *t*, an individual of a population exists in one of the three states – susceptible state, infected state, or recovered state. The sum of susceptible, infected, and the recovered populace is assumed to be equal to the entire population under study, *N*.

The 'Susceptible' populace is at risk of either contracting the virus or being asymptotic carriers. A portion of the susceptible population that becomes infected with the disease advances to the 'Infected' compartment. The infected from the prevalence pool either recover with immunity or meet with un-

Figure 1. The flow within SIR model. It is linear, and cannot be reversed (a recovered person cannot return to the prevalence pool)

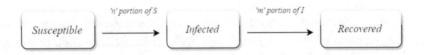

timely death; regardless of the cause, the subjects progress into the next block - the 'Recovered' state. Recovered subjects are excluded from the susceptible population hereafter, as the probability of being infected twice is extremely low.

In a classic SIR model, the two consistent variables defined for estimating the disease's growth and fatality are β (contact rate) and γ (recovery rate). 'β' gives an approximate value on the number of people contacted by an infected subject (i.e., number of individuals likely to contract an infection, γ specifies the rate at which an infected person recovers. In the initial stages of an epidemical spreading, the β and γ are hypothetical and remain constant until sizeable and meaningful data about the spread of infection surfaces. β and γ are parameters which are intangibly associated with the population size. Jong, Diekmann, and Heesterbeek researched the dependence of transmission on population size – under the assumption that contact between individuals occur at random, i.e., through mass-action kinetics (Jong et al., 1994). The authors coined true-mass action models with transmission term $\beta XY/N$, where X is susceptible population and Y is infected population.

A parameter of prime importance is R_0 (also known as the Basic Reproduction Number), a function defined through β and γ. It indicates the transmissibility of the disease and is formulated by taking into account, the number of people an infected person has contacted, number of days a person takes to contract and recovered from the disease. In the initial outspread of an epidemic, if $R_0 > 1$ - the disease continues to spread, and if $R_0 < 1$ - the disease can be curbed with minimal fatalities. The governing equations are outlined below –

$$\frac{dS}{dt} = -\frac{\beta SI}{N}$$

$$\frac{dI}{dt} = \frac{\beta NI}{N} - \gamma I$$

$$\frac{dR}{dt} = \gamma I$$

SIR	(Hyeontae J., et al., 2020) (Nesteruk & Benlagha, 2021) (Xiaowei et al., 2020) (Boudrioua & Boudrioua, 2020) (Fuminori et al., 2011) (Ndiaye et al., 2020)	(Novara et al., 2020) (Caccavo, 2020) (Lalwani et al., 2020) (Chatterjee et al., 2020) (Jahanshahia et al., 2021) (Sedaghat et al., 2020) (Lounis & Al-Raeei, 2021)	SIRD
SIQR	(Tovissodé et al., 2021) (Pedersen & Meneghini, 2020) (Zhang & Liu, 2020) (Abdalla et al., 2021) (Mahrouf et al., 2020) (Kuniya, 2020) (Odagaki, 2020) (Pedersen & Meneghini, 2021) (Cordelli et al., 2021) (Malik et al., 2021)	(Bajaña et al., 2020) (Li et al., 2020) (Wickramaarachchi & Perera, 2020) (Allahi et al., 2021) (Abolmaal, 2021) (Gruyter, 2021) (Malhotra & Kashyap, 2020) (Kushta & Prenga, 2021) (Shastri et al., 2021)	SIER
SIRV	(Sugiyanto & Abrori, 2020) (Harizi et al., 2020) (Chen et al., 2020) (Sen & Ibeas, 2021) (Chattopadhyay et al., 2021) (Rahardiantoro & Sakamoto, 2020) (Katal et al., 2021)	(Nevesac & Guerrero, 2020) (Sun et al., 2020) (Maki, 2020)	Miscellaneous Models (A-SIR, v-SIR, SEIQR)

The equations defined above can be expanded to include vaccinated, quarantined, and asymptotic individuals. The SIR model can be modified to incorporate the compartments mentioned before to precisely predict the rise in cases. Its variations have been widely used to model the spread of the Novel Corona Virus amongst people.

Table 2. A compilation of stochastic and deterministic SIR models built for Covid-19

| (Priyanka & Verma, 2020)
(Zhang et al., 2004)
(Sato et al., 2015)
(Malim & Shaadan, 2020)
(Kaur & Goyal, 2021)
(Ideris, 2016)
(Saito et al., 2014)
(Aguiar et al., 2011)
(Brune, 2008)
(Jaćimovski & Kekić, 2010) | Stochastic Models |
| (Chuo et al., 2008)
(Ledzewicz & Schattler, 2011)
(Khalid & Khan, 2016)
(Perra et al., 2011)
(Omar & Hassan, 2013)
(Hota, 2014)
(Ren, 2014) | Deterministic Models |

The processes in SIR models are presumed to be deterministic or stochastic in nature. Deterministic models are built and guided by the parameter values and primary conditions, while stochastic models possess some degree of intrinsic randomness. The same set of parameter values and initial conditions lead to an ensemble of different outputs. Practically, stochasticity is best suited for the real world. But, due to its complex nature, stochastic models are considerably harder to model.

The use of machine learning modules to predict the spread of disease, has been extensively popularized post the contagion of Covid-19 globally. Ndiaye used Facebook's Prophet [15, 18] to analyse and predict the rise of Covid-19 cases. The model utilizes an algorithm based on an additive model, where trends are fit with natural seasonality and include the effects of holidays while dealing with outliers and missing data (Ndiaye et al., 2020a). Baldé (2020) implemented a Neural Network to predict rise in cases for France and Senegal, while using China's present data to train the model; China's model was used for comparison as well as for prototypical purposes. Ndiaye built various versions of a deterministic SIR model by including compartments such as Deaths(SIRD) and fatalities(SIR-F) and analysed the data descriptively on Python, using statistical packages and functions such as scipy.optimize.curve_fit (Ndiaye et al., 2020b). In this chapter, a deterministic SIR model is deployed, which is built in Jupyter Notebook using differential packages supported by Python.

Logistic Regression

In this chapter, the logistic regression model fits data points of the pandemic using a sigmoid function, whose resultant curve is a regressed line between confirmed and recovered cases; this logistic regression model is built to predict recovered cases when confirmed cases are known. The model does not consider the change of rate of transmission concerning time (like SIR does) and is solely built to understand the relationship between confirmed and recovered cases. To elucidate further, for 'k' independent variables, the general logistic model is defined by the mathematical equation –

$$y_i = \beta_0 + \beta_1 x_{i1} + \beta_2 x_{i2} + \ldots + \beta_k x_{ik} + \varepsilon_i$$

Kleinbaun and Klein discussed two salient qualities of logistic regression models - they emphasized on the model's indispensability in diseased environments, especially in scenarios where the measure of illness is dichotomous in nature (Kleinbaum & Klein, 2010a). The first point throws light on the usage of probabilities in epidemical logistic models. Exposure probabilities utilized in logistic models describe the likeliness of the spread of disease. The value derived from p(X) (the logistic model which is defined below) denotes the chance of a person being infected with the disease. A probabilistic axiom of Andrey Kolmogorov states that probability lies between 0 and 1, and it won't exceed unity. In this case, the probability of a person being infected will not be greater than one. Another aspect that makes the logistic model appealing is the S-shaped curve, which illustrates the combined effect of multiple risky characteristics on the plausible spread of disease. A simple logistic model for epidemic cases is formulated as (Kleinbaum & Klein, 2010b) –

$$P(X) = \frac{1}{1 + e^{-(x + \beta_1 E)}}$$

Kleinbaum and Klein (2010b) introduced an exposure variable 'E' to the classic logistic regression model. E equals 0 for unexposed individuals, while it is 1 for exposed individuals.

An alternate way of defining the logistic model is through a logit function - it is defined as logit of logistic model equals α (which is a simple linear sum) plus β_1 times E (exposure variable), i.e. ***logit*** $P(X) = \pm + {}^2{}_1E$. The logit function is essential as it has many beneficial features that a classic linear regression model would have; it has linear parameters, could be continuous, and lies between – infinity and +infinity (Hosmer, Jr. et al., 2013).

Ideally, logistic regression is used for dichotomous variables. To transform non-dichotomous values, sigmoid function is used. It converts population values and fits them into a logistic regression model. The sigmoidal logistic function is an inverse of the logit function and lies between 0 and 1. Devi et al. (2020) stated that "Logit is defined as the logarithm of the ratio of frequencies of two different categorical and mutually exclusive outcomes such as healthy and sick". The logit function is converted into predictions using Linear Regression techniques. The sigmoid function is given as follows (Li et al., 2021) –

$$sigmoid(z) = \frac{1}{1 + e^{-z}}$$

Precision Metrics: Precision metrics consist of methods that check the accuracy of a developed data model. A trained predictive model whose precision isn't leveraged might prove to be inefficient or provide unproductive predictions. Popular measurements for binary classification models like logistic regression consist of Confusion Matrix (sensitivity, specificity, and Overall Accuracy), AUC-ROC Curve, RMSE, and R^2.

AUC-ROC is an abbreviation for Area under the ROC (Receiver Operating Characteristic) curve. The ROC curve is a graph between True Positive rate (Sensitivity) and False Positive Rate (1- Specificity). A desirable quality of the ROC curve is that it is independent of the change in size (of responders).

Root Mean Squared Error (RMSE) is the root of sum of squared residuals divided by N (Size). This metric gives us a rough idea about the distribution of residual data points around the best fit line. R^2 denotes the goodness of fit of the regression model. Mathematically, it is equal to 1 - (Total sum of squares/ Total sum of Residuals). Confusion Matrix, a matrix of N x N dimension, is a table that weighs the relationship between predicted positive/negative values against the actual test points. Sensitivity/ Recall and Specificity are key metrics of the confusion matrix - Sensitivity is the proportion between True Positives and (True Positives + False Negatives). Specificity is the ratio between True Negatives and (False Positives + True Negatives).

Table 3. Specificity and Sensitivity are computed utilizing true positives, true negatives, false positives, and false negatives. The overall accuracy of the model is given by (true positive + true negative) divided by (true positives + true negative + false positive + false negatives)

	Positive	Negative
Positive	True Positive	False Positive
Negative	False Negative	True Negative
	$Sensitivity = \dfrac{True\ Positive}{True\ Positive + False\ Negative}$	$Specificity = \dfrac{True\ Negative}{False\ Positive + True\ Negative}$

Table 4 is a collection of research papers in the field of medical and epidemical sciences which employ logistic regression for predictive purposes. Various metrics are used to measure the predictive ability of the model across these papers. Confusion Matrix and R^2 are utilized frequently.

Table 4. Different types of metrics are used for disparate scenarios. Cross-validation through suitable metrics aids in better understanding of the accuracy in predictions.

Authors	Country, Sample Size	Disease	Precision Metrics
Terence D. Valenzuela, Denise J. Roe, Shan Cretin, Daniel W. Site, and Mary P. Larsen, 1997	Two regions from United States of America (n=205 and n=1667)	Cardiac Arrests	*ROC*: 0.664
A. L. Mila, A. L. Carriquiry, and X. B. Yang, 2007	United States of America (n= 1545) *(Two models were built - Model I with Spring (April) factors and Model II with Summer (July and August) factors.)*	*Sclerotinia* stem rot	Metric: R^2 Model I - 0.65 Model II - 0.71
Shaoyan Zhang & Christos Tjortjis & Xiaojun Zeng & Hong Qiao & Iain Buchan & John Keane, 2009	United Kingdom (n = 16,653)	Child Obesity	*Data recorded at 8 months*: Sensitivity – 13.3% Specificity – 98.1% Overall Accuracy – 83.7% *Data recorded after 2 years*: Sensitivity – 29.1% Specificity – 97.1% Overall Accuracy – 83.2%
Hon-Yi Shi, King-Teh Lee, Hao-Hsien Lee, Wen-Hsien Ho, Ding-Ping Sun, Jhi-Joung Wang, Chong-Chi Chiu, 2012	Taiwan (n = 22,926)	In Hospitality after Liver Cancer Surgery	*Accuracy Rate – 88.29% AUCROC – 0.76*
Emmanuel P. Mwanga, Elihaika G. Minja, Emmanuel Mrimi, Mario González Jiménez, Johnson K. Swai, Said Abbasi, Halfan S. Ngowo, Doreen J. Siria, Salum Mapua, Caleb Stica, Marta F. Maia, Ally Olotu, Maggy T. Sikulu-Lord, Francesco Baldini, Heather M. Ferguson, Klaas Wynne, Prashanth Selvaraj, Simon A. Babayan & Fredros O. Okumu, 2019	Tanzania (n = 296)	Malaria	*For predicting P. falciparum infections*: Overall Accuracy – 92% Specificity = 91.7% Sensitivity = 92.8% *For predicting mixed infections of P. falciparum and Plasmodium ovale:* Overall Accuracy – 85% Specificity = 85% Sensitivity = 85%
Abdullah M. Almeshal, Abdulla I. Almazrouee, Mohammad R. Alenizi and Saleh N. Alhajeri, 2020	Kuwait (From 24th February to 19th April 2020)	Covid-19	R^2 - 0.992

Crude Mortality Rate and Infection Fatality Rate

Crude Mortality Rate is the ratio of deaths (due to Covid-19) to the total population present in that region. It indicates the lethality of the disease. The Crude Death Rate can be computed by the formula–

Infection Fatality Rate is a ratio between Covid-19 deaths to the infected cases, which are symptomatic and asymptomatic.

For cases of early onset of a disease, distinguishing between asymptomatic and uninfected subjects is a tricky task when data is limited. Infection Fatality rate cannot be greater than Case Fatality Rate; in this chapter, Case Fatality Rate is computed instead of Infection Fatality Rate.

ANALYSIS FOR TAMIL NADU

Data Source

Data used in analysis was forked from a public resource - https://www.covid19india.org/

To visualize confirmed cases from the clusters, CMR graphs, and IFR report data used is from 30th January – 30th June, and for the SIR and Logistic regression model data used is from 15th June – 30th July.

Timeline of Events

The trajectory of rise in Covid-19 cases took a steep rise from the month of June. The increase in confirmed cases occurred after Unlock 1.0 was announced by the Government – it is a key event that led to the tripling of cases in less than a month. In this Chapter, the SIR and logistic model are built after the curve peaked (i.e., 15th June).

Susceptible-Infected-Recovered (SIR) Model

To implement the model, a Python code that encapsulates the governing equations into a user-defined function and integrates it with respect to time was developed in Jupyter Notebook. A sample function for the equations is defined below –

```
def sir(model, time, N, beta, gamma):
    Sus, Inf, Rec = model
    dSdt = (-beta * Sus * Inf)/ N
    dIdt = (beta * Sus * Inf) / (N - gamma * Inf)
    dRdt = gamma * Inf
    return dSdt, dIdt, dRdt
```

Scipy.integrate package holds functions such as odeint, which integrate the equations above into a predictive model for the susceptible, infected, and recovered.

Figure 2. A timeline summarizing the key events in Tamil Nadu, related to Covid-19

7th March 2020		First case of Covid-19 detected from an individual who returned from Oman
18th March 2020		Second case identified from a person who travelled in train from Chennai to Delhi
22nd March 2020		Three positive Covid-19 cases declared
		Lockdown(Phase 1)
23rd March 2020		Declaration of lockdown till 31st March
25th March 2020		Five new cases detected (from four Indonesians and their travel guide)
31st March 2020		Extension of Lockdown to 14th April
5th April – 14th April 2020		50+ confirmed cases were reported everyday
		Lockdown(Phase 2)
14th April 2020		Extension of lockdown till 3rd May
		Lockdown(Phase 3)
4th May – 17th May 2020		300+ confirmed cases recorded everyday
		Lockdown(Phase 4)
18th May – 31st May 2020		500 + confirmed cases recorded everyday
		Unlock 1.0
1st June – 30th June 2020		1000+ confirmed cases reported every day until 17th June
	17th June 2020	2000+ confirmed cases recorded everyday
	26th June 2020	3000+ confirmed cases reported everyday
30th June 2020		*Unlock 2.0*
	3rd July – 14th July 2020	3500+ confirmed cases recorded everyday

```
model0 = Sus0, Inf0, Rec0
deriv = odeint(sir, model0, time, args=(N, beta, gamma))
S, I, R = deriv.T
```

The model deployed is normalized and deployed, considering the values of 'S' as the total population in Tamil Nadu, 'I' as the total infected cases on 14th July, and 'R' as the total recovered cases as of 14th July. The R_0 was found to be 1.22, and gamma = 1/10. The outcome from the SIR model is plotted using the matplotlib.pylot package; the resultant curves are shown below -

The line graphs of the deployed model indicated a peak of 5000 confirmed cases daily around the 10th day after its' (model) deployment, after which the curve would start to flatten. The predicted proportion of recovered patients soared to 7000 cases every day. If transmission rate remains constant, i.e., 1.22, confirmed cases would subside, and eventually, the transmission of Covid-19 would cease in the next 60 days.

Figure 3. An SIR predictive model for Tamil Nadu, predictions made for 160 days after 11ᵗʰ July

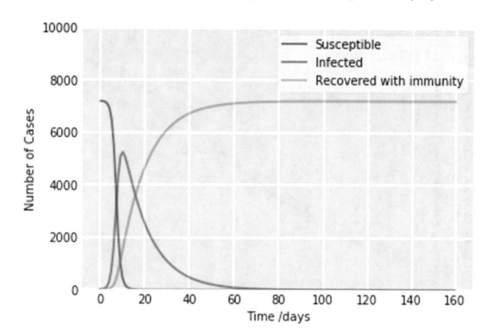

Logistic Regression Model

Splitting data into train/test sets in an 8:2 or 7:3 ratio and assigning them to a variable is a standard measure for most machine learning models; 8:2 ratio is considered for this model. The initial step for building a non-linear (logistic) regression model is to define an activation function for introducing non-linearity to the model. A sigmoid function assigns predictions for recovered cases to probabilities and determines which values to pass output. The mathematical expression for the sigmoid function is-

Provided below is the sample code for a user-defined sigmoid function -

```
def sigmoid(x_VAR, Beta1, Beta2):
    y_VAR = 1 / (1 + np.exp(- Beta1*(X_VAR - Beta2)))
    return y_VAR
```

From scipy.optimize, the function curve_fit() utilized to fit the data points into the sigmoid curve gives the values of β_1 and β_2; elimination of probabilities corresponding data points that fail to fall between the range 0 to 1 happens in this process. The respective values of β_1 and β_2 are 6.021007 and 0.541678.

The normalized data is trained through the logistic regression model. R^2 score between the test and trained data is 0.9452, with Mean Absolute Error of 0.05; Residual Sum of Squares (MSE) is 0.

Figure 4. Graph between fit sigmoid values and observed values

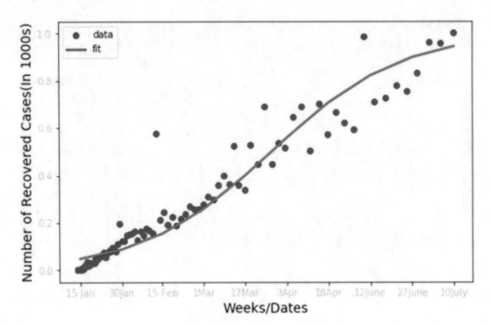

Exploratory Analysis

For visual analysis, the state of Tamil Nadu is segmented into four hypothetical clusters, based on their geographic location. Grouping districts in Tamil Nadu into four zones facilitates an easier understanding of the data.

- *Kongu Nade* (Western districts of Tamil Nadu) -
- Krishnagiri, Dharmapuri, Salem, Namakkal, Karur, Dindigul, Tiruppur, Coimbatore, Nilgiris, Erode
- *Pandy Nadu* (Southern districts of Tamil Nadu) -
- Sivaganga, Madurai, Theni, Virudhunagar, Tenkasi, Thoothukkudi, Tirunelveli, Kanyakumari, Ramanathapuram
- *Chola Nadu* (Mid districts of Tamil Nadu) -
- Viluppuram, Kallakurichi, Cuddalore, Perambalur, Ariyalur, Tiruchirappalli, Thanjavur, Thiruvarur, Nagapattinam, Pudukkottai
- *Tondaimalam* (Northern districts of Tamil Nadu) -
- Thiruvallur, Ranipet, Vellore, Tirupathur, Tiruvannamalai, Chengalpattu, Kanchipuram, Chennai

Covid-19 cases confirmed daily in the four Tamil partitions were visualized through a Scatter Facet-Grid (using seaborn).

Majority of the cases in Tamil Nadu arose from Tondaimalam, the Northern segment that houses the capital city, Chennai. The range of confirmed cases in Tondaimalam osclatess between (0, 2500). Other clusters of Tamil Nadu recorded ≥ 500 cases every day, indicating that most of the cases from Tamil Nadu originated from the Northern districts. This indicates that most of the cases from Tamil

Figure 5. Map of the four hypothesized clusters in Tamil Nadu

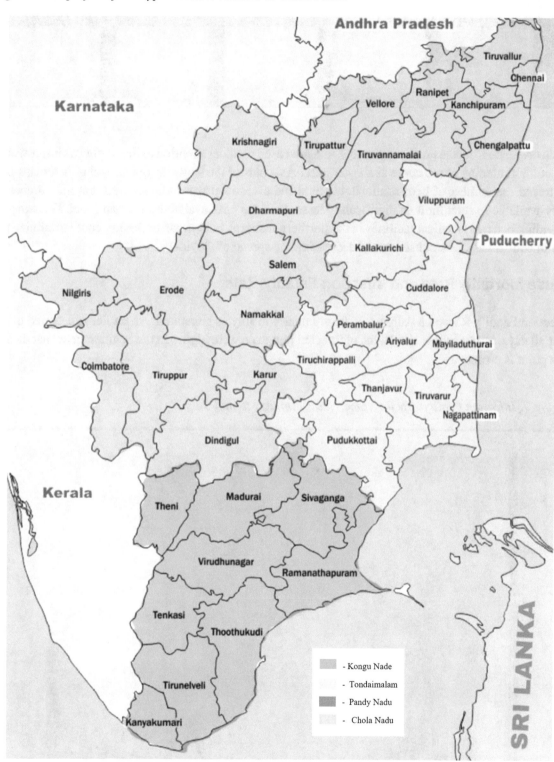

Figure 6. Facet grid of confirmed cases in Tamil Nadu (till 11ᵗʰ July).

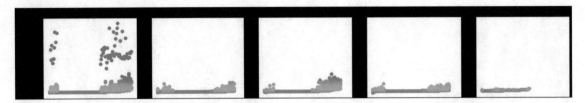

Nadu originate from the northern districts, and increased medical attention to the northern cluster would aid in the flattening of the curve at a faster pace. As a part of the study, a comparison of heatmaps that portrayed the number of beds available in Rural India versus urban India showed that the number of beds available in rural India is significantly lesser than the ones available in Urban India. Focusing on providing beds and medical facilities in the northern districts, both urban and rural, could minimize the rise in confirmed cases, subsequently, decreasing the spread of Covid-19.

Crude Mortality Rate and Infection Fatality Rate

Infection Fatality Rate on a daily basis, from January to July, is generated. An outlier is detected in the first 30 days, implying that the deaths of infected populace were higher in the beginning, or that data at that point is erroneous.

Figure 7. Infection fatality rate for Tamil Nadu, January to mid-July.

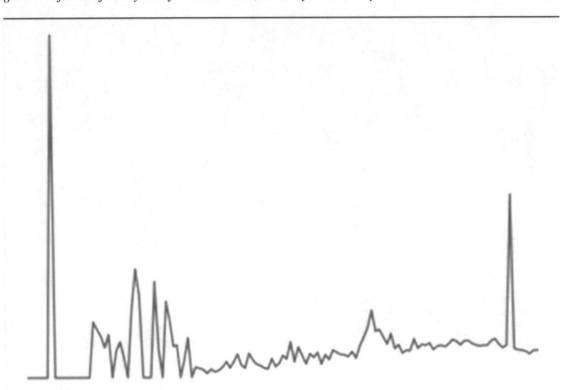

Figure 8. Crude mortality rate for Tamil Nadu, January to mid-July.

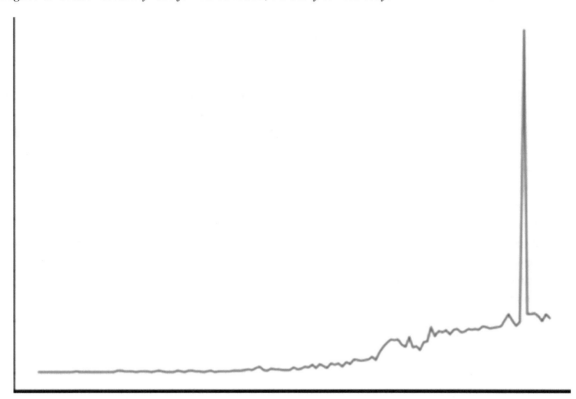

Crude Mortality rate spikes around the 130th day, which could signal an incorrect data entry, or a rise in deaths on that particular day. Excluding the outlier, mortality rate in Tamil Nadu is < 0.0002. Less than 0.3% of the total population turn into Covid-19 fatalities and eventually, die.

DISCUSSIONS

To summarize the findings of the exploratory study - In a scenario where the transmission rate remains constant at 1.22, the spread of Covid-19 would have ceased in the next 60 days. However, the real-world simulation consists of randomness and unpredictable circumstances that make the transmission rate fluctuate. In the early stages of a pandemic, a model built on stochastic processes prove to more adaptable to change in the transmission rate. In contrast, the logistic regression model yielded an R^2 score of 0.9452 with Mean Absolute Error of 0.05 and Residual Sum of Squares (MSE) is 0. The infection fatality curve is unstable, and often fluctuates between 0 and 5.00, whereas the crude mortality rate has remained below 0.0002 until the mid of July (precisely, 15th July). The spread of Covid-19 is prevalent in the northern segment of Tamil Nadu than other hypothesized parts.

FUTURE RESEARCH SCOPE

The SIR model can be extended to most diseased environments; for example, the aftereffects of medical anomalies caused after recovering from Covid-19, such as the spread of black fungi (a secondary infection affecting recovered Covid-19 patients) or the spread of Covid-19 after vaccination has been administered are intriguing issues to investigate. Employing machine learning algorithms to examine diseased environments simplifies model-building and provides multiple devices (such as functions and packages) to decrease computation time (useful for large datasets). Regression models prove to be beneficial in scenarios where the correlation between two variables is high. A regression model between normalized values of vaccinations administered and the consumption/sales of Favipiravir could provide insights on the question, "Would an increase in vaccinated individuals lead to a decrease or increase the consumption of Favipiravir?". Another issue that could be implored scientifically through regression models is whether social media posts amplify the reach of Covid-19 drugs available in the market. For the situations proposed above, an extension to the models discussed in this paper would produce illuminating results. An extension of the SIR model by including an Exposed compartment (SIER model) for the state of Tamil Nadu would increase accuracy in terms of predictions. The logistic regression model could provide more information by examining residuals between the predicted and observed values. These models are helpful for contagious and non-contagious diseases alike, proven in studies by (Engels et al., 2006) and (Amundsen et al., 2004)

Visual analysis through charts like heat maps and facet grids facilitates easier understanding and segmenting data into smaller parts by clubbing them into smaller groups - this yields more manageable and interpretable results.

CONCLUSION

In this chapter, implementation of the SIR model aided by data visualization has brought forth the results stated above; the said model disregards exposed and vaccinated individuals, but it can further extend to do the same. The model predicted a peak in daily cases around the 10th day after its deployment and provided an insight on the recovered individuals, which was 40 times greater (7000+ cases every day) than that of the confirmed cases. A non-linear regression (logistic regression) model employed to predict recovered figures reported an R^2 score of 94.52 between the predicted and test values. A brief visual analysis of the state pointed to a cluster of cases in the northern districts of Tamil Nadu (Tondaimalam); illustrations and codes of the study are interpreted in the chapter. This chapter is centred around a descriptive and predictive analysis on the state of Tamil Nadu, which revealed a decline in the confirmed curve around the 60th day after 11th July if the R_0 remained constant at 1.22. This study could further be extended to various states in India, using models such as SEIR, SIS, and SI.

REFERENCES

Abolmaali, S. (2021). A comparative study of SIR Model, Linear Regression, Logistic Function and ARIMA Model for forecasting COVID-19 cases. doi:10.1101/2021.05.24.21257594

Aguiar, M., Stollenwerk, N., Kooi, B. W., Simos, T. E., Psihoyios, G., Tsitouras, C., & Anastassi, Z. (2011). *The Stochastic Multi-strain Dengue Model: Analysis of the Dynamics.* Academic Press.

Al-Raeei, M., El-Daher, M., & Solieva, O. (2021). Applying SEIR model without vaccination for CO-VID-19 in case of the United States, Russia, the United Kingdom, Brazil, France, and India. *Epidemiologic Methods*, *10*(s1), 20200036. doi:10.1515/em-2020-0036

Allahi, F., Fateh, A., Revetria, R., & Cianci, R. (2021). The COVID-19 epidemic and evaluating the corresponding responses to crisis management in refugees: A system dynamic approach. *Journal of Humanitarian Logistics and Supply Chain Management*, *11*(2), 347–366. doi:10.1108/JHLSCM-09-2020-0077

Almeshal, A. M., Almazrouee, A. I., Alenizi, M. R., & Alhajeri, S. N. (2020). Forecasting the Spread of COVID-19 in Kuwait Using Compartmental and Logistic Regression Models. *Applied Sciences (Basel, Switzerland)*, *10*(10), 3402. doi:10.3390/app10103402

Amundsen, E. J., Stigum, H., Rottingen, J. A., & Aalen, O. O. (2004). Definition and estimation of an actual reproduction number describing past infectious disease transmission: application to HIV epidemics among homosexual men in Denmark, Norway and Sweden. *Epidemiology and Infection*.

Atkeson, A., Kopecky, K., & Zha, T. (2020). *Estimating and Forecasting Disease Scenarios for CO-VID-19 with an SIR Model.* doi:10.3386/w27335

Baldé, M. A. (2020). Fitting SIR model to COVID-19 pandemic data and comparative forecasting with machine learning. doi:10.1101/2020.04.26.20081042

Basu, M. (2020, 7 July). India's R value increases for the first time in 3 months – at 1.19 from 1.11 a week ago. *The Print India.* https://www.theprint.in/

Berkane, S., Harizi, I., & Tayebi, A. (2021). Modeling the Effect of Population-Wide Vaccination on the Evolution of COVID-19 Epidemic in Canada. doi:10.1101/2021.02.05.21250572

Boudrioua, M. S., & Boudrioua, A. (2020). Predicting the COVID-19 epidemic in Algeria using the SIR model. doi:10.1101/2020.04.25.20079467

Brune, R. (2008). *A Stochastic Model for Panic Behaviour in Disease Dynamics.* Academic Press.

Caccavo, D. (2020). Chinese and Italian COVID-19 outbreaks can be correctly described by a modified SIRD model. doi:10.1101/2020.03.19.20039388

Calafiore, G. C., Novara, C., & Possieri, C. (2020). A time-varying SIRD model for the COVID-19 contagion in Italy. *Annual Reviews in Control*, *50*, 361–372. doi:10.1016/j.arcontrol.2020.10.005 PMID:33132739

Chatterjee, S., Sarkar, A., Chatterjee, S., Karmakar, M., & Paul, R. (2020). Studying the progress of COVID-19 outbreak in India using SIRD model. doi:10.1101/2020.05.11.20098681

Chattopadhyay, A. K., Choudhury, D., Ghosh, G., Kundu, B., & Nath, S. K. (2021). Infection kinetics of Covid-19 and containment strategy. *Scientific Reports*, *11*(1), 11606. doi:10.103841598-021-90698-2 PMID:34078929

Chen, M., Kuo, C., & Chan, W. K. (2021). Control of COVID-19 Pandemic: Vaccination Strategies Simulation under Probabilistic Node-Level Model. *2021 6th International Conference on Intelligent Computing and Signal Processing (ICSP)*.

Chen, X., Li, J., Xiao, C., & Yang, P. (2020). Numerical solution and parameter estimation for uncertain SIR model with application to COVID-19. *Fuzzy Optimization and Decision Making*, *20*(2), 189–208. doi:10.100710700-020-09342-9

Chuo, F., Tiing, S., & Labadin, J. (2008). A Simple Deterministic Model for the Spread of Hand, Foot and Mouth Disease (HFMD) in Sarawak. *2008 Second Asia International Conference on Modelling & Simulation (AMS)*.

Cordelli, E., Tortora, M., Sicilia, R., & Soda, P. (2020). Time-Window SIQR Analysis of COVID-19 Outbreak and Containment Measures in Italy. *2020 IEEE 33rd International Symposium on Computer-Based Medical Systems (CBMS)*.

Covid19India. (2020). Available from https://www.covid19india.org/

Crokidakis, N. (2020). COVID-19 spreading in Rio de Janeiro, Brazil: Do the policies of social isolation really work? doi:10.1101/2020.04.27.20081737

Devi, M. N., Balamurugan, A., & Kris, M. R. (2016). Developing a Modified Logistic Regression Model for Diabetes Mellitus and Identifying the Important Factors of Type II Dm. *Indian Journal of Science and Technology*.

Engels, E. A., Pfeiffer, R. M., Goedert, J. J., Virgo, P., McNeel, T. S., Scoppa, S. M., & Biggar, R. J. (2006). Trends in cancer risk among people with AIDS in the United States 1980–2002. *AIDS (London, England)*, *20*(12), 1645–1654. doi:10.1097/01.aids.0000238411.75324.59 PMID:16868446

Hattori, A., & Sturm, R. (2013). The obesity epidemic and changes in self-report biases in BMI. *Obesity (Silver Spring, Md.)*, *21*(4), 856–860. doi:10.1002/oby.20313 PMID:23712990

Hosmer, D. W., Lemeshow, S., & Sturdivant, R. X. (2013). *Applied Logistic Regression*. Wiley Series in Probability and Statistics. doi:10.1002/9781118548387

Hota, A. (2014). *Development and Validation of Statistical and Deterministic Models Used to Predict Dengue Fever in Mexico* [Bachelors Dissertation]. Harvard University.

ICMR COVID Study Group, COVID Epidemiology & Data Management Team, COVID Laboratory Team, & VRDLN Team. (2020). Laboratory surveillance for SARS-CoV-2 in India: Performance of testing & descriptive epidemiology of detected COVID-19. *The Indian Journal of Medical Research*, *151*, 424–437. doi:10.4103/ijmr.IJMR_1896_20

Ideris, S. H., Malim, M. R., & Shaadan, N. (2021). Relative Risk Estimation for Human Leptospirosis Disease in Malaysia Based on Existing Models and Discrete Space-Time Stochastic Sir Model. *Pertanika Journal of Science & Technology*, *29*(2). Advance online publication. doi:10.47836/pjst.29.2.20

Ideris, S. H. B. (2016). *The development of stochastic SIR and S(I^m I^f) R models for heterosexual HIV and AIDS disease mapping in Malaysia* [Masters Dissertation, Universiti Pendidikan Sultan Idris]. UPSI Digital Repository.

Jacimovski, S., & Kekić, D. (2010). A mathematical SIR model for epidemic emergency. *NBP - Journal of Criminalistics and Law, 15*, 65-76.

Jahanshahi, H., Munoz-Pacheco, J. M., Bekiros, S., & Alotaibi, N. D. (2021). A fractional-order SIRD model with time-dependent memory indexes for encompassing the multi-fractional characteristics of the COVID-19. *Chaos, Solitons, and Fractals, 143*, 110632. doi:10.1016/j.chaos.2020.110632 PMID:33519121

Jo, H., Son, H., Hwang, H. J., & Jung, S. Y. (2020). *Analysis of COVID-19 spread in South Korea using the SIR model with time-dependent parameters and deep learning.* Academic Press.

Jong, M.C.M., & de., Diekmann, O., & Heesterbeek, H. (1995). How Does Transmission of Infection Depend on Transmission Size*? Publications of the Newton Institute, 5*, 84–94.

Katal, S., Pouraryan, A., & Gholamrezanezhad, A. (2021). COVID-19 vaccine is here: Practical considerations for clinical imaging applications. *Clinical Imaging, 76*, 38–41. doi:10.1016/j.clinimag.2021.01.023 PMID:33548891

Kato, F., Tainaka, K., Sone, S., Morita, S., Iida, H., & Yoshimura, J. (2011). Combined effects of prevention and quarantine on a breakout in SIR model. *Scientific Reports, 1*(1), 10. doi:10.1038rep00010 PMID:22355529

Kaur, N., & Goyal, K. (2021). Uncertainty Quantification of Stochastic Epidemic SIR Models Using B-spline Polynomial Chaos. *Regular and Chaotic Dynamics, 26*(1), 22–38. doi:10.1134/S1560354721010020

Kermack, W. O., & McKendrick, A. G. (1927). A contribution to the mathematical theory of epidemics. *Proceedings of the Royal Society of London. Series B, Containing Papers of a Biological Character, 115*, 700–721.

Khalid, M., & Khan, F. (2016). Stability Analysis of Deterministic Mathematical Model for Zika Virus. *British Journal of Mathematics & Computer Science, 19*(4), 1–10. doi:10.9734/BJMCS/2016/29834

Kleinbaum, D. G., & Klein, M. (2010a). Introduction to Logistic Regression. *Logistic Regression,* 1–39.

Kleinbaum, D. G., & Klein, M. (2010b). Important Special Cases of the Logistic Model. Logistic Regression. *Logistic Regression,* 41–71.

Kuniya, T. (2020). Evaluation of the effect of the state of emergency for the first wave of COVID-19 in Japan. *Infectious Disease Modelling, 5*, 580–587. doi:10.1016/j.idm.2020.08.004 PMID:32844135

Kushta, E., & Prenga, D. (2021). Extended log periodic approach in analysing local critical behaviour–case study for Covid -19 spread in Albania. *Journal of Physics: Conference Series, 1730*(1), 012056. doi:10.1088/1742-6596/1730/1/012056

Lalwani, S., Sahni, G., Mewara, B., & Kumar, R. (2020). Predicting optimal lockdown period with parametric approach using three-phase maturation SIRD model for COVID-19 pandemic. *Chaos, Solitons, and Fractals, 138*. PMID:32834574

Ledzewicz, U., & Schattler, H. (2011). On optimal singular controls for a general SIR-model with vaccination and treatment. *Conference Publications 2011.*

Li, J., Wang, Y., Wu, J., Ai, J., Zhang, H., Gamber, M., Li, W., Zhang, W.-H., & Sun, W. (2020). Do Stay at Home Orders and Cloth Face Coverings Control COVID-19 in New York City? Results From a SIER Model Based on Real-world Data. *Open Forum Infectious Diseases*, 8(2), ofaa442. doi:10.1093/ofid/ofaa442 PMID:33553466

Li, S., Lin, Y., Zhu, T., Fan, M., Xu, S., Qiu, W., Chen, C., Li, L., Wang, Y., Yan, J., Wong, J., Naing, L., & Xu, S. (2021). Development and external evaluation of predictions models for mortality of CO-VID-19 patients using machine learning method. *Neural Computing & Applications*. PMID:33424133

Lounis, M. (2021). Estimation of epidemiological indicators of COVID-19 in Algeria with an SIRD model. *Eurasian Journal of Medicine and Oncology*.

Mahrouf, M., Boukhouima, A., Zine, H., Lotfi, E. M., Torres, D. F., & Yousfi, N. (2021). Modeling and Forecasting of COVID-19 Spreading by Delayed Stochastic Differential Equations. *Axioms*, *10*(1), 18. doi:10.3390/axioms10010018

Maki, K. (2020). A delayed SEIQR epidemic model of COVID-19 in Tokyo. doi:10.1101/2020.08.18.20177709

Malhotra, B., & Kashyap, V. (2020). Progression of COVID-19 in Indian States - Forecasting Endpoints Using SIR and Logistic Growth Models. doi:10.1101/2020.05.15.20103028

Malik, A., Kumar, N., & Alam, K. (2021). Estimation of parameter of fractional order COVID-19 SIQR epidemic model. *Materials Today: Proceedings*.

Mila, A. L., Carriquiry, A. L., & Yang, X. B. (2004). Logistic Regression Modeling of Prevalence of Soybean Sclerotinia Stem Rot in the North-Central Region of the United States. *Phytopathology*, *94*(1), 102–110. doi:10.1094/PHYTO.2004.94.1.102 PMID:18943826

Mohamed, I. A., Aissa, A. B., Hussein, L. F., Taloba, A. I., & Kallel, T. (2021). A new model for epidemic prediction: COVID-19 in kingdom Saudi Arabia case study. *Materials Today: Proceedings*. Advance online publication. doi:10.1016/j.matpr.2021.01.088 PMID:33520671

Mwanga, E. P., Minja, E. G., Mrimi, E., Jiménez, M. G., Swai, J. K., Abbasi, S., . . . Okumu, F. O. (2019). Detection of malaria parasites in dried human blood spots using mid-infrared spectroscopy and logistic regression analysis. doi:10.1101/19001206

Ndiaye, B., & Tendeng, L., & Seck, D. (2020). *Analysis of the COVID-19 pandemic by SIR model and machine learning technics for forecasting*. ResearchGate database.

Nesteruk, I., & Benlagha, N. (2021). Predictions of COVID-19 Pandemic Dynamics in Ukraine and Qatar Based on Generalized SIR Model. *Innovative Biosystems and Bioengineering*, *5*(1), 37–46. doi:10.20535/ibb.2021.5.1.228605

Odagaki, T. (2021). Exact properties of SIQR model for COVID-19. *Physica A*, *564*, 125564. doi:10.1016/j.physa.2020.125564 PMID:33250562

Omar, A. H., & Hasan, Y. A. (2013). Numerical simulations of an SIR epidemic model with random initial states. *ScienceAsia*, *39S*(1), 42. doi:10.2306cienceasia1513-1874.2013.39S.042

Pedersen, M., & Meneghini, M. (2020a). *Quantifying undetected COVID-19 cases and effects of containment measures in Italy: Predicting phase 2 dynamics.* . doi:10.13140/RG.2.2.11753.85600

Pedersen, M. G., & Meneghini, M. (2020b). Data-driven estimation of change points reveals correlation between face mask use and accelerated curtailing of the COVID-19 epidemic in Italy. doi:10.1101/2020.06.29.20141523

Pedersen, M. G., & Meneghini, M. (2020c). A simple method to quantify country-specific effects of COVID-19 containment measures. doi:10.1101/2020.04.07.20057075

Perra, N., Balcan, D., Gonçalves, B., & Vespignani, A. (2011). Towards a Characterization of Behavior-Disease Models. *PLoS One*, *6*(8), e23084. Advance online publication. doi:10.1371/journal.pone.0023084 PMID:21826228

Rahardiantoro, S., & Sakamoto, W. (2021). Clustering Regions Based on Socio-Economic Factors Which Affected the Number of COVID-19 Cases in Java Island. *Journal of Physics: Conference Series*, *1863*(1), 012014. doi:10.1088/1742-6596/1863/1/012014

RenZ. (2013). *A Case Study of Using Refined Epidemic SIR Model to Analyse Bad Takeover and the Distributions of Well-Performed, Bad-Performed and Bankrupt Companies.* Available at https://ssrn.com/abstract=2513691

Rodas, F., Paredes, M., Celis, G., & Pullas-Tapia, G. (2020). *Use of mathematical models for epidemiological simulation of Covid-19 in Ecuador.* Academic Press.

Saito, M. M., Imoto, S., Yamaguchi, R., Miyano, S., & Higuchi, T. (2014). Parameter estimation in multi-compartment SIR model. *17th International Conference on Information Fusion (FUSION)*, 1-5.

Sato, A., Ito, I., Sawai, H., & Iwata, K. (2015). An epidemic simulation with a delayed stochastic SIR model based on international socioeconomic-technological databases. *2015 IEEE International Conference on Big Data (Big Data)*. 10.1109/BigData.2015.7364074

Sedaghat, A., Alkhatib, F., Mostafaeipour, N., & Oloomi, S. A. (2020). Prediction of COVID-19 Dynamics in Kuwait using SIRD Model. *International Journal of Medical Sciences*, *7*. Advance online publication. doi:10.15342/ijms.7.170

Sen, M. D., & Ibeas, A. (2021). On an SE(Is)(Ih)AR epidemic model with combined vaccination and antiviral controls for COVID-19 pandemic. *Advances in Difference Equations*, *2021*(1). doi:10.118613662-021-03248-5

Shastri, S., Singh, K., Kumar, S., Kour, P., & Mansotra, V. (2020). Time series forecasting of Covid-19 using deep learning models: India-USA comparative case study. *Chaos, Solitons, and Fractals*, *140*, 110227. doi:10.1016/j.chaos.2020.110227 PMID:32843824

Shi, H., Lee, K., Lee, H., Ho, W., Sun, D., Wang, J., & Chiu, C. (2012). Comparison of Artificial Neural Network and Logistic Regression Models for Predicting In-Hospital Mortality after Primary Liver Cancer Surgery. *PLoS One*, *7*(4), e35781. doi:10.1371/journal.pone.0035781 PMID:22563399

Sugiyanto, S., & Abrori, M. (2020). A Mathematical Model of the Covid-19 Cases in Indonesia (Under and Without Lockdown Enforcement). *Biology, Medicine, & Natural Product Chemistry*, *9*(1), 15–19. doi:10.14421/biomedich.2020.91.15-19

Sun, H., Qiu, Y., Yan, H., Huang, Y., Zhu, Y., Gu, J., & Chen, S. (2021). Tracking Reproductivity of COVID-19 Epidemic in China with Varying Coefficient SIR Model. *Journal of Data Science: JDS*, 455–472. doi:10.6339/JDS.202007_18(3).0010

Tovissodé, C. F., Doumatè, J. T., & Kakaï, R. G. (2021). A Hybrid Modeling Technique of Epidemic Outbreaks with Application to COVID-19 Dynamics in West Africa. *Biology (Basel)*, *10*(5), 365. doi:10.3390/biology10050365 PMID:33922834

Valenzuela, T. D., Roe, D. J., Cretin, S., Spaite, D. W., & Larsen, M. P. (1997). Estimating Effectiveness of Cardiac Arrest Interventions. *Circulation*, *96*(10), 3308–3313. doi:10.1161/01.CIR.96.10.3308 PMID:9396421

Verma, V., & Priyanka. (2020). *Study of lockdown/testing mitigation strategies on stochastic sir model and its comparison with South Korea, Germany and New York data.* arXiv preprint arXiv:2006.14373.

Wickramaarachchi, W. P. T. M., & Perera, S. S. (2021). An SIER model to estimate optimal transmission rate and initial parameters of COVD-19 dynamic in Sri Lanka. *Alexandria Engineering Journal*, *60*(1), 1557–1563. doi:10.1016/j.aej.2020.11.010

Zhang, G., & Liu, X. (2020). Prediction and control of COVID-19 infection based on a hybrid intelligent model. doi:10.1101/2020.10.22.20218032

Zhang, S., Tjortjis, C., Zeng, X., Qiao, H., Buchan, I., & Keane, J. (2009). Comparing data mining methods with logistic regression in childhood obesity prediction. *Information Systems Frontiers*, *11*(4), 449–460. doi:10.100710796-009-9157-0

Zhang, Z., Sheng, C., Ma, Z., & Li, D. (2004). The outbreak pattern of the SARS cases in Asia. *Chinese Science Bulletin*, *49*(17), 1819–1823. doi:10.1007/BF03183407 PMID:32214712

KEY TERMS AND DEFINITIONS

β **(Contact Rate):** Average number of people contacted by an infected person before isolation.

γ **(Recovery Rate):** Parameter for number of days taken to recover from a disease; helps in computing the reproduction number.

Crude Mortality Rate: Ratio of deaths to active infected cases; reports mortality amongst the infected.

Epidemic Model: A predictive model that estimates the probable spread of disease for contagious and non-contagious diseases.

Infection Fatality Rate: Ratio of deaths to total population in a country/region.

Logistic Regression: A regression model built using exponential functions for dichotomous variables; usually non-linear in nature.

R_0 **(Basic Reproduction Number):** A value that denotes the transmissibility of a disease; if $R_0 > 1$, there is an outbreak of disease.

Sigmoid: An activation function that introduces non-linearity into a regression model

SIR Model: Susceptible-Infected-Recovered model is an epidemic model that uses differential equations to shift from one state to the other.

Chapter 3
Predicting Daily Confirmed COVID–19 Cases in India:
Time Series Analysis (ARIMA)

Sudip Singh

Uttar Pradesh Rajya Vidyut Utpadan Nigam, India

ABSTRACT

India, with a population of over 1.38 billion, is facing high number of daily COVID-19 confirmed cases. In this chapter, the authors have applied ARIMA model (auto-regressive integrated moving average) to predict daily confirmed COVID-19 cases in India. Detailed univariate time series analysis was conducted on daily confirmed data from 19.03.2020 to 28.07.2020, and the predictions from the model were satisfactory with root mean square error (RSME) of 7,103. Data for this study was obtained from various reliable sources, including the Ministry of Health and Family Welfare (MoHFW) and http://covid19india.org/. The model identified was ARIMA(1,1,1) based on time series decomposition, autocorrelation function (ACF), and partial autocorrelation function (PACF).

INTRODUCTION

Coronavirus disease (COVID-19) is an infectious disease caused by a Novel Coronavirus discovered in 2019. COVID-19 virus is primarily transmitted through droplets discharged when an infected person coughs, sneezes, or exhales. India has seen significant increase in daily confirmed cases despite initiating stringent lockdown measures across the country.

Time Series is a collection of data points collected at constant time intervals. These are analyzed to determine the long term trend so as to forecast the future or perform some other form of analysis. Since covid-19 spreads from person to person, the basic assumption of a linear regression model that the observations are independent doesn't hold making a case for time series analysis. Covid-19 daily confirmed data series has an increasing trend, while seasonality trends may also exist, i.e. variations specific to a particular time frame.

DOI: 10.4018/978-1-7998-7188-0.ch003

Various authors have applied ARIMA and other time series models to predict cases for other diseases like Ebola virus disease in west African countries (Manikandan et al., 2016), incidence of dengue in Rajasthan (Bhatnagar et al., 2012), hemorrhagic fever with renal syndrome in China (Liu et al., 2011). Zhang X, Zhang T, Young AA, Li X provided for comparisons of four time series models in epidemiological surveillance data in his paper (Zhang et al., 2014). In the context of covid-19 cases in India, Santanu Roy, Gouri Sankar Bhunia, Pravat Kumar Shit have used Geographic Information System based approach to apply ARIMA(2,2,2) and predicted which Indian district are highly vulnerable for COVID-2019 (Roy & Bhunia, n.d.).

In this paper we have applied simple prediction of daily Covid-19 confirmed cases in India. In further paper we will apply other time series methodologies like Seasonal ARIMA (SARIMA), Vector Auto Regression (VAR) and Vector Error Correction Model (VECM) to predict Daily Confirmed, Active and Recovered Cases respectively and compare the predictions with ARIMA(1,1,1).

ARIMA MODEL

A Time Series is said to be stationary if its statistical properties such as mean, variance remain constant over time. Time Series models are based on the assumption that the Time Series is stationary. Various techniques like differencing, log-differencing etc. are employed to make a non-stationary Time Series stationary. ARIMA model is a combination of differencing with auto-regression and a moving average model. ARIMA is an acronym for Auto-Regressive Integrated Moving Average (in this context, "integration" is the reverse of differencing).

We call this a non-Seasonal ARIMA(p, d, q) model, where

'p' is the order of the AR term. it refers to the number of Y lags which should be used as predictors.

'd' is the number of differencing required to make the time series stationary. It is the minimum amount of differentiation needed to render the sequence stationary, and if the time series is stationary already, then $d = 0$.

'q' is the order of the MA term. it refers to the number of lagged errors in the forecast that should go into the ARIMA model.

The objective of this paper is to fit a non-stationary ARIMA model to correctly recognize the stochastic mechanism of the time series of Covid-19 Daily Confirmed cases and forecast future values for the same.

METHODOLOGY

The best parameters of the ARIMA Model (suitable lags for the components of the AR and MA and the number of differencing required to induce stationarity) is determined for the Daily Confirmed Covid-19 Time Series data. The Auto Correlation (ACF) function and the Partial Auto Correlation (PACF) function are used to determine the best model.

Simple plot of the Daily Confirmed Covid-19 Time Series data is given (Figure 1). It is visually evident from the lag plot of Daily Confirmed Covid-19 Time Series data that there is strong correlation (Figure 2). Further, we observe some significant correlation between t=1 and t=28 (roughly) with significant decline in correlation after that timeframe (Figure 3). It is clearly evident that there is an overall increasing trend in the data along with some possible seasonal variations. First we plot rolling statistics for our data. We have plotted the moving average or moving variance and see if it varies with time. This is more of a visual technique. Subsequently, we have used Dickey-Fuller Test for formally checking stationarity (Figure 4). The null hypothesis is that the Time Series is non-stationary. The test results comprise of a Test Statistic and some Critical Values for difference confidence levels. If the 'Test Statistic' is less than the 'Critical Value', we can reject the null hypothesis and say that the series is stationary.

From Figure 4, it can be seen that the variation in standard deviation is small, mean is clearly increasing with time and thus it is not a stationary series. The test statistic from Dickey-Fuller Test is way more than the critical values.

```
Results of Dickey-Fuller Test:
Test Statistic                    3.366267
p-value                           1.000000
#Lags Used                        8.000000
Number of Observations Used     123.000000
Critical Value (1%)              -3.484667
Critical Value (5%)              -2.885340
Critical Value (10%)             -2.579463
```

Figure 1.

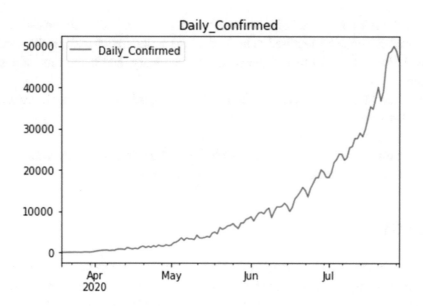

Figure 2.

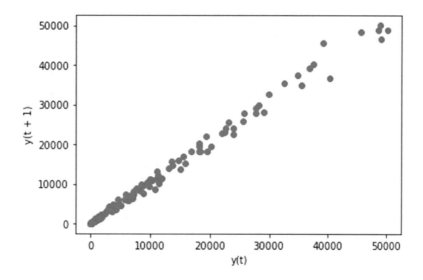

Figure 3.

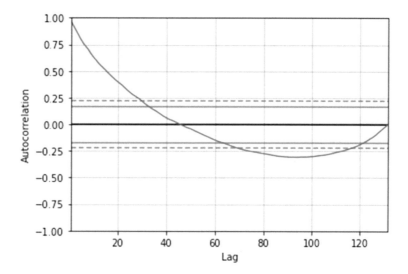

Figure 4.

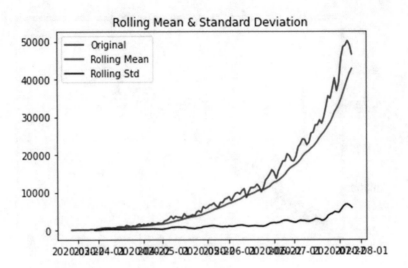

The Corresponding Python Code

```
import numpy as np
import pandas as pd
import matplotlib.pyplot as plt
%matplotlib inline
#plt.style.use('seaborn')
import cufflinks as cf
# Import Statsmodels
from statsmodels.tsa.api import VAR
from statsmodels.tsa.stattools import adfuller
from statsmodels.tools.eval_measures import rmse, aic
CovidDF = pd.read_csv("DailyCovidIndia.csv")
CovidDF.head()
PredAG  = CovidDF[['Date','Daily_Confirmed']].set_index('Date')
PredAG.index = pd.to_datetime(PredAG.index)
PredAG.plot(title="Daily_Confirmed")
pd.plotting.lag_plot(PredAG['Daily_Confirmed'])
pd.plotting.autocorrelation_plot(PredAG['Daily_Confirmed'])
```

Estimating and Eliminating Trend

We have first explored log transform with the intention to penalize higher values more than smaller values (Figure 5). We have then taken rolling averages - taking average of 12 consecutive values (Smoothening) to visualize forward trend in the data given the presence of noise (Figure 5). We have then subtracted the rolling average time series with the log time series and test it for stationarity (Fig 5.0). The Dickey-Fuller test statistic is smaller than 10% critical value; thus the Time Series is stationary with approximately 90% confidence. However, a drawback of this approach is that the time-period needs to be decided that may be a complex task for forecasting models.

```
Results of Dickey-Fuller Test:
Test Statistic                  -2.810926
p-value                          0.056730
#Lags Used                       1.000000
Number of Observations Used    119.000000
Critical Value (1%)             -3.486535
Critical Value (5%)             -2.886151
Critical Value (10%)            -2.579896
```

Figure 5.

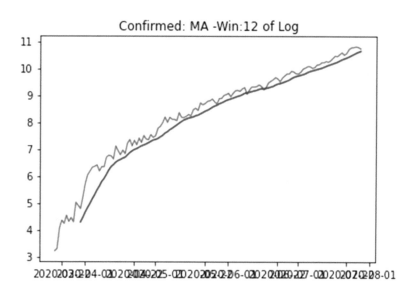

We thus further explore using exponentially weighted moving average where weights are assigned to all the previous values with a decay factor instead of simple rolling moving average. We give recent values a higher weight. We proceed as before: differencing exponentially weighted moving average of the log series with the log series itself and testing the result for stationarity (Fig. 6.0 and Figure 8).

Figure 6.

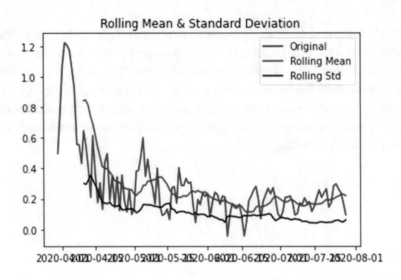

The parameter 'half-life' defines the amount of exponential decay and we have set it to 12. We observe that the test static is smaller than the 1% critical value so we can say with 99% confidence that this is a stationary series.

```
Results of Dickey-Fuller Test:
Test Statistic                    -3.573040
p-value                            0.006298
#Lags Used                         1.000000
Number of Observations Used      130.000000
Critical Value (1%)               -3.481682
Critical Value (5%)               -2.884042
Critical Value (10%)              -2.578770
```

The rolling moving average and exponential weighted moving average methods discussed above deal fairly with trend reduction. However, to deal with both trend and seasonality we finally explore, test for stationarity and apply log differencing taking the difference with a particular time lag and decomposing (modeling both trend and seasonality and removing them from the model). First order differencing of the log series is shown (Figure 9). We can observe that trend and seasonality reduces considerably. Also, the Dickey-Fuller test statistic is much less than the 1% critical value, thus the TS is stationary with 99% confidence (Figure 10). Thus we need not take 2nd or more order of differencing.

```
Results of Dickey-Fuller Test:
Test Statistic                    -1.405142e+01
p-value                            3.172418e-26
#Lags Used                         0.000000e+00
```

Figure 7.

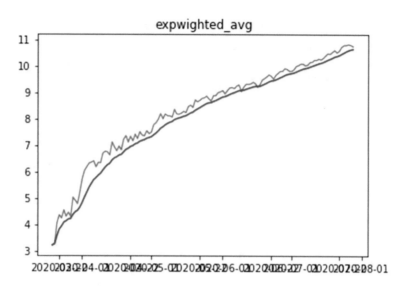

Number of Observations Used	1.300000e+02
Critical Value (1%)	-3.481682e+00
Critical Value (5%)	-2.884042e+00
Critical Value (10%)	-2.578770e+0

Figure 8.

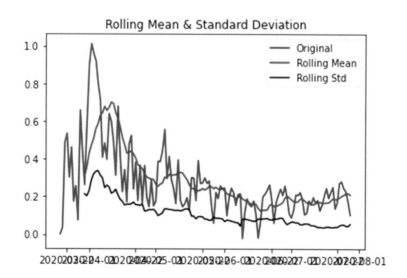

Figure 9.

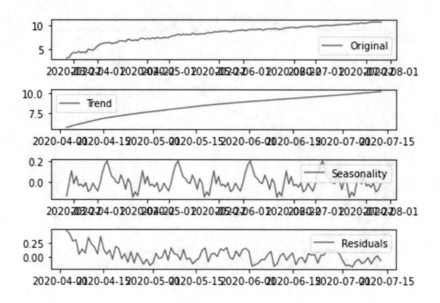

By using Decomposition technique (Figure 11), the trend and seasonality are separated out from data series and we model the residuals. The Dickey-Fuller test statistic is significantly lower than the 1% critical value. Thus the residual time series is also stationary with 99% confidence (Figure 12).

```
Results of Dickey-Fuller Test:
Test Statistic                     -4.923028
p-value                             0.000031
#Lags Used                          1.000000
Number of Observations Used       100.000000
Critical Value (1%)                -3.497501
Critical Value (5%)                -2.890906
Critical Value (10%)               -2.582435
```

The Corresponding Python Code

```python
PredAG['Daily_Confirmed'].corr(PredAG['Daily_Confirmed'].shift(28))
#The above command gives us a correlation value of 0.99 which is high
PredAG['I1']=PredAG['Daily_Confirmed'].diff()
PredAG['I1'].plot()
from statsmodels.tsa.ar_model import AR
#create train/test datasets
X = PredAG['I1'].dropna()
train_data = X[1:len(X)-22]
```

Figure 10.

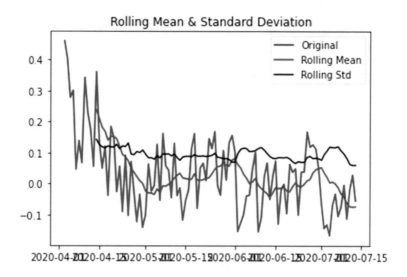

Figure 11.

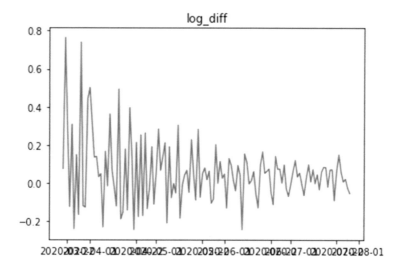

```
test_data = X[X[len(X)-22:]]
#train the autoregression model
model = AR(train_data)
model_fitted = model.fit()
print('The lag value chose is: %s' % model_fitted.k_ar)
print('The coefficients of the model are:\n %s' % model_fitted.params)
```

Figure 12.

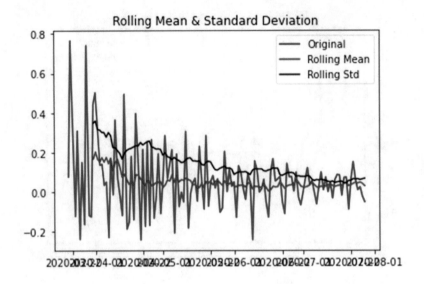

```
from statsmodels.tsa.stattools import adfuller
def test_stationarity(timeseries):
    #Determing rolling statistics
    rolmean =pd.Series(timeseries).rolling(window=12).mean()
    rolstd =pd.Series(timeseries).rolling(window=12).std()
    #Plot rolling statistics:
    orig = plt.plot(timeseries, color='blue',label='Original')
    mean = plt.plot(rolmean, color='red', label='Rolling Mean')
    std = plt.plot(rolstd, color='black', label = 'Rolling Std')
    plt.legend(loc='best')
    plt.title('Rolling Mean & Standard Deviation')
    plt.show(block=False)
    #Perform Dickey-Fuller test:
    print('Results of Dickey-Fuller Test:')
    dftest = adfuller(timeseries, autolag='AIC')
    dfoutput = pd.Series(dftest[0:4], index=['Test Statistic','p-value','#Lags
Used','Number of Observations Used'])
    for key,value in dftest[4].items():
        dfoutput['Critical Value (%s)'%key] = value
    print(dfoutput)
test_stationarity(PredAG['Daily_Confirmed'])
ts_log = np.log(PredAG['Daily_Confirmed'])
plt.plot(ts_log)
plt.title('Confirmed: log chart')
```

```
plt.show()
moving_avg = pd.Series(ts_log).rolling(window=12).mean()
plt.plot(ts_log)
plt.plot(moving_avg, color='red')
plt.title('Confirmed: MA -Win:12 of Log')
plt.show()
ts_log_moving_avg_diff = ts_log - moving_avg
ts_log_moving_avg_diff.tail(12)
ts_log_moving_avg_diff.dropna(inplace=True)
test_stationarity(ts_log_moving_avg_diff)
expwighted_avg = pd.DataFrame.ewm(ts_log, span=12).mean()
plt.plot(ts_log)
plt.plot(expwighted_avg, color='red')
plt.title('expwighted_avg')
plt.show()
ts_log_ewma_diff = ts_log - expwighted_avg
test_stationarity(ts_log_ewma_diff)
ts_log_diff = ts_log - ts_log.shift()
plt.plot(ts_log_diff)
plt.title('log_diff')
plt.show()
ts_log_diff.dropna(inplace=True)
test_stationarity(ts_log_diff)
from statsmodels.tsa.seasonal import seasonal_decompose
decomposition = seasonal_decompose(ts_log, period=30)
trend = decomposition.trend
seasonal = decomposition.seasonal
residual = decomposition.resid
plt.subplot(411)
plt.plot(ts_log, label='Original')
plt.legend(loc='best')
plt.subplot(412)
plt.plot(trend, label='Trend')
plt.legend(loc='best')
plt.subplot(413)
plt.plot(seasonal,label='Seasonality')
plt.legend(loc='best')
plt.subplot(414)
plt.plot(residual, label='Residuals')
plt.legend(loc='best')
plt.tight_layout()
plt.show()
ts_log_decompose = residual
```

```
ts_log_decompose.dropna(inplace=True)
test_stationarity(ts_log_decompose)
```

ESTIMATING THE MODEL

We have chosen ARIMA(p,d,q) model for prediction of Daily Confirmed Cases in India. The predictors depend on the parameters (p,d,q) of the ARIMA model. We have already analyzed parameter 'd' for the ARIMA model to be 1and it represents the number of non-seasonal differences. For selecting p and q we use PACF (Partial Autocorrelation Function) and ACF (Autocorrelation Function) respectively. ACF measures the correlation between the Time Series with a lagged version of itself while PACF measures the correlation between the Time Series with a lagged version of itself but after eliminating the variations already explained by the intervening comparisons. For instance, at lag 5, ACF would compare series at time instant 't1'…'t2' with series at instant 't1-5'…'t2-5' (t1-5 and t2 being end points) whereas PACF will check the correlation but remove the effects already explained by lags 1 to 4. It is clear from ACF (Figure 13) and PACF plots (Figure 14) that both PACF and ACF charts cross the upper confidence interval for the first time at lag value of 1. Thus we select p and q as 1.

Figure 13.

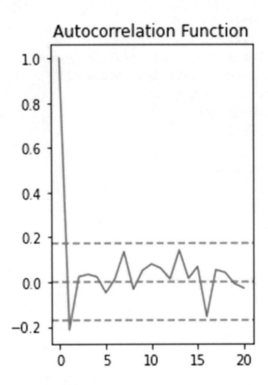

Figure 14.

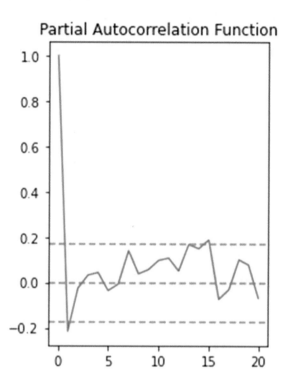

We have made three different ARIMA models considering individual as well as combined effects i.e. ARIMA(1,1,0), ARIMA(0,1,1) and, finally, ARIMA(1,1,1). The corresponding plots are Fig 13.0, 14.0 and 15.0 respectively. Residual Sum of Squares (RSS), which is a measure of the discrepancy between

Figure 15.

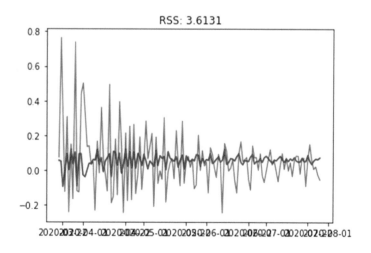

the data and the estimation model, obtained for ARIMA(1,1,0), ARIMA(1,1,0) and ARIMA(1,1,0) are 3.6131, 3.6155 and 3.6115 respectively (lowest for ARIMA(1,1,1).

Finally, we revert the prediction generated from our model to the orginal scale (Figure 18). The predictions from the model are obtained with a Root Mean Square Error (RMSE) of 7103.

Figure 16.

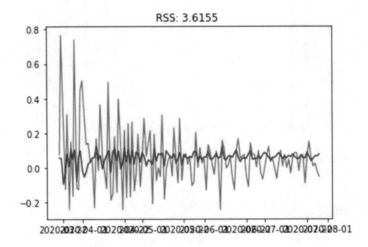

Figure 17.

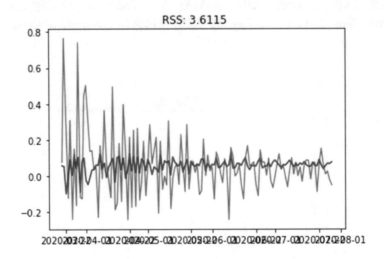

Figure 18.

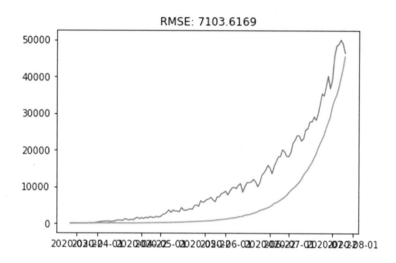

The Corresponding Python Codes

```
#ACF and PACF plots:
from statsmodels.tsa.stattools import acf, pacf
lag_acf = acf(ts_log_diff, nlags=20)
lag_pacf = pacf(ts_log_diff, nlags=20, method='ols')
#Plot ACF:
plt.subplot(121)
plt.plot(lag_acf)
plt.axhline(y=0,linestyle='--',color='gray')
plt.axhline(y=-1.96/np.sqrt(len(ts_log_diff)),linestyle='--',color='gray')
plt.axhline(y=1.96/np.sqrt(len(ts_log_diff)),linestyle='--',color='gray')
plt.title('Autocorrelation Function')
plt.show()
#Plot PACF:
plt.subplot(122)
plt.plot(lag_pacf)
plt.axhline(y=0,linestyle='--',color='gray')
plt.axhline(y=-1.96/np.sqrt(len(ts_log_diff)),linestyle='--',color='gray')
plt.axhline(y=1.96/np.sqrt(len(ts_log_diff)),linestyle='--',color='gray')
plt.title('Partial Autocorrelation Function')
plt.tight_layout()
plt.show()
from statsmodels.tsa.arima_model import ARIMA
```

```
model = ARIMA(ts_log, order=(1, 1, 0))
results_MA = model.fit(disp=-1)
plt.plot(ts_log_diff)
plt.plot(results_MA.fittedvalues, color='red')
plt.title('RSS: %.4f'% sum((results_MA.fittedvalues-ts_log_diff)**2))
plt.show()
model = ARIMA(ts_log, order=(0, 1, 1))
results_MA = model.fit(disp=-1)
plt.plot(ts_log_diff)
plt.plot(results_MA.fittedvalues, color='red')
plt.title('RSS: %.4f'% sum((results_MA.fittedvalues-ts_log_diff)**2))
plt.show()
model = ARIMA(ts_log, order=(1, 1, 1))
results_ARIMA = model.fit(disp=-1)
plt.plot(ts_log_diff)
plt.plot(results_ARIMA.fittedvalues, color='red')
plt.title('RSS: %.4f'% sum((results_ARIMA.fittedvalues-ts_log_diff)**2))
plt.show()
model = ARIMA(ts_log, order=(1, 1, 1))
results_ARIMA = model.fit(disp=-1)
plt.plot(ts_log_diff)
plt.plot(results_ARIMA.fittedvalues, color='red')
plt.title('RSS: %.4f'% sum((results_ARIMA.fittedvalues-ts_log_diff)**2))
plt.show()
predictions_ARIMA_diff = pd.Series(results_ARIMA.fittedvalues, copy=True)
print(predictions_ARIMA_diff.head())
print(predictions_ARIMA_diff.tail())
predictions_ARIMA_diff_cumsum = predictions_ARIMA_diff.cumsum()
print(predictions_ARIMA_diff_cumsum.head())
print(predictions_ARIMA_diff_cumsum.tail())
predictions_ARIMA_log = pd.Series(ts_log.iloc[0], index=ts_log.index)
predictions_ARIMA_log = predictions_ARIMA_log.add(predictions_ARIMA_diff_
cumsum,fill_value=0)
predictions_ARIMA_log.sort_index(inplace=True)
print(predictions_ARIMA_log.head())
print(predictions_ARIMA_log.tail())
predictions_ARIMA_log.plot()
predictions_ARIMA = np.exp(predictions_ARIMA_log)
plt.plot(PredAG['Daily_Confirmed'])
plt.plot(predictions_ARIMA)
plt.title('RMSE: %.4f'% np.sqrt(sum((predictions_ARIMA-PredAG['Daily_Con-
firmed'])**2)/len(PredAG['Daily_Confirmed'])))
plt.show()
```

CONCLUSION AND DISCUSSION

In this study we analyzed Time Series Daily Confirmed Cases data for Covid-19 from 10.03.2020 to 28.07.2020. The ARIMA model predictions are more and more closer to actual values for recent data points. The predictions for the model should further improve with addition of new daily data. Further to this study, we would consider seasonality aspect of the Time Series by applying SARIMA (Seasonal – ARIMA). Also, we would consider other methodologies –Vector Auto Regression (VAR) and Vector Error Correction Model (VECM) to predict Daily Confirmed, Active and Recovered Cases respectively and compare the predictions with ARIMA(1,1,1). The ARIMA model captures past values through the AR component and current lagging residual series through the MA component. Thus, ARIMA(1,1,1) model used in the paper could efficiently account for the linear pattern of the COVID-19 pandemic data. However, this linearity dependency is a constraint of the ARIMA(1,1,1) model presented in this paper. There are "trigger events" that characterize sudden bursts in total covid-19 cases that are influenced by several factors like social events etc. For such scenarios long-term decomposition models would give far better results with generalized models that incorporate non-linear functions in the time series.

Furthermore, autoregressive models like AR, ARMA or ARIMA are uni-directional, where, the predictors influence the Y and not vice-versa. A better model to predict for covid-19 would be provided by Vector Auto Regression (VAR) which is bi-directional - that is, the variables influence each other. Vector Autoregression (VAR) is a multivariate forecasting algorithm that is used when two or more time series influence each other. Further, Vector Error Correction Model (VECM) that utilizes the co-integration restriction information into its specifications can be deployed to make superior covid-19 predictions like Daily Recovered, Daily active etc (multiple time-series).

REFERENCES

Bhatnagar, S., Lal, V., Gupta, S. D., & Gupta, O. P. (2012). Forecasting incidence of dengue in Rajasthan, using time series analyses. *Indian Journal of Public Health*, *56*(4), 281. doi:10.4103/0019-557X.106415 PMID:23354138

Liu, Q., Liu, X., Jiang, B., & Yang, W. (2011). Forecasting incidence of hemorrhagic fever with renal syndrome in China using ARIMA model. *BMC Infectious Diseases*, *11*(1), 218. doi:10.1186/1471-2334-11-218 PMID:21838933

Manikandan, M., Velavan, A., & Singh, Z. (2016). Forecasting the trend in cases of Ebola virus disease in west African countries using auto regressive integrated moving average models Int. *Journal of Community Medicine & Public Health*, *3*, 615–618.

Roy, S., & Bhunia, G. S. (n.d.). Spatial prediction of COVID-19 epidemic using ARIMA techniques in India. *Data in Brief*, *29*, 105340.

Zhang, X., Zhang, T., Young, A. A., & Li, X. (2014). Applications and comparisons of four time series models in epidemiological surveillance data. *PLoS One*, *9*(2), e88075. doi:10.1371/journal.pone.0088075 PMID:24505382

Chapter 4

A Study on COVID-19 Prediction and Detection With Artificial Intelligence-Based Real-Time Healthcare Monitoring Systems

Sonia Rani

School of Computer Applications, Lovely Professional University, India

ABSTRACT

COVID-19 is a major pandemic disease exploited in this century in the whole world. COVID-19 was started om Wuhan, China in November 2019. The main reason for spreading this disease was that test kits were not available in huge amounts to diagnose the COVID-19, and no vaccine was available to cure this disease. Many researchers are trying to make a vaccine for the treatment of this disease. Prevention is better than cure. Therefore, prevention from this epidemic disease is diagnosis at early stages, and treatment should be given to the patient at an accurate time so that patient can escape death. Millions of people were infected by this disease, and most of them lost their lives after suffering from this disease. As we all know, this disease diagnosis test is complicated. Therefore, many smart apps like Siri, Cova App, Arogya Setu App, etc. and digital systems are used to detect and diagnose cases of infected people. These systems are embedded with artificial intelligence techniques. For diagnosis, the COVID-19 computer tomography is based on deep learning convolutional neural network.

OBJECTIVES OF THIS REVIEW

1. To identify use of Deep learning methods to detect the computer tomography of covid patients.
2. To Analysis of Artificial Intelligence based Apps are used to detect the covid symptoms.
3. To identify the maximum use of machine learning methods used to develop the real-time health monitoring system.

DOI: 10.4018/978-1-7998-7188-0.ch004

INTRODUCTION

Covid-19 is also called coronavirus is an epidemic disease of this century. This disease started in China. Now it is spread in the whole world. Due to the increase in positive cases, Governments of every country has ordered the lockdown, social distancing, curfews, and done work from home to decrease the virus diseased rate. The first case of covid-19 was founded in Wuhan city of China. WHO (world health organization) declared on Jan 31, 2020, this covid-19 virus as PHEIC (public health emergency of international concern). Presently, most of the citizens from several countries with China shown their serious concerns about the diagnosis, estimate, and rectify of the virus infection (Ping, 2020). The Wuhan centre's Epidemiological investigators exposed the covid-19 from that patient who worked in the local seafood market, admitted to the central hospital on 26 Dec 2019. Investigators suggested that the covid-19 outbreak-related is with a seafood market in Wuhan. After investigation, founded that SARS-like COVS categorize into RBD sequences and amino acid. The receptor ACE2 of the human body affected by the 3 Bats SARS- with COVS (Wu, 2020). SARS-COVS was recognized in animal marketplaces, authors developed a method to quickly screen ancestry B beta coronaviruses, such as SARS-COVS and the current SARS-COV-2. Firstly, it appeared in humans in 2003 afterward spreading from animals in open-air markets in China. Afterward, numerous natively related viruses were identified in Chinese horseshoe bats, which directed in wild animals everywhere in the world (Letko and Marzi, 2020). The covid-19 is credentialed and classified by an extensive of grave respirational disease in humans of Wuhan, China. which started on 12 Dec 2019, had produced 2,794 laboratory-confirmed cases with 80 deaths by 26 Jan 2020. This virus epidemic and that started from a seafood local market has full-grown considerably to contaminate 2,761 people in China. Distinctive clinical indications of these patients are temperature, dry cough, breathing problems, pneumonia, and headache. Seven patients suffered from which six are sellers from the seafood market. They were sent to the laboratory at the Wuhan Institute of virology for the treatment. 2019-CoVID equals to 96% with the genome-wide level to a bat coronavirus. This virus exists to types of SARSr-CoV confirmed by pairwise protein system study of 7 preserved non-structural proteins. "It is quarantined from the bronchoalveolar lavage liquid of a critically ill patient could be deactivated by sera from several patients and also established that 2019-nCoV routines the similar cell entry receptor ACE2 (angiotensin-converting enzyme II) as SARS-CoV" (Zhou, et al. (2020). At present medical tests of covid-19 are not available at high scale because of time, health care specialists, testing kits are limited (Subirana, et al. 2020).

ARTIFICIAL INTELLIGENCE INITIATION

A machine and human mind could be a connection between behaviour and experience, rather than on the specific behaviour of a human. A machine works like as human thinks. "Artificial intelligence" also substituted by "computer intelligence" or "machine intelligence". "Intelligence is the capacity of an information-processing system to adapt to its environment while operating with insufficient knowledge and resources" (Wang, 2019). A conference of artificial intelligence at Dartmouth College was introduced in 1956. They developed the idea in 1975-1980 that AI can use in many branches of science like psychology and several areas (Mijwel, 2015). Artificial Intelligence was coined out by the "British logician and computer pioneer Alan Turing in 1936 digital computing machine is called the universal Turing machine. The first AI program code run in Britain in Manchester and Cambridge in 1951-1952.

'nouvelle AI' was founded by the roboticist Rodney Brooks in 1980 at the MIT AI Laboratory (Copeland and Proudfoot, 2007). Artificial intelligence is an area that supports the computer system to be smart and make conclusions. Machine learning assisted to apply AI on the system and deep learning supports to attain the output on the system. Machine learning is a subset of AI that trained the machines on how to learn. Deep learning is a narrower subset of machine learning. It supports the growth of the high values of the learning environment (Chahal and Gulia, 2019).

Figure 1. Subsets of artificial intelligence

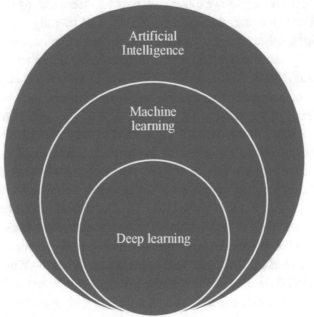

Machine Learning

In medical decisions used machine learning tools designed independently to assist the doctors. Physicians predicted and analyzed big-data with these ML tools. A medical system is moved to advance with research articles in healthcare with AI. But surely, the physician is more educated for used the systems to work with machine learning (Char, Shah, and Magnus, 2018). Smart expert systems are developed with Artificial intelligence algorithms and computation methods. It includes procedures that think, act, and implement tasks using procedures that are outside of the human scope. Machine learning algorithms can be supervised, unsupervised, semi-supervised, reinforcement. In supervised learning imitates an algorithm to specify the features and labels, it is used for classified the output by decision tree and linear regression model. The unsupervised learning algorithms implemented on those problems where labels are not presented earlier and categorized output into cluster grouped data by PCA and k-means algorithms. So that algorithm can be used in further to estimate the new unlabelled cases. In reinforcement learning identified data and patterns through the environment (Alloghani, 2020). Machine learning is a multidisciplinary field which derives and build upon concepts from "statistics, computer science, engineering, cognitive science, optimization" model and several disciplines of mathematical and science. It is also used in several fields like clinical, business, education and agriculture (Ghahraman, 2004). Afterwards splitting data in to training and testing then applied the machine learning algorithms on data and used the cross- validation technique for divide trained data into different subsets (Domingos, 2012).

Figure 2. Types of machine learning

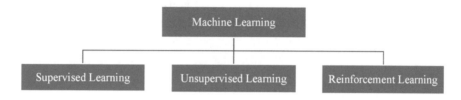

Supervised, Unsupervised Learning, and Reinforcement Learning

Machine learning enforced as connotation study concluded supervised learning, unsupervised learning, and reinforcement Learning for pathophysiological testing of a disease. However, the complete representation of any disease can be understood by considering the behaviour changes with any condition. Class labels are predicted by features through a concise supervised learning model. Example of supervised learning methods knn, DT, RBF. Mostly knn is used for classified the target when there is less knowledge about data distribution. These features can be categorical, continuous, or binary. If cases are given with known output, then supervised learning is used. Though if examples are unlabelled then the unsupervised learning approach is used. In the reinforcement learning information of training given to the knowledge system by the environment. In this type of learning outside a mentor is in the form of a scalar reinforcement signal that established a quantity of how well the system works. A deep convolutional neural network is used for pattern recognition. The deep learning model consists of many hidden convolutional layers, so it is complex. It effected on numerous applications such as computer-vision, speech-recognition, natural-language processing (Muhammad and Zhu, 2015). AI-based computer tomography medical imaging. The computer-aided platform used to assist the radiologists to make medical decisions, i.e., for disease analysis, pursuing, and diagnosis with image procurement, separation, diagnosis. These techniques use supervised deep learning methods (Shi and Wang, 2020). Semi-supervised learning is used when inputs are partly presented in particular cases or limited to the superior response. These are used to progress the mathematical model after inadequate training data, where a bit of the sample data doesn't contain labels. This learning is beneficial when the charge of labelling is too high. Reinforcement learning is used when a software agent yields actions in an environment to exploit the growing prize and feedback is to be given in the form of confident or negative reinforcement in an active environment. This is frequently used in self-driving cars or in learning to play the game compared to human rivals. Q-learning is an example of reinforcement learning. Unsupervised learning methods do not use any internal parameters to adjust the data. In fact, Supervised learning methods use the weight and threshold parameters to explore the data. Semi-supervised learning methods are only use the portion of the data for optimize the parameters, for example, a subset of Identified network connections (Maetschke et al, 2013).

Deep Learning Era

Deep learning use more complex neural network models with several stages of features that predict results. In this model, many hidden layers or features are present, which are exposed by the quick filtered by cloud architectures and graphics processing units (Davenport and Kalakota, 2019). Deep learning in supervised or unsupervised used with a gradient-based search method to guess, observe, encrypt, and categorize the patterns (Schmidhuber, 2014). Deep learning is a mathematical model that contained multiple layers to study hidden levels of data. Deep CNN is used for image, video, pattern, activity, speech, audio, text, visual object detection, and recognition. Several levels of depiction of data composed simple but in non-linear segments. It defined a set of approaches that permits a machine to be fed with raw data and to automatically learn the techniques that are needed for detecting or classify an object (Cun, Bengio and Hinton, 2015).

ROLE OF ARTIFICIAL INTELLIGENCE-BASED TECHNIQUES IN THE HEALTH SECTOR

Computer Analysis systems are used to access a variety of fields studying models of diseases, neuroscience, immunology, etc (Gris, Coutu and Gris, 2017). AI methods comprise the support vector machine, an artificial neural network designed for structure data and unstructured data processed by deep learning with convolutional neural network and natural language processing. AI is used for many diseases diagnosis mainly it contained cancer, cardiovascular, neurology. AI used the supervised and unsupervised machine learning for clinical purpose. Mostly used supervised rather than unsupervised learning methods in medical areas. Occasionally k-means clustering and PCA (principal component analysis) unsupervised learning methods used in medical outcomes in grouping data. Presently maximum used deep learning with a large number of network layers, which is improbable for classical artificial neural networks. Deep learning can be traversed more composite non-linear patterns in the data (Jiang et al, 2017). "Integrating AI systems into clinical practice necessitates building a mutually beneficial relationship between AI and clinicians". For example, if AI classified the type2 diabetes in a patient it takes less time, but if it diagnoses by blood tests then reports are must read by clinicals. It takes more time and efforts of patient. In this AI could inevitably prepare all records. In future, AI will must give assistance to clinicals, patients, radiologist. So that improve the efficiency of medical experience (Maruthappu et al, 2018).

ROLE OF ARTIFICIAL INTELLIGENCE-BASED MACHINE LEARNING TECHNIQUES IN THE HEALTH SECTOR

A medical system is moved to advance with research articles in healthcare with AI. But surely, the physician is more educated to use the systems to work with machine learning (Char, Shah, and Magnus, 2018). Machine learning is also used in several fields like clinical, business, education, and agriculture (Ghahraman, 2004). Computer Analysis systems are used to access a variety of fields studying models of diseases, neuroscience, immunology, etc (Gris, Coutu, and Gris, 2017). AI used the supervised and unsupervised machine learning for clinical purpose. Deep learning can be traversed more composite non-linear patterns in the data (Jiang et al, 2017). The Recurrent or convolutional neural networks have increased the performance with the use of composite and improved parameters to classify the images and videos (Gibbons1 and Gibbons2, 2019). AI systems influenced healthcare specialists with excellent care, and patient results come in the most productive form (Kelly, Suleyman, and Corrado, 2019). The computer-aided platform used to assist the radiologists to make medical decisions, i.e., for disease analysis, pursuing, and diagnosis with image procurement, separation, diagnosis. These techniques used supervised deep learning methods (Shi and Wang, 2020). In the future, AI will assist clinicians, patients, radiologists. So there will be improvement in the efficiency of medical experience (Maruthappu et al, 2018).

SUPERVISED, UNSUPERVISED MACHINE LEARNING, DEEP LEARNING METHODS USED TO PREDICTION

Machine learning enforced as a connotation study concluded supervised learning, unsupervised learning, and reinforcement Learning (Alloghani et al, 2020). Semi-supervised learning methods only use the portion of the data to optimize the parameters (Maetschke et al, 2013). The unsupervised learning algorithm SOM(Self-organizing-map) classifies secreted patterns without labelled data and mentions the capability to acquire and establish info without providing an error sign to estimate the possible result (Sathya and Abraham, 2013). Deep learning use more complex neural network models with more hidden layers as stages of features that predict results and it is exposed by the quick filtered by cloud architectures and graphics processing units (Davenport and Kalakota, 2019). Deep learning in supervised or unsupervised used with a gradient-based search method to guess, observe, encrypt, and categorize the patterns (Schmidhuber, 2014). The deep learning model is affected on numerous applications such as computer-vision, speech-recognition, natural-language processing (Muhammad and Zhu, 2015). Deep CNN is used for image, video, pattern, activity, speech, audio, text, visual object detection, and recognition. It defined a set of approaches that permits a machine to be fed with raw data and to automatically learn the techniques that are needed for detecting or classify an object (Cun, Bengio and Hinton, 2015).

MAINTAIN A REAL-TIME DATABASE OF COVID-19 IN GITHUB, GOOGLE DRIVE THROUGH AI TECHNIQUES

A real-time system and data collected from many sources to maintain a database from peer-reviewed scientific papers, hospitals, news channels, govt or public health institutions, government sources, and websites of health commissions. A covid-19 database of CSV file in the GitHub repository in which, explained every source of data. In this database collected information about cases of death confirmation infected by corona, any travel history about these cases, age and sex, mainly symptoms of patients, and geographic district information and of patients. This database updated regularly live version of this database in a format of CSV file that can be download from GitHub and google drive (Xu et al, 2020).

Diagnosis the Covid-19 with Artificial Intelligence Methods and Real Time Systems

Artificial Intelligence based methods SRLSR (sparse rescaled linear square regression), GFS (Gradient boosted feature selection), RFE (recursive feature elimination) were practical to deal this problem. All categorize values of variables labelled with median, percentages, frequency rates, and range of inter-quartile standards. SPSS 25.0 version software is used for statistical studies (Peng et al., 2020). The cross-validation technique is used to divide trained data into different subsets (Domingos, 2012). The cost-effective software based on a mobile-based survey would be simply used to classify and monitored those persons who have any slight signs and indications of covid-19 (Rao, 2020). Real-time RT-PCR system for users to diagnose the covid-19 affected Positive cases and 85 negative cases of this viral (Peng et al., 2020). An epidemiological and medical study on 10 paediatrics SARS-CoV-2 contagion cases confirmed by real-time converse record PCR examine of SARS-CoV-2 RNA (Xu et al, 2020). An IHiS (integrated health information systems) developed for fever screening solution using iThermo to diagnosis the covid-19. AI with CT image examines help to diagnose and measurable the cases of covid-19 (Dr. Kapoor et al, 2020).

Different Android Apps used for Classified the Covid-19

Siri App is developed forgave the guidance of related symptoms of an epidemic in a simple natural language voice message to the public. Alexa App is mainly assisted to elder persons who can be most affected by covid-19, told the symptoms of an epidemic, and replied most of the questions. Apple health check app developed by teamwork with Apple, the CDC. It provided consistent information on measures and increasing the infection. Arogya Setu App is a mobile application app launched by the Government of India to link important health facilities with the public to explain them of risks related to covid-19, and also traced the suspected patient nearby you. Digital DHIS2 This digital app solutions helped to express the information related to passenger's time of entered in the country from at-risk countries to help covid-19 investigation. Appropriate info passed to health majors in their particular geographic areas. These systems also help fast-track finding, broadcasting, energetic observation, and fast response for cases of Covid-19, it can be installed as a separate Covid-19 package or combined into a country's current virus surveillance systems (Kapoor et al, 2020). Cough is classified into 3 classes: 1) normal cough 2) covid-cough 3) non-covid, but viral cough with machine learning and deep learning classifier approach using artificial intelligence engine. An app named AI4 covid-19 for initially diagnosis the covid-19 from listening to sounds of all types of cough. This app engine runs with a front-end framework programmed like an easy and adaptable mobile app. The app listens to the cough and recorded it as pertussis and bronchitis. To trained and test the diagnosis system the dataset had accessed in types as pertussis-131 and bronchitis-102, covid-19 is 48, normal cough sounds samples-76. Then this data trained by machine learning algorithm deep learning convolutional neural network. For recognize the type of cough brute force algorithm is used. Then send it to the AI engine server wirelessly. This app useful at community places such as airports and rushy areas like shopping malls if a cough is detected, it is passed on to the diagnosis portion to the AI engine. After analysis of the AI engine, it gave possible results. 1) covid-19 2) Not covid-19. This app also defined the cough caused by a normal person with no disease 2) pertussis 3) bronchitis 4) COVID-19. It mainly classified the cough problem into different categories (Ali et al, 2020). A smart app that diagnoses the covid-19 based on speech recognition. A linear audio test to check the patients who are infected from covid-19 and stayed at home. For the most serious patients of covid-19 an achievement ratio to order the ICU (intensive care unit) allocation. Thus, authors have found a process to gather short audio recordings the word "Ommmmmmm", with the "m" sound sections of 12 seconds for covid-19 patients and received them by what's app, web, email or using a mobile app developed by MIT. Sigma rapid progress method used, where data and code are shared in real-time.

DIAGNOSE COVID-19 WITH COMPUTER TOMOGRAPHY BASED ON AI TECHNIQUES

Machine learning algorithms used to convert CT images into predictors. Covid-19 is diagnosed with symptoms and infection is the prognosis in patients (Wynants et al, 2020). Diagnostic conduct was evaluated by the ROC curve, sensitivity, and specificity. The dataset is contained of 4356 chest CT exams from 3,322 patients. The average age between 15 to 49 years and there were more male patients than female patients (Li et al, 2020). CT study of AUC 0.996 and CT 95% datasets with 98.2% sensitivity, 92.2% specificity high sensitivity 96.4% sensitivity, 98% specificity. Progression and regression of cases could be supervised additional quantitatively and constantly (Gozes, 2020). Regression analysis is used for comparing the confirmed cases with variations of day-to-day weather parameters (wind, average temperature, and moisture). It is found that weather parameters ought to maximum influence on positive cases. This model gave accuracy 95.7% for trained data and 85.7% for tested data. The investigation committed that the GMDH method could be a suitable technique to predict and classify the confirmed cases of covid-19 and examine the probable pattern of a dataset (Pirouz et al., 2020).

Notify the Death Cases by Real-Time System

A research study was done by Joseph on cases and notified that death rate increased by1.4% after emerging symptoms of covid-19 in Wuhan, and recovery of cases had 11% of recovery cases till Feb 2020. The death cases are mostly aged less than 30 and greater than 59 years. This data Intended through using statistical methods and MATLAB (Joseph et al, 2020).

DEEP LEARNING MODEL USED TO IDENTIFY COVID-19 AND PNEUMONIA

A 2d and 3d deep learning algorithm to identify pneumonia and covid-19 with chest CT exams. Statistical analysis is done by using R (ver-3.6.3). A huge number of CT tests from several hospitals, which comprised 1296 covid-19 CT tests. Sample of 1325 non-pneumonia and 1735 CAP CT tests were also gathered to confirm the finding robustness seeing that alike image features might be detected in Covid-19 and additional types of lung diseases. (Li, et al., 2020). To classify the text, images, videos, and sounds use the Deep CNN. It is mainly used for pattern, face, and image recognition. Deep learning model use to detect the covid-19 on x-rays. The testing of this model is done by 260 images which are available on GitHub and Kaggle repository database. From these images, 130 are normal images. This model has given the 100% accuracy, specificity, sensitivity (Salman et al, 2020). Optimized blockchain method used for better positioning and attain better performance solving outbreak corona associated tracking. This system gave the 5 significant solutions 1) with epidemic tracking, protection with the privacy of the user, safely day-to-day operations, medical stream chain, tracing of donation (Peng et al., 2020). The authors presented probable focuses on the expansion of drugs and vaccines for SARS-CoV-2. Full-length S proteins of SARS-CoV-2 and SARS-CoV S share virtually 76% characteristics in amino acid orders, the NTDs demonstration only 53.5% of homology (Ou et al., 2020). An improved skewed SEIR (showing an epidemiological infected-removed) model developed to predict the SARS covid-19 epidemic data. The authors tested this model with a machine-learning algorithm of artificial intelligence (Yang, 2020). The Deep Learning model has given the 100% accuracy, specificity, sensitivity to classify the x-rays images of covid-19. It has also shown equivalent performance with a professional radiologist, and it will expand the proficiency of radiologists in medical practice (Salman et al., 2020).

Figure 3. Different machine learning methods use for diagnosis Covid-19

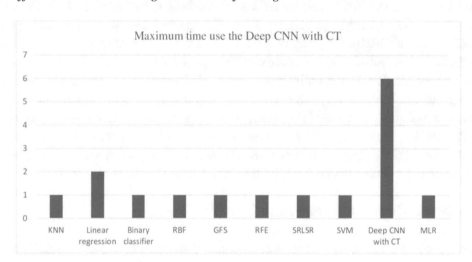

CONCLUSION

Covid-19 is such an epidemic disease of this century. This disease has shaken the whole world completely. Day by day many people have suffered from this disease and some of them lost their lives. Till there is no permanent solution available of this disease, and no maximum testing kits are available to diagnose this disease so death cases of suffered from epidemic are increasing rapidly. Thus, the diagnosis of this disease at the exact time is compulsory. After doing a detailed study it is found that artificial intelligence-based tests are doing to identify and classify this disease. Various apps are used for identifying the covid-19 patients are nearby you and some android apps are used for classifying the covid-19 with symptoms and audios of cough also used for prediction and diagnosis covid-19 patients through classifications of cough, cold, and sound. These apps are embedded with many machine learning algorithms based on artificial intelligence technology. Presently the deep learning with a convolutional neural network is maximumly used to diagnose several diseases. Computer tomography scan is a medical imaging procedure is used to diagnose this disease and other lung infections. Thus, artificial intelligence-based many smart healthcare digital systems and medical imaging scan systems are exploited in the future and it will surely assist physicians, radiologists, and patients.

REFERENCES

Ali, I. (2016). AI4COVID-19: AI-Enabled Preliminary Diagnosis for COVID-19 from Cough Samples via an App. *IEEE Access, 4*, 1–12.

Allam, Z., & Jones, D. S. (2020). On the Coronavirus (COVID-19) Outbreak and the Smart City Network: Universal Data Sharing Standards Coupled with Artificial Intelligence (AI) to Benefit Urban Health Monitoring and Management. *Healthcare MDPI, 8*(1), 46. doi:10.3390/healthcare8010046

Alloghani, M. (2020). A Systematic Review on Supervised and Unsupervised Machine Learning Algorithms for Data Science. In *Unsupervised and Semi-Supervised Learning.* Springer Nature Switzerland AG 2020.

Butt, C., Gill, J., Chun, D., & Babu, B. A. (2020). Deep learning system to screen coronavirus disease 2019 pneumonia. *Applied Intelligence, Springer, 2020*, 1–7.

Chahal, A., & Gulia, P. (2019). Machine Learning and Deep Learning. *International Journal of Innovative Technology and Exploring Engineering, 8*(12), 4910-4914.

Chahal, A., & Gulia, P. (2019). Machine Learning and Deep Learning. *International Journal of Innovative Technology and Exploring Engineering, 8*(12).

Char, D.S. (2018). Implementing Machine Learning in Health Care — Addressing Ethical Challenges. *N Engl J Med, 378*(11), 981–983.

Copeland, B. J., & Proudfoot, D. (2007). Artificial Intelligence: History, Foundations, And Philosophical Issues. Handbook of the Philosophy of Science. Philosophy of Psychology and Cognitive Science, 429-485.

Cun, Y.L., Bengio, Y., & Hinton, G. (2015). Deep Learning. *Nature, 521*, 438-444.

Davenport, T., & Kalakota, R. (2019). The potential for artificial intelligence in healthcare. *Future Healthcare Journal, 6*(2), 94–98. doi:10.7861/futurehosp.6-2-94 PMID:31363513

Domingos, P. (2012). A Few Useful Things to Know About Machine Learning. *Communications of the ACM, 55*(10), 1–10. doi:10.1145/2347736.2347755

Domingos, P. (2012). A Few Useful Things to Know About Machine Learning key insights. *Communications of the ACM, 55*(10), 1–10. doi:10.1145/2347736.2347755

Ghahraman, Z. (2004). Unsupervised Learning. *Machine Learning, LNAI, 3176*, 72–112.

Gibbons, J.A. (2019). Machine learning in medicine: a practical introduction. *BMC Medical Research Methodology*, 19-64.

Gris, K. V., Coutu, J. P., & Gris, D. (2017). Supervised and Unsupervised Learning Technology in the Study of Rodent Behavior. *Frontiers in Behavioral Neuroscience, Vol, 11*, 141–143. doi:10.3389/fnbeh.2017.00141 PMID:28804452

Jiang, F. (2017). Artificial intelligence in healthcare: past, present, and future. *Stroke and Vascular Neurology, 2*, 230-243.

Jiang, F. (2017). Artificial intelligence in healthcare: Past, present and future. Stroke and Vascular Neurology. *BMJ (Clinical Research Ed.), 2017*, 230–243.

Kapoor, A., Guha, S., Kanti Das, M., Goswami, K. C., & Yadav, R. (2020). Digital healthcare: The only solution for better healthcare during COVID-19 pandemic? *Indian Heart Journal, 72*(2), 61–64. doi:10.1016/j.ihj.2020.04.001 PMID:32534691

Kelly, C. (2019). Key challenges for delivering clinical impact with artificial intelligence. *BMC Medicine, 17*(195), 1–9.

Letko, M., Marzi, A., & Munster, V. (2020). Functional assessment of cell entry and receptor usage for SARS-CoV-2 and other lineage B beta coronaviruses. *Nature, 5*, 562–569. PMID:32094589

Li, L. (2020). Artificial Intelligence Distinguishes COVID-19 from Community-Acquired Pneumonia on Chest CT. *Radiology*. Advance online publication. doi:10.1148/radiol.2020200905

Maetschke, S. R., Madhamshettiwa, P. B., Davis, M. J., & Ragan, M. A. (2013). Supervised, semi-supervised and unsupervised inference of gene regulatory networks. *Briefing in Bioinformatics, Vol, 15*(2), 195–211. doi:10.1093/bib/bbt034 PMID:23698722

Maruthappu, M. (2018). Debate & Analysis Artificial intelligence in medicine: Current trends and future possibilities. *The British Journal of General Practice*, 143–144.

Muhammad, I., & Ya, Z. (2015). *Supervised machine learning approaches A survey.* State Journal on Soft Computing. doi:10.21917/ijsc.2015.0133

Ou. (2020). Characterization of spike glycoprotein of SARS-CoV-2 on virus entry and its immune cross-reactivity with SARS-CoV. *Nature Communications, 2*,16-20.

Peng, M. (2020). Artificial intelligence application in COVID-19 diagnosis and prediction. SSRN *Electronic Journal*, 1-17. doi:10.2139srn.3541119

Pirouz, B. (2020). Investigating a serious challenge in the sustainable development process: Analysis of confirmed cases of COVID-19 (New Type of Coronavirus) Through a Binary Classification Using Artificial Intelligence and Regression Analysis. *Sustainability*.

Rao, A. S. R. (2020). Identification of COVID-19 Can be Quicker through Artificial Intelligence framework using a Mobile Phone-Based Survey in the Populations when Cities/Towns Are Under Quarantine. *Infection Control and Hospital Epidemiology*, 1–18.

Salman, F. M. (2020). COVID-19 Detection using Artificial Intelligence. *International Journal of Academic Engineering Research, 4*(3), 18–25.

Sathya, R., & Abraham, A. (2013). Comparison of Supervised and Unsupervised Learning Algorithms for Pattern Classification. *International Journal of Advanced Research in Artificial Intelligence, Vol, 2*(2), 34–38. doi:10.14569/IJARAI.2013.020206

Schmidhuber, J. (2015). Deep learning in neural networks: An overview. *Neural Networks, 61*, 85–117.

Wang, P. (2019). On Defining Artificial Intelligence. *Journal of Artificial General Intelligence, 10*(2), 1-37.

Wu, F., Zhao, S., Yu, B., Chen, Y.-M., Wang, W., Song, Z.-G., Hu, Y., Tao, Z.-W., Tian, J.-H., Pei, Y.-Y., Yuan, M.-L., Zhang, Y.-L., Dai, F.-H., Liu, Y., Wang, Q.-M., Zheng, J.-J., Xu, L., Holmes, E. C., & Zhang, Y.-Z. (2020). 'A new coronavirus associated with human respiratory disease in china'. *Nature, 579*(7798), 265–284. doi:10.103841586-020-2008-3 PMID:32015508

Wu, J. T., Leung, K., Bushman, M., Kishore, N., Niehus, R., de Salazar, P. M., Cowling, B. J., Lipsitch, M., & Leung, G. M. (2020). Estimating the clinical severity of COVID-19 from the transmission dynamics in Wuhan, China. *Nature Medicine, Vol, 26*(4), 506–510. doi:10.103841591-020-0822-7 PMID:32284616

Wynants, L. (2020). Prediction models for diagnosis and prognosis of covid-19 infection: a systematic review and critical appraisal. *BMJ Open, 369*, 1-11.

Xu, B. (2020). Epidemiological data from the COVID-19 outbreak, real-time case information. Nature, 7(106), 1-6.

Xu, B. (2020). Epidemiological data from the COVID-19 outbreak, real-time case information. *Scientific Data, 7*,106.

Xu, Y., Li, X., Zhu, B., Liang, H., Fang, C., Gong, Y., Guo, Q., Sun, X., Zhao, D., Shen, J., Zhang, H., Liu, H., Xia, H., Tang, J., Zhang, K., & Gong, S. (2020). Characteristics of pediatric SARS-CoV-2 infection and potential evidence for persistent fecal viral shedding. *Nature Medicine, Vol, 26*(4), 502–505. doi:10.103841591-020-0817-4 PMID:32284613

Yang, Z. (2020). Modified SEIR and AI prediction of the trend of the epidemic of COVID-19 in China under public health interventions. *Journal of Thoracic Disease,* 1-18.

Zhou, P., Yang, X.-L., Wang, X.-G., Hu, B., Zhang, L., Zhang, W., Si, H.-R., Zhu, Y., Li, B., Huang, C.-L., Chen, H.-D., Chen, J., Luo, Y., Guo, H., Jiang, R.-D., Liu, M.-Q., Chen, Y., Shen, X.-R., Wang, X., ... Shi, Z.-L. (2020). A pneumonia outbreak associated with a new coronavirus of probable bat origin. *Nature, 579*(7798), 270–289. doi:10.103841586-020-2012-7 PMID:32015507

Chapter 5
Landmark Recognition Using Ensemble-Based Machine Learning Models

Kanishk Bansal
Lovely Professional University, India

Amar Singh Rana
Lovely Professional University, India

ABSTRACT

Recognizing landmarks in images with machine learning is an excellent topic for research today. Landmark recognition is an important field in computer vision. In this field, we train the machine learning models to identify and recognize the closed distinctly distinguishable objects in a digital image. In general, if we consider a digital image to be a set of coordinates of different pixels, a landmark is said to be enclosed in that closed polygon formed by the pixels that may be considered as a distinct and distinguishable thing in one or the other sense. Landmark recognition is an important subject area of image classification since it is considered as one of the first steps towards reaching complete computer vision. The extremely broad definition of a landmark makes it eligible to be considered as one of the leading problems in image classification tasks. Since the task is considered to be a very broad one, the solutions to the task hold no easy procedures. This chapter explores landmark recognition using ensemble-based machine learning models.

INTRODUCTION

Recognizing landmarks in images with machine learning is an excellent topic for research today. Landmark recognition is an important field in computer vision (Noh, 2017). In this field, we train the machine learning models to identify and recognize the closed distinctly distinguishable objects in a digital image. In general, if we consider a digital image to be a set of coordinates of different pixels, a landmark is

DOI: 10.4018/978-1-7998-7188-0.ch005

said to be enclosed in that closed polygon formed by the pixels that may be considered as a distinct and distinguishable thing in one or the other sense (Magliani et al., 2019).

Landmark Recognition is an important subject area of image classification since it is considered as one of the first steps towards reaching complete computer vision (Zheng, 2009). The extremely broad definition of a landmark makes it eligible to be considered as one of the leading problems in image classification tasks (Chen et al., 2014). Since the task is considered to be a very broad one, the solutions to the task hold no easy procedures.

Today, many Machine Learning techniques have been developed to handle the process of image classification (Weyand, 2020). However, landmark recognition remains a difficult task due to its broadness. The datasets available for landmark recognition continue to grow exponentially and with the increase in sizes of datasets, the accuracies tend to fall. But with the continuous efforts of people working in Artificial Intelligence (AI), accuracies, too, have seen a considerable jump (Chen, 2011).

Figure 1. An overview of machine learning models

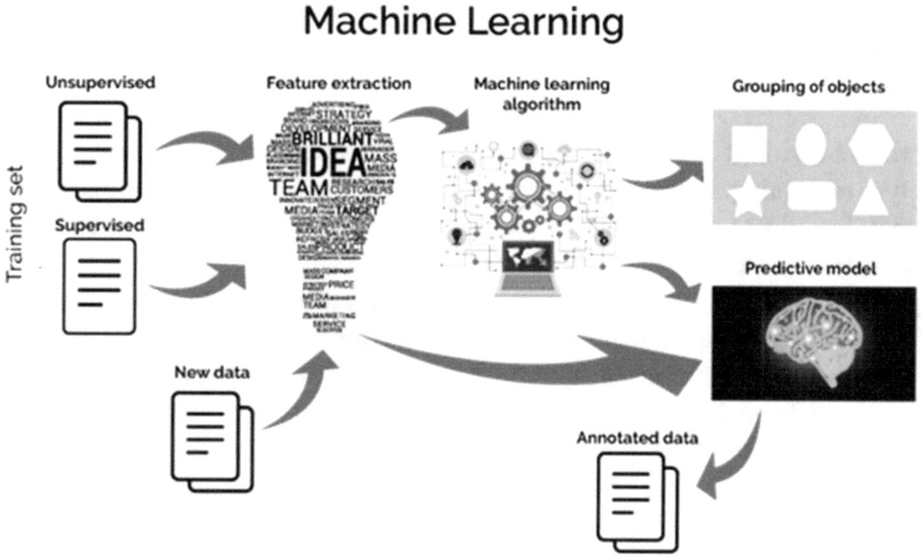

MACHINE LEARNING AND ITS TECHNIQUES

Machine Learning can be defined as the field of Artificial Intelligence (AI) that deals with training machines to determine patterns in the data that is fed to it and based on the patterns that the machine determines, making acceptable decisions on the new data which may be used to further carry out different other tasks. Machine learning (ML) algorithms are mostly thought to work well only on very crisp and clean data. Moreover, the lesser the data needed for generalization, the better is an ML model expected to work (Jordan & Mitchell, 2015).

Machine Learning models are trained on various types of data. Based on the type of data, ML techniques are classified into the following categories:

Figure 2. Different types of machine learning

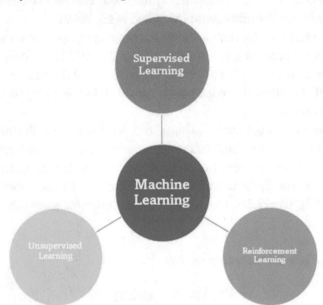

1. **Supervised Learning:** This type of learning is the "Help would be appreciated" type of learning. In this type of learning, we provide data for training that is already labeled. A dataset that includes both inputs for training and their real outputs is given. Then, the model is trained which can predict the outcomes of new data to be given (Caruana & Niculescu-Mizil, 2006).
2. **Unsupervised Learning:** This is the "Help is not needed" type of learning. In this type, we do not provide a labeled data for training. The ML models are trained on datasets without outputs and then other parameters determine how well the model has been trained (Barlow, 1989).
3. **Reinforcement Learning:** This is the "I'm learning from the environment" type of learning. In this type of learning, we do not provide data with labeled outputs, but the models are made to learn from external sources. This type of model can train itself over longer periods and get better without worrying about overfitting (Sutton & Barto, 2018).

IMAGE CLASSIFICATION TECHNIQUES

Image classification mostly includes a supervised learning paradigm only. The labeled training set is given to the machine to learn and train itself for new prediction. Models are generated via sophisticated algorithms that have been developed by scientists and researchers over time.

Landmark recognition is an image classification problem that is solved using Supervised Learning techniques. These techniques include:

1. **Convolutional Neural Networks –** Convolutional Neural Networks or CNNs are a type of Deep Learning technique. In this technique, digital images undergo a convolution operation and then

Figure 3. Different types of image classification

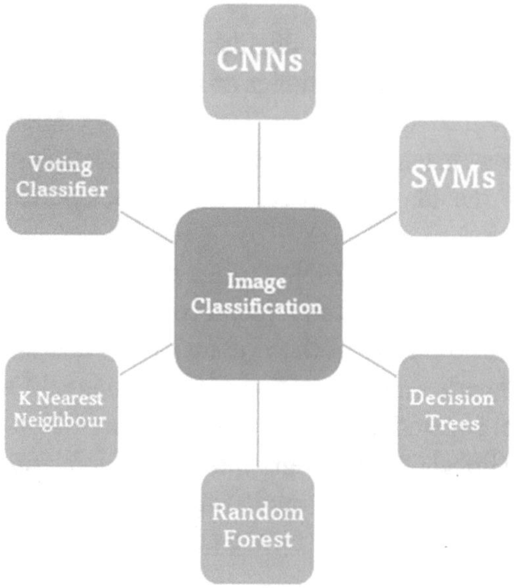

convolved images are fed into a network of activation functions which are then trained to behave in a way similar to the working of neurons in our body (Albawi et al., 2017).

2. **Support Vector Machines** – Support Vector Machines or SVMs are used to classify labeled data by introducing hyperplanes in the existing multidimensional data. A support vector, also known as a hyperplane, is introduced in the data space to separate various classes from each other, and then the data points are classified (Vishwanathan & Narasimha Murty, 2002).

3. **Decision Tree Classifier** – Decision trees work as a tree hierarchy. Data points in a decision tree classifier are modeled like the branches in a tree. The data points with maximum information gain are put into one class and those with more entropy are put in different classes (Brijain, 2014).

4. **Random Forest Classifier** – Random Forest Classifier is based on the concept of a forest. Just like Decision trees, it creates a hierarchical structure. However, unlike the former, it creates many trees instead of just one. The data points with more information gain are put together and those with more entropy are put in different classes (Belgiu & Drăguţ, 2016).

5. **K Nearest Neighbours** – In this technique, no new model from the data points is created. It just plots a Euclidean multi-dimensional graph and calculates the distance of a new data point from the previous data points and based on the value of K, it classifies new datapoint into one class or another (Zhang, 2017).

6. **Voting Classifier** – It works on the concept of the process of voting. Some hyperparameters are pre-designed to make the procedure work. The probability of voting of these hyperparameters decides which class the new data point should belong to (Ruta & Gabrys, 2005).

TECHNIQUES FOR LANDMARK RECOGNITION

Landmarks are defined as the distinct and distinguishable objects enclosed in a closed polygon, if formed, on a digital image. Landmark recognition is of high importance since it is considered the first step towards realizing a complete computer vision. Today, mostly CNNs are used for the identification of landmarks in the vast datasets that are available with us for this task.

The various types of CNNs that have been used over time for landmark recognition include:

1. **ResNets:** Residual neural networks (ResNets) are a type of Artificial Neural Networks (ANNs). These work like the pyramidal cells in the cerebral cortex of our brains. These networks use some sort of skipped connections in the network to get maximum benefit (Balduzzi, 2017).
2. **DELF:** Deep Local Features is a transformation of Convolutional Neural Networks that are trained only with the image-level annotations on a landmarks dataset (Noh, 2017).
3. **DELG:** Deep Local and Global Features is an approach that combines two approaches namely Deep Local Features and Global Features. This approach makes models that combine mean pooling for global features and attentive selection for local features (Zhu, 2018).

Figure 4. Different CNN architectures for landmark recognition

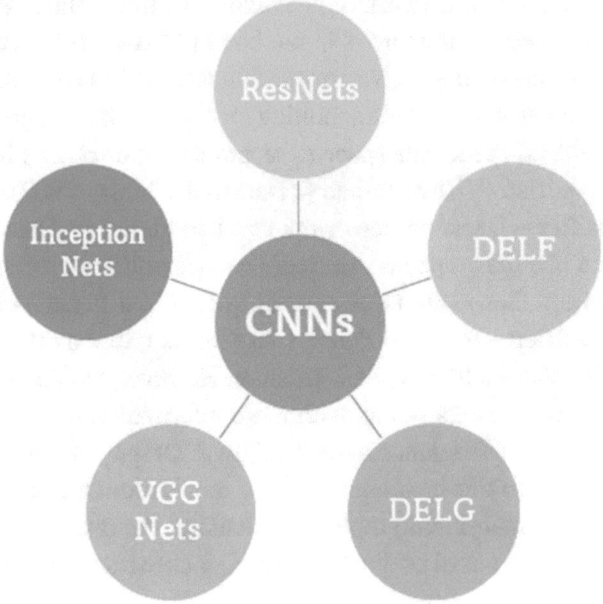

4. **VGGNets:** Visual Geometry Group Neural Networks or VGGNets is one of the most widely used CNN architectures used today for image classification tasks. VGG is an object-recognition technique that supports up to 19 layers. Built as a deep CNN, VGG outperforms many architectures out there (He, 2016).
5. **Inception Nets:** Inception Neural Networks are 27 level layers deep convolutional neural networks (CNN) which use three different sizes of filters namely (1x1, 3x3, 5x5). Then max-pooling is done

and resulting outputs are concatenated and sent to the next layer. This type of network is used by Google for image classification tasks (Szegedy, 2016).

IMPLEMENTATION OF SOME ML TECHNIQUES

In this section, we discuss the implementation of some machine learning algorithms on the task of landmark recognition. We use a publicly available dataset taken from the renowned machine learning platform Kaggle. The dataset named Qutub Complex Monuments' Images Dataset consisted of 1286 image files belonging to 5 classes. Out of these 1286 image files, 1270 images had a 3-color coding. We used only the 3 color-coded images (RGB) for the sake of uniformity (Bhatt & Patalia, 2017).

So, our dataset was appropriately cleaned for being fed to various machine learning models. We trained 4 machine learning models with this dataset. These models were namely:

1.   Convolutional Neural Network
2.   Support Vector Machine
3.   K Nearest Neighbours
4.   Decision Tree Classifier

A generalized algorithmic approach for the implementation of a Machine Learning Technique for image classification can be drawn as follows:

Figure 5. Implementation of various ML techniques on landmark recognition

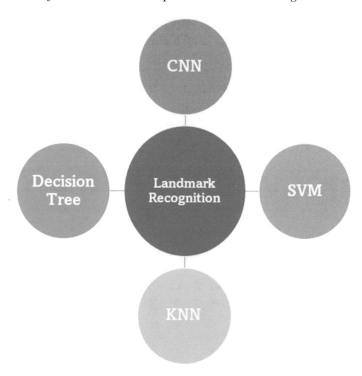

On implementing the above-mentioned ML techniques, we found the training and test accuracies as mentioned in Table 1. Where all the training accuracies were quite high, the test accuracies were considerably lower than the training accuracy, thereby, indicating overfitting of the models.

Figure 6. Process of training an ML model.

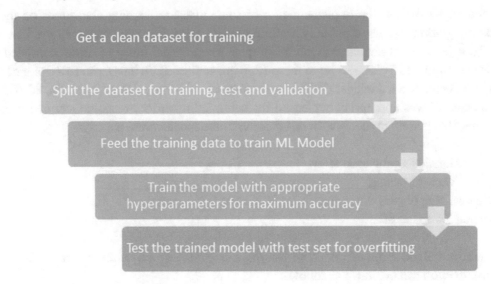

All the ML models were run in their most basic form without any changes in hyperparameters. The convolutional neural network was run with a single layer. In SVM too, no kernel or hyperparameters were changed. Similarly, KNN and Decision tree were also run in their default form. As it is imperative from Table 1, Convolutional Neural Networks fared better than all other Machine Learning techniques.

Table 1. Summarising training and test accuracies for various ML models

ML Technique	Training Accuracy (in %)	Test Accuracy (in %)
Support Vector Machine (SVM)	89	64
K-Nearest Neighbour	74	54
Decision Tree Classifier	99	49
Convolutional Neural Network	98	73

It should not be difficult to understand that CNNs belong to a whole new class of Machine Learning algorithms named the "Deep Learning" techniques. In Deep Learning, instead of a single model being trained to classify data, we have a whole network of activation functions that work like a neuron in our body. The deep learning paradigm may also be thought of as a model trained from numerous models (Goodfellow, 2016).

Figure 7. Summarising training and test accuracies for various ML models

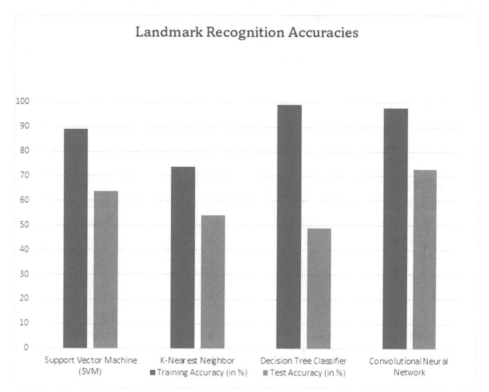

As we can see from Table 1, CNN performs the best on our dataset both in terms of training and test accuracy. Though the test accuracy is a little lower than the training accuracy, thereby, indicating over-fitting; the accuracies are much better than the rest of the techniques. Out of the rest of the techniques known as the classical machine learning techniques, Support Vector Machines fare the best.

Out of the classical machine learning approaches, SVMs are known to fare the best. It is also thought that SVMs can achieve a 100% training accuracy if appropriate parameters are changed (Vishwanathan & Narasimha Murty, 2002). However, a 100% training accuracy does not imply that our model is good enough to be generalized. Also, the other two algorithms do not seem to fare that well. Though decision trees seem to give a training accuracy of 99%, test accuracy of 49% makes it inappropriate to be used for practical uses.

FUTURE SCOPE

As the name suggests, Convolutional Neural Networks are based on the working of Neural Networks in a living being. No wonder, it has been seen that Artificial Intelligence performs best when it has inspiration from nature in it (Binitha & Sathya, 2012; He et al., 2009; Rafiq et al., 2001; Yang, 2010). Neural Networks are inspired by the mechanisms of neurons, the spinal cord, and the brain in our body (Singh et al., 2015). However, every living being has a different set of neural networks in its body.

We believe that neural networks can be optimized for even better performances if we optimize them with the so-called Nature-Inspired-Computing (NIC) Algorithms. NIC algorithms are the evolutionary algorithms that use inspiration from a natural phenomenon while their execution (Kumar et al., 2018; Singh et al., 2019). Evolutionary algorithms in Soft-Computing derive their working from the evolutionary processes in our environment.

It is believed today that the evolutionary algorithms just like the normal evolution of any body part in a living being can optimize the existing Machine Learning Techniques for better accuracies. It is believed that these algorithms, inspired from nature can evolve the currently existing techniques. Significant work has been done in this field to establish this fact (Singh et al., 2020) and a lot more opportunities currently hold.

Today, there exist many NIC algorithms like Genetic Algorithm, Ant Colony Algorithm, and Particle Swarm Optimization, etc. which are used to optimize existing AI techniques to get the best results for problems. We believe, using more of such algorithms, we would be able to optimize CNNs to get the best outcomes (Singh et al., 2020).

CONCLUSION

In this chapter, we discussed the types of machine learning paradigms, machine learning for image classification, and focusing especially on Landmark Recognition. We discuss the implementation of four Machine Learning approaches including the Convolutional Neural Networks on the classification of landmarks in an image. We have seen that there are three types of machine learning out of which the supervised learning paradigm is used for tasks of image classification. We performed image classification for the task of recognizing landmarks in an image. The task of landmark recognition is at the heart of computer vision due to its fundamental nature. We saw that for image classification, today mostly the convolutional neural networks are deployed. The convolutional neural nets or the CNNs belong to the newly developed category of deep learning and work differently from the classical machine learning models. We trained the four different types of machine learning models with a proper training set and a test set. We saw that training accuracies are achieved greatly by classical machine learning models but the test accuracies fail miserably making way for the CNNs. CNNs performed way better than classical ML approaches implying that classical ML approaches cannot and should not be used for image classification. Then we discuss about the Nature Inspired Computing techniques which use the inspirations from nature to optimize the currently existing techniques. We find out that CNNs are much more capable for variations in them making them highly flexible for better usages. Classical ML approaches like SVMs, Decision Tree, and KNN fared poorly on the task of image classification plus they are not much flexible for variations. Varying parameters in a CNN, we have achieved milestones that could not have been expected earlier. Deploying Nature Inspired Computing along with evolution of architectures is expected to be the trend in the near future. Researchers are working on these footsteps and new researches expect to follow.

REFERENCES

Albawi, S., Mohammed, T. A., & Al-Zawi, S. (2017). Understanding of a convolutional neural network. In *2017 International Conference on Engineering and Technology (ICET)*. IEEE. 10.1109/ICEngTechnol.2017.8308186

Balduzzi, D. (2017). The shattered gradients problem: If resnets are the answer, then what is the question? In *International Conference on Machine Learning*. PMLR.

Barlow, H. B. (1989). Unsupervised learning. *Neural Computation*, *1*(3), 295–311. doi:10.1162/neco.1989.1.3.295

Belgiu, M., & Drăguţ, L. (2016). Random forest in remote sensing: A review of applications and future directions. *ISPRS Journal of Photogrammetry and Remote Sensing*, *114*, 24–31. doi:10.1016/j.isprsjprs.2016.01.011

Bhatt & Patalia. (2017). Indian monuments classification using support vector machine. *International Journal of Electrical and Computer Engineering*, *7*(4), 1952.

Binitha, S., & Sathya, S. S. (2012). A survey of bio inspired optimization algorithms. *International Journal of Soft Computing and Engineering*, *2*(2), 137–151.

Brijain, M. (2014). *A survey on decision tree algorithm for classification*. Academic Press.

Caruana, R., & Niculescu-Mizil, A. (2006). An empirical comparison of supervised learning algorithms. *Proceedings of the 23rd international conference on Machine learning*. 10.1145/1143844.1143865

Chen, D. (2011). Residual enhanced visual vectors for on-device image matching. In *2011 Conference Record of the Forty Fifth Asilomar Conference on Signals, Systems and Computers (ASILOMAR)*. IEEE. 10.1109/ACSSC.2011.6190128

Chen, T., Yap, K.-H., & Zhang, D. (2014). Discriminative soft bag-of-visual phrase for mobile landmark recognition. *IEEE Transactions on Multimedia*, *16*(3), 612–622. doi:10.1109/TMM.2014.2301978

Erol, O. K., & Eksin, I. (2006). A new optimization method: Big Bang-Big Crunch. *Advances in Engineering Software*, *37*(2), 106–111. doi:10.1016/j.advengsoft.2005.04.005

Goodfellow, I. (2016). Deep learning: Vol. 1. *No. 2*. MIT Press.

He, K. (2016). Deep residual learning for image recognition. *Proceedings of the IEEE conference on computer vision and pattern recognition*.

He, S., Wu, Q. H., & Saunders, J. (2009). Group search optimizer: An optimization algorithm inspired by animal searching behavior. *IEEE Transactions on Evolutionary Computation*, *13*(5), 973–990. doi:10.1109/TEVC.2009.2011992

Jordan, M. I., & Mitchell, T. M. (2015). Machine learning: Trends, perspectives, and prospects. *Science*, *349*(6245), 255–260. doi:10.1126cience.aaa8415 PMID:26185243

Kumar, S., Singh, A., & Walia, S. S. (2018). Parallel Big Bang - Big Crunch Global Optimization Algorithm: Performance and its Applications to routing in WMNs. *Wireless Personal Communications, Springer, 100*(4), 1601–1618. doi:10.100711277-018-5656-y

Magliani, F., Fontanini, T., & Prati, A. (2019). Landmark recognition: From small-scale to large-scale retrieval. Springer.

Noh, H. (2017). Large-scale image retrieval with attentive deep local features. *Proceedings of the IEEE international conference on computer vision.* 10.1109/ICCV.2017.374

Rafiq, M. Y., Bugmann, G., & Easterbrook, D. J. (2001). Neural network design for engineering applications. *Computers & Structures, 79*(17), 1541–1552. doi:10.1016/S0045-7949(01)00039-6

Ruta, D., & Gabrys, B. (2005). Classifier selection for majority voting. *Information Fusion, 6*(1), 63–81. doi:10.1016/j.inffus.2004.04.008

Singh, Kumar, Walia, & Chakravorty. (2015). Face Recognition: A Combined Parallel BB-BC & PCA Approach to Feature Selection. *International Journal of Computer Science & Information Technology, 2*(2), 1-5.

Singh, A., Kumar, S., Singh, A., & Walia, S. S. (2019). Three-parent GA: A Global Optimization Algorithm. *Journal of Multiple-Valued Logic and Soft Computing, 32,* 407–423.

Singh, A., Kumar, S., & Walia, S. S. (2020). Parallel 3-Parent Genetic Algorithm with Application to Routing in Wireless Mesh Networks. In *Implementations and Applications of Machine Learning* (pp. 1–28). Springer. doi:10.1007/978-3-030-37830-1_1

Sutton, R. S., & Barto, A. G. (2018). *Reinforcement learning: An introduction.* MIT Press.

Szegedy, C. (2016). Rethinking the inception architecture for computer vision. *Proceedings of the IEEE conference on computer vision and pattern recognition.* 10.1109/CVPR.2016.308

Vishwanathan, S. V. M., & Narasimha Murty, M. (2002). SSVM: a simple SVM algorithm. In *Proceedings of the 2002 International Joint Conference on Neural Networks. IJCNN'02* (Cat. No. 02CH37290). IEEE. 10.1109/IJCNN.2002.1007516

Weyand, T. (2020). Google landmarks dataset v2-a large-scale benchmark for instance-level recognition and retrieval. *Proceedings of the IEEE/CVF Conference on Computer Vision and Pattern Recognition.*

Yang, X.-S. (2010). A new metaheuristic bat-inspired algorithm. Nature inspired cooperative strategies for optimization (NICSO 2010), 65–74. doi:10.1007/978-3-642-12538-6_6

Zhang, S. (2017). Learning k for knn classification. *ACM Transactions on Intelligent Systems and Technology, 8*(3), 1–19.

Zheng, Y.-T. (2009). Tour the world: building a web-scale landmark recognition engine. In *2009 IEEE Conference on Computer Vision and Pattern Recognition.* IEEE. 10.1109/CVPR.2009.5206749

Zhu, Q. (2018). A deep-local-global feature fusion framework for high spatial resolution imagery scene classification. *Remote Sensing, 10*(4), 568.

Chapter 6
Image Classification Using Deep Neural Networks:
Emotion Detection Using Facial Images

Sukanta Ghosh

https://orcid.org/0000-0002-7715-7669
Lovely Professional University, India

Amar Singh
Lovely Professional University, India

ABSTRACT

Facial expression recognition is an activity that is performed by every human in their day-to-day lives. Each one of us analyses the expressions of the individuals we interact with to understand how people interact and respond with us. The malicious intentions of a thief or a person to be interviewed can be recognized with the help of his facial features and gestures. Face recognition from picture or video is a well-known point in biometrics inquiry. Numerous open places, for the most part, have reconnaissance cameras, and these cameras have their noteworthy security incentives. It is generally recognized that face recognition has assumed a significant job in reconnaissance framework. The genuine favorable circumstances of face-based distinguishing proof over different biometrics are uniqueness. Since the human face is a unique item having a high level of inconstancy in its appearance, face location is a troublesome issue in computer vision. This chapter explores emotion detection using facial images.

INTRODUCTION

Emotions enable a form of communication among human beings. Complex social communication come into context with the understanding of Emotion. Emotion Detection can be done via voice, body gestures and other complex methods. There are many practical methods to examine facial emotions too. There are seven types of human emotions that are universally recognized. The seven we are talking about includes happiness, sadness, fear, surprised, anger, disgust and neutral. A service that detects emotion from facial

DOI: 10.4018/978-1-7998-7188-0.ch006

emotions would be widely applicable, as such a service can bring advancement in various applications of gaming, marketing, consumer product satisfaction and entertainment. Emotion Detection has attracted significant attention in the advancement of human behavior and machine learning. Various applications related to face and emotion detection include: Personal Credentials and Access Control, Video Phone and Tele conferencing, Medica land Forensic Applications, Gaming and Applications, analyzing human behavior to ascertain work satisfaction (Franco & Treves, 2001).

Face recognition is a method of identifying or verifying the identity of an individual using their face. There are various algorithms that can do face recognition but their accuracy might vary. Here I am going to describe how we do face recognition using deep learning. In computer vision, one essential problem we are trying to figure out is to automatically detect objects in an image without human intervention. Face detection can be thought of as such a problem where we detect human faces in an image. There may be slight differences in the faces of humans but overall, it is safe to say that there are certain features that are associated with all the human faces. There are various face detection algorithms but Viola-Jones Algorithm is one of the oldest methods that is also used today. Face detection is usually the first step towards many face-related technologies, such as face recognition or verification. However, face detection can have very useful applications. The most successful application of face detection would probably be photo taking. When you take a photo of your friends, the face detection algorithm built into your digital camera detects where the faces are and adjusts the focus accordingly.

There are four categories of methods that are used to detect human face, namely: Feature Method: Based on facial features like placement of eyes, nose, contour; Knowledge Method: Pre-Trained Models as we instill our model with datasets; Appearance Method: Based on Neural Networks approach; Template Method: Checks for the correlation between standard image and input image face pattern. These methods if used separately, cannot solve all the problems of face detection like orientation, pose and expression. The difficulty one face with the emotion recognition is basically due to the following: There is a moderate size database for training images, based on input image whether it is a static frame or it is a transition frame it becomes difficult to classify the emotion (Saaidia et al., 2014).

For real-time detection in which facial expressions differs dynamically, it is very difficult to detect emotions. In the present emotion detection application examine static images of facial emotions. We will inspect the system that will do the emotion recognition in real time with a live video streaming. Computation of frame-by-frame classification is necessary for live detection. So, we have developed a system for detecting emotions in real time. The result we achieved is an innovative system where an emotion-indicating text is displayed on screen.

The aim of the project is to come up with a solution to problem of emotion detection by dividing it into sub-problems. The scope of project does not only the two problems which will tell us whether a human face is detected or not, but also the multi-class problems that will take the user input, to start detecting the face and afterwards starts with a live emotion detection. For this different methodologies and techniques for dataset training, selection and classification, solutions to the problems as well as taking the computational complexity and timing issues has been considered (Busso et al., 2004). The major objective of the project is to implement emotion detection in terms of run time on the embedded system. Various Hardware Resources has been used to achieve the goal. Also, various algorithms and methodologies are studied to attain the desired goals. Such type of emotion detection system can be useful for our day to day tasks. This system may would help the human life in near future. The typical application for this system is listed here: Business Meetings, Social Gatherings, Teaching Assistant, Education, Audio-Visual Speech Recognition, Gaming Experience, Multimedia (Kotsia et al., 2007).

STUDY OF LITERATURE

Research endeavors in human–machine connection is centered around the way to enable machines (robots and different machines) to comprehend human aim, for example discourse acknowledgment and signal acknowledgment frameworks (Franco & Treves, 2001). Despite extensive accomplishments right now the previous a very long while, there are still a ton of issues, and numerous specialists are attempting to unravel them. Plus, there is another significant however disregarded method of correspondence that might be significant for increasingly common cooperation: feeling assumes a significant job in logical comprehension of messages from others in discourse or visual structures.

There are various territories in human–machine connection that could viably utilize the capacity to comprehend feeling (Saaidia et al., 2014), (Busso et al., 2004). For instance, it is acknowledged that enthusiastic capacity is a fundamental factor for the cutting-edge individual robot, for example, the Sony AIBO (Kotsia et al., 2007). It can likewise assume a critical job in intelligent room (Katsis et al., 2008) and affective machine coach (Yang et al., 2018). Albeit restricted in number contrasted and the endeavors being made towards expectation interpretation implies, a few specialists are attempting to acknowledge man–machine interfaces with a feeling getting ability.

The vast majority of them are centered around outward appearance acknowledgment and discourse signal investigation (Pérez et al., 2020). Another conceivable methodology for feeling acknowledgment is physiological sign investigation. We accept this is an increasingly regular methods for feeling acknowledgment, in that the impact of feeling on outward appearance or discourse can be stifled generally effectively, and enthusiastic status is characteristically reflected in the action of the sensory system. In the field of psychophysiology, conventional devices for the examination of human passionate status depend on the chronicle and measurable investigation of physiological signs from both the focal and autonomic sensory systems (Arkin et al., 2001).

Another issue with current frameworks is the necessary length of signs. At present, at any rate 2–5 min of sign checking is required for a choice (Ghosh & Singh et al., 2020). For down to earth purposes, the necessary checking time ought to be diminished further. Right now, novel feeling acknowledgment framework dependent on the handling of physiological signs is introduced. This framework shows an acknowledgment proportion a lot higher than chance likelihood, when applied to physiological sign databases got from tens to several subjects.

REQUIREMENT FOR THE STUDY

Emotion Detection is a very essential research topic for psychologists. Current advancements in image processing and emotion recognition has motivated research work on Automated Emotion Recognition. In past, to detect facial emotions from still images, lots of effort were dedicated. To fulfil this need of emotion detection, many techniques have been applied and neural networks, Gabor wavelets, and active appearance models are one of them. The only limitation that was caught with this strategy is that the still images only captures the apex of emotion from expression, that is the instant at which the indicators of emotion are most marked. People rarely show this apex of their Facial Emotions during normal communication. It can be captured for very precise cases and is short-term.

Technical Requirement:

The aspects of our technical requirements are:

- Determining our budget
- Create our work break down schedule
- Develop the project DFDs
- Initiate a communication plan
- Define risk-management aspects

Economical Requirements:

The Economic requirement here deals with the Economic Assessment. It is a very important tool for achieving results like value for money and user satisfaction. Economical Assessment is a process for making alternative use of resources such as Raspberry Pi or PC. We are also focusing on analysis of customer needs, goal of project, options available, costing, various benefits and affordability.

1. Wide Scope of Economic Requirements.
2. Covers the cost and benefits.

Environmental Requirements:

1. Our project work is not creating any disastrous effect on environment.
2. We can say that our project is eco-friendly.

IMPLEMENTATION PROCESS

After going through various literature reviews, it is found that Facial Emotion Recognition is a procedure that is implemented by both machines and human beings.
Computer needs to follow the following process that consist the following:

1. Finding or locating various faces in a live stream captured by camera. This is a step known as Face Detection.
2. From detected regions on the face, extracting various facial features like facial components, skin texture of face, etc. This step is called Facial Feature Extraction.
3. Analyzing changes in appearance of facial features and categorizing these features into categories that can interpret Facial Expressions into various emotions like angry, happy, sad, etc. This step is called Facial Expression Interpretation.

On the basis of some systems that has already been designed in this arena, we found that this project can be implemented with four steps.

1. Identifying and Pre-processing
2. Registering Face
3. Extracting Facial Features
4. Emotion Detection

These processes are described here:

Identifying and Pre-Processing:

Operations with the image at the entry level of abstraction is known as Preprocessing. Steps involved in Pre-processing are as follows:

1. Noise Reduction
2. Converting image to gray scale
3. Pixel Transformation
4. Geometric Transformation

Registering Face

Identification of Human Faces as Digital Images make use of Face Registration. During the process of Face Registration, first we locate the image with the help of predefined set that contains landmark points. This is known as "Face Localization" or "Face Detection". Faces that are detected have been Geometrically Normalized so that it can match the dataset images also known as template image. This is called as Face Registration.

Extracting Facial Features

Process of locating specific facial regions, points, curves, landmarks and contours in a given 2D image or a 3D image is known as Facial Feature Extraction. For Face Extraction, Registered Image generate a numerical vector of facial features. We can extract following features: Eyes, Nose Tip, Lips, Eyebrows.

Emotion Detection

At this step, algorithm classifies the face on the basis of emotions and data images. Emotion Detection can be done using various approaches.

1. **Neural Network Approach:** Artificial Neural Network Approach is based on the biological neural networks that constitute brains. In this approach neural networks are trained independently. Neural Network is a framework for various Machine Learning Algorithms to process complex data inputs. Learning of these systems is based on examples, and they are not programmed for rules specific to the task. For example, they learn to identify images with happy faces by evaluating images that were labelled "happy" manually (Zhang et al., 2017). They will automatically generate characteristics from the material they processed and it can help them with identification.

2. **Gabor Filter:** A linear filter, called Gabor Filter, has its uses in texture analysis. It will analyses the content of image for specific frequency that will be fixed for directions in a local region also known as region of analysis. According to vision scientists Human Visual System and Gabor Filters are similar. They are suitable for representing texture and discriminating textures (Yan et al., 2020). Some scientists also claim that Gabor Functions can model the cells in the cortex of mammal brain. Perception in human visual system is also on the same lines with Process of image analysis using Gabor Filter.

3. **Support Vector Machine:** Support Vector Network (SVMs) are supervised learning models. They have associated learning algorithms. These algorithms analyses data for analyzing regression and classification. If we provide SVM with set of training examples and they are marked which category they will either belong category one or to category two. SVMs will itself build a model. This model will assign various new examples to both categories. SVM perform linear as well non-linear classification. If there is unavailability of Labelled data, supervised learning cannot be possible. Thus, we need an unsupervised learning approach. Hava Siegelmann and Vladimir Vapnik created Support-Vector Clustering algorithm. Statistics of support vectors are applied by this algorithm. Support Vectors are developed in Support Vector Machines Algorithm. They are used to categorize unlabeled data.

4. **Training Database and Testing Database:** We can design algorithms in machine learning that learns from the data and make predictions on similar set of data. These algorithms follow data-driven approach by constructing a mathematical model from the data, to make predictions and decisions.

The final model of algorithm is based on data that comes from Multiple Datasets shown in Figure 1. For creating such algorithms following three datasets are used in different stages:

1. **Training Dataset:** Training dataset contains set of examples that help in accommodating various parameters of the algorithm. Using supervised learning we train the model with training dataset. Training Dataset consists of an input vector and the corresponding answer that can be scalar or vector and is indicated as target. The present model is kept running with the training dataset and produces an outcome, which is then differentiated with the target, for each input vector in the training dataset. In view of the result of the evaluation and the particular learning algorithm that has been used, the parameters of the model are balanced. The model fitting can incorporate both variable choice and parameter estimation.

2. **Validation Dataset:** Progressively, the fitted model is utilized to foresee the reactions for the observations in a second dataset called the Validation dataset. The Validation Dataset gives an impartial evaluation of a model fit on the Training dataset while tuning the model's hyper parameters (for example the quantity of hidden units in a neural system). Validation datasets can be utilized for regularization by early halting: quit training when the error on the Validation Dataset increases, as this is an indication of overfitting to the Training dataset. This straightforward method is complicated by the fact that the Validation Dataset error may change amid training, delivering numerous local minima. This inconvenience has prompted the production of some especially decided rules for choosing while over fitting has started.

3. **Test Dataset:** This dataset provides an impartial assessment of a final model fit on Training Dataset.

Figure 1. Work flow of the system

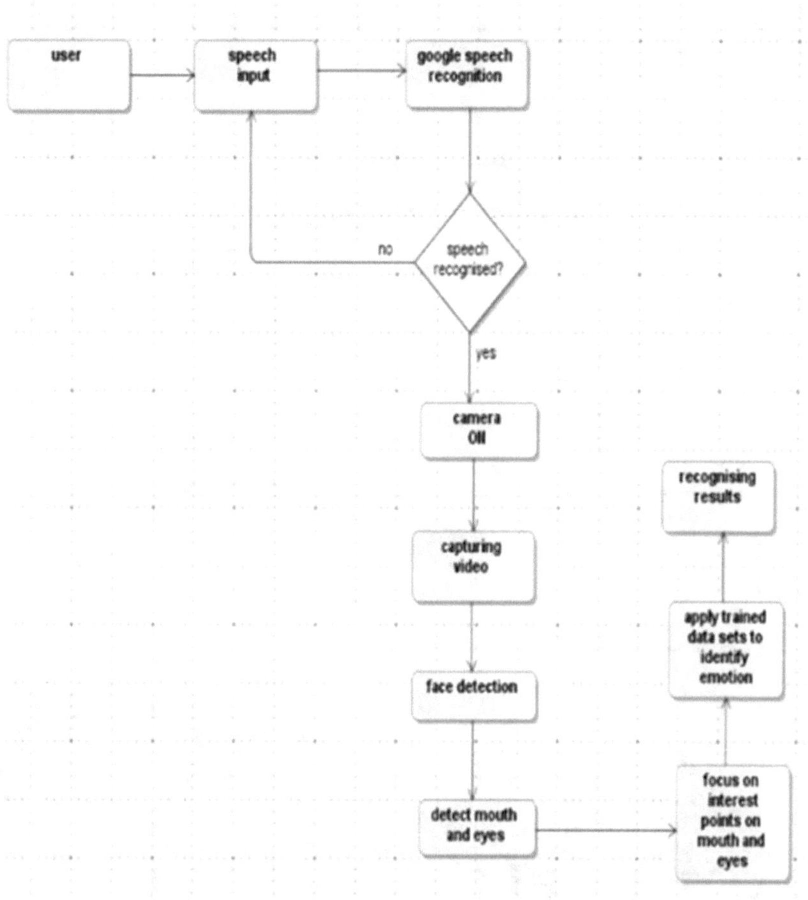

RESULT AND ANALYSIS

We have used IDLE to code in Python Programming Language. Our front-end code is developed using Tkinkter which is used to build Graphical User Interface. We have used multiple libraries in this article. gTTS abbreviated from Google-Text-to-Speech is aPython library and CLI tool to interact with Google Translate's text-to-speech API. OpenCV stands for Open Source Computer Vision. As a library of programming functions, the main aim of OpenCV is Real Time Computer Vision. Numpy is a core library and adds support for multi-dimensional arrays, matrices, high level mathematical functions for operation on arrays to the Python Programming Language. PyAudio provides Python bindings for Port Audio, the cross-platform audio I/O library. Tensorflow is a machine learning open-source software library. It can be used for research as well as production. It is also used for Machine Learning Applications e.g. CNN (Convolutional Neural Network) and DNN (Deep Neural Network). Tensorflow framework will help train the model for Emotion Recognition shown in Figure 2.

Test Case 1: Testing with spectacles shown in Figure 3
Expected Outcome: Detects Emotion with Spectacles
Final Result: Pass

Figure 2. System design

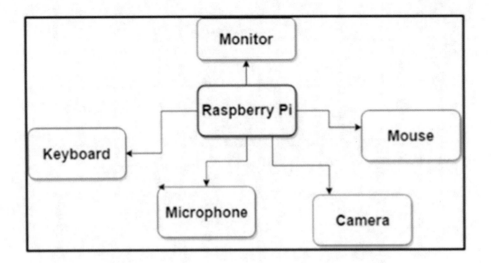

Figure 3. Human face

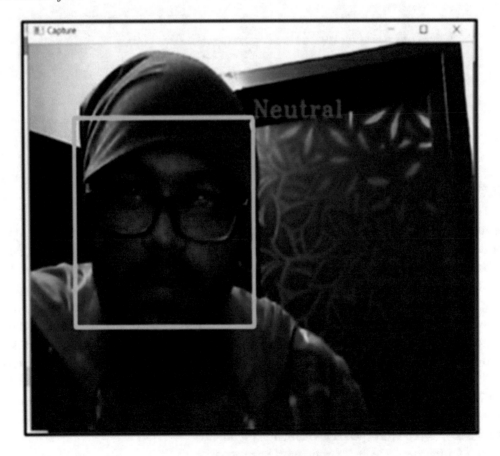

Figure 4. Animal face

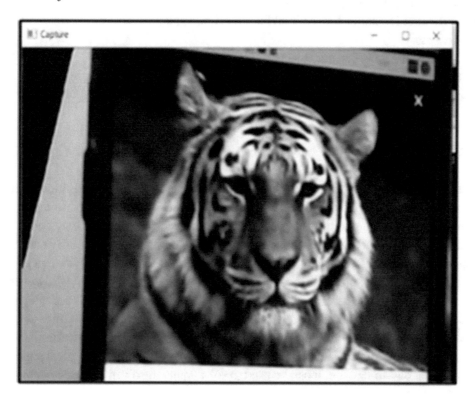

Figure 5. Non-living object

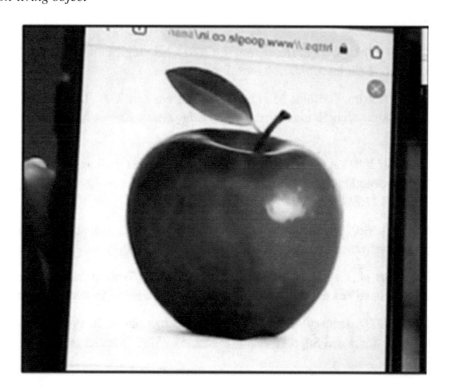

Test Case 2: Detecting Emotion on Animals shown in Figure 4
Expected Outcome: Do not Detect Animal Face as Human Face
Final Result: Pass
Test Case 3: Detecting Non-Living Objects shown in Figure 5
Expected Outcome: Do not detect any non-living object
Final Result: Pass

CONCLUSION

Further into the future? There are almost limitless applications of emotion recognition technology if we think outside the box. One of the good uses is of using it in a retail environment. Imagine a world in which the faces of people waiting in line in a store are scanned and analyzed. Not only could we reduce the need for customer experience surveys about a store visit but retailers could identify staff who make customers happy or stores that perform well and conduct A/B testing on any number of elements. Spooky? Perhaps. But exciting! Facial expression recognition is an activity that is performed by every human in our day to day lives. Each one of us analyses the expressions of the individuals we interact with, to understand how people interact and respond with us. The malicious intentions of a thief or a person to be interviewed can be recognized with the help of his facial features and gestures. Another best place to use facial expression recognition is in medical terms. It can be used on psychological patient to track their emotions of their day-to-day life. It can be used to solve many unsolved mysteries in medical field where it's hard to understand the emotion of a patient.

REFERENCES

Arkin, R. C., Fujita, M., Takagi, T., & Hasegawa, R. (2001), Ethological modeling and architecture for an entertainment robot. *IEEE Int. Conf. Robotics & Automation*.

Busso, C., Deng, Z., Yildirim, S., Bulut, M., Lee, C. M., Kazem Zadeh, A., Lee, S. B., Neumann, U., & Narayanan, S. (2004). *Analysis of Emotion Recognition using Facial Expression, Speech and Multimodal Information*. ICMI.

Franco, L., & Treves, A. (2001). A neural network facial expression recognition system using unsupervised local processing. In *Proceedings of the 2nd International Symposium on Image and Signal Processing and Analysis*. IEEE. 10.1109/ISPA.2001.938703

Ghosh, S., & Singh, A. (2020). The scope of Artificial Intelligence in mankind: A detailed review. *Journal of Physics: Conference Series*, *1531*, 012045.

Katsis, C. D., Katertsidis, N., Ganiatsas, G., & Fotiadis, D. I. (2008). Toward Emotion Recognition in Car Racing Drivers: A Bio signal Processing Approach. *IEEE Transactions on Systems, Man, and Cybernetics*.

Kotsia, I., & Pitas, I. (2007, January). Facial Expression Recognition in Image Sequences Using Geometric Deformation Features and Support Vector Machines. *IEEE Transactions on Image Processing*, *16*(1), 172–187.

Pérez, Aguilar, & Dapena. (2020). MIHR: A Human-Robot Interaction Model. *IEEE Latin America Transactions, 18*(9), 1521-1529.

Saaidia, M., Zermi, N., & Ramdani, M. (2014). Facial Expression Recognition Using Neural Network Trained with Zernike Moments. *2014 4th International Conference on Artificial Intelligence with Applications in Engineering and Technology*, 187-192. 10.1109/ICAIET.2014.39

Yan, Y., Huang, Y., Chen, S., Shen, C., & Wang, H. (2020). Joint Deep Learning of Facial Expression Synthesis and Recognition. *IEEE Transactions on Multimedia, 22*(11), 2792–2807.

Yang, B., Cao, J., Ni, R., & Zhang, Y. (2018). Facial Expression Recognition Using Weighted Mixture Deep Neural Network Based on Double-Channel Facial Images. *IEEE Access: Practical Innovations, Open Solutions, 6*, 4630–4640.

Zhang, K., Huang, Y., Du, Y., & Wang, L. (2017). Facial Expression Recognition Based on Deep Evolutional Spatial-Temporal Networks. *IEEE Transactions on Image Processing, 26*(9), 4193–4203.

Chapter 7
Pandemic Management Using Artificial Intelligence–Based Safety Measures:
Prediction and Prevention

Megha Nain

https://orcid.org/0000-0003-1592-652X

Manipal University Jaipur, India

Shilpa Sharma

https://orcid.org/0000-0002-6013-820X

Manipal University Jaipur, India

Sandeep Chaurasia

Manipal University Jaipur, India

ABSTRACT

The pandemic corona virus disease (COVID-19) caused by the virus 'SARS-CoV-2' continues affecting the health and affluence of the worldwide population. The role of artificial intelligence in improving safety and health conditions has been studied in the chapter. The various fields of artificial intelligence such as machine learning, computer vision, deep learning, and natural language processing are contributing to almost every field ranging from healthcare, agriculture, automotive, astronomy, and many others. For overcoming a global outbreak such as COVID-19, conventional approaches are not feasible enough, and therefore the requirement for the more robust and automated techniques for making predictions in advance is essential. The vision of this chapter is to assess and survey the impact of artificial intelligence-based approaches in the management of pandemics and recommend procedures for the enhancement of the currently used techniques along with the imminent research areas in artificial intelligence for controlling pandemics.

DOI: 10.4018/978-1-7998-7188-0.ch007

INTRODUCTION

The pandemic COVID-19 has disturbed the worldwide population. Roads are deserted, shops are shut, and individuals are out of employment, open social meetings have been prohibited in numerous regions, travel limitations have been forced and the entirety of this is majorly affecting the worldwide economy. With 165,158,285 confirmed cases globally and 26,031,991 cases in India as of 21 May 2021 (World Health Organization, 2020). As of May 2021, a total of 14448,242,899 vaccine doses have been administered globally to World Health Organization, however, inevitably it is going to continue to spread but how far and rapid that is going to occur and what can be done to control is still in question. Artificial Intelligence (AI) plays a vital part in providing the answers to all such questions and maybe even improving the outcome. AI has an indispensable role in the prime understanding of the outcome.

Numerous actions and mitigation measures are implemented globally for the COVID-19 pandemic, which involves total lockdowns, social distancing, compulsory face masks and hand-wash recommendations. These measures are based on the mathematical and prediction analysis of the virus spread (Alvarez FE et al. 2020), ((IHME) 2020), (Das S et al. 2020). From controlling through the platform of social media to interpreting the root of COVID-19, AI is employed to battle the COVID-19 pandemic in all diverse ways. For example, from the inception of the episode, when China first started giving reaction to COVID-19, China concentrated on AI using cameras for facial recognition to check the contaminated individuals having a history of travel, robots for the grocery delivery, sanitization using drones, announcements airing for urging people to stay home. With currently employed technologies in AI, firms require determining an optimized plan to unsettle COVID-19 (Jo Best, 2020). An extensive study of AI technologies that would help people to diminish and stifle the huge impacts of the pandemic have been presented in this chapter. Ongoing enhancements in AI have added substantially to the development and improvement of our health and safety and, with the usage of an appropriate framework of AI techniques, this difficult coronavirus fight could be vanquished (Estrada et al., 2020). A variety of researchers and scientists are using AI for finding out new prescriptions and remedies to concentrate on detecting infected persons through medical imaging techniques such as 'X-rays' and 'CT scans' ((Nguyen TT et al., 2020).

There are several contributions of AI techniques enlightened in this chapter which is not just limited to the current pandemic but also for any future outbreaks. With that objective, AI is conferred comprehensively to bring attention towards the existing technologies in AI for improved assistance in healthcare. For instance, AI in Radiology for detecting COVID-19 or AI in the Intensive Care Unit (ICU) advancement, for the smooth diagnosis and treatment. In the next section, Computer Vision (CV) techniques have been examined for monitoring the safety measures like detection of face masks, social distancing violations, thermal vision cameras for the inspection of the body temperature of an individual for controlling the spread of coronavirus. A list of CV approaches has been addressed in terms of their accuracy of treatment. Apart from this, Mathematical models based on deep learning (DL) are analyzed to obtain predictions about the spread where Natural Language Processing (NLP) has also been brought up as extensive support in creating an enhanced mathematical model and in identifying the key symptoms of the coronavirus. Proceeding ahead, Machine Learning (ML) based methodologies have been recognized for the usage in contact tracing applications for knowing the contaminated patients as well as **locations** that would aid in monitoring the virus spread. Several contact tracing applications are discussed which are getting employed worldwide. Thorough matters concerning the present technologies in AI and an in-depth review of the model accuracy are presented in the discussion.

The author's purpose is to study the applications of artificial intelligence as a firm approach to interpret, develop controlling parameters, and challenge the COVID-19 and other future outbreaks. The methodology includes the swift literature survey on the database of Scopus, PubMed, and Google Scholar with the usage of the keyword of artificial intelligence or AI, machine learning, computer vision, deep learning, natural language processing and hybrid model along with the COVID -19 pandemic or coronavirus. Gathered the most updated records regarding COVID-19 with artificial intelligence and examined those to evaluate the viable usage for the COVID-19 virus. Authors have recognized the vital role of artificial intelligence applications in controlling the COVID-19 pandemic. Artificial intelligence plays an enormous part in identifying the cluster in the present cases and predicting where the COVID-19 virus will hit next by gathering and studying the existing data. To conclude, healthcare needs prediction-based technologies to deal with the COVID-19 and assist by getting concrete ideas continuously to prevent the virus spread and additionally works as a key role for the understanding and advising of the formulation of vaccines. Artificial intelligence operates efficiently to imitate human intelligence and this decision-oriented technology is employed for different purposes to manage and control the virus spread which includes interpretation of the usage of artificial intelligence applications for diagnosing, screening, detecting, predicting the present infected patients and further tracking of the individuals who might be affected in future. For tracking the COVID-19 confirmed patients, recovered cases and cumulative deaths, necessary artificial intelligence applications are implemented.

The usage of the Artificial Intelligence (AI) domains such as Computer Vision (CV), Deep Learning (DL), Natural Language Processing (NLP), and Machine Learning (ML) have been reviewed for innovating a better framework for the safety and prevention from COVID-19 or any future pandemic circumstances. Therefore, the chapter is structured in a way that section 2 is about AI in general to challenge the COVID-19 outbreak, section 3 is focusing on CV based methods in combating the COVID-19, section 4 illustrates the usage of DL and NLP based models for COVID-19, section 5 illuminates ML-based applications for COVID-19, section 6 constitutes authors observations and Section 7 establishes the conclusion.

ARTIFICIAL INTELLIGENCE TO CHALLENGE COVID-19 OUTBREAK

AI is one of those advances that is making this world a better place by benefitting humanity in different manners. The field of AI has gotten in various applications contributing an incredible bit of benefits to several fields. AI, being a conclusion based quantifiable tool has the power to improve the treatment and planning to overcome the revealed outcome of the COVID-19 patient. High accuracy decreased unpredictability and duration can be achieved by associating AI in the treatment (Haleem et al., 2020).

With AI, most emerging fields like CV, Robotics, ML, NLP, and DL are present. These technologies are used to produce a substantial difference in overcoming COVID-19 by taking correct safety measures, for instance, AI-based monitoring bracelets could help in the checking of people breaking isolation (Aishwarya Kumar et al., 2020), (Maghdid HS et al., 2020). Likewise, AI-enabled thermal cameras were employed for dissecting affected individuals. With the help of the data from the immigration and custom records, countries like Taiwan also imparted its national health insurance database (Wang CJ et al., 2020), (Broga et al., 2020) for checking travel history and symptoms of the individuals to separate the coronavirus patients. To fight coronavirus, AI significantly centres on the treatment and diagnosis by using medical imaging techniques and finding outpatients from the emergency clinic and clinical database who can be inclined to infection later built on their sickness history.

Radiologists using AI to Detect COVID-19

AI-based models have precisely helped in diagnosing and classifying COVID-19 from community-acquired pneumonia (CAP) from different lung disorders. A detection model "COVNet" based on deep neural networks (DNNs) for COVID-19, created to eliminate the visual highlights from 4,356 computed tomography scans from 3,322 patients for the identification of COVID-19. The preciseness of the model could be analysed by understanding CAP and other CT scan tests (Lin Li et al., 2020). Covid-19 could be interpreted on 'chest X-ray' and 'CT scans'.

To encourage CT imaging diagnosis, AI-based software has been employed. AI built software is not only helpful in arranging the disease into various severity, incorporating the organized report but also helps in an arrangement by abstract contemplation, with quantifiable, objective estimations of the degree of an abscess (Maria Paola Belfiore et al., 2020). 'Gradient weighted-class activation mapping method' ("GRAD-CAM") could be retrieved for intensifying the interpretability of a DL model, which could be utilized to picture out the key elements/areas that would promote the decision of the DL based model. **Figure (1)**, **Figure (2)** and **Figure (3)** below shows suspected areas of COVID-19, CAP, and non-pneumonia cases respectively with the help of heat maps. More consideration is on the anomalous regions using the algorithm heat maps and that ignored the normal regions as in the case of **Figure (3)**. CT scanned images of COVID-19 cases are distinguished from the CAP and other non-pneumonia disorders using the DL-based framework model (Lin Li et al., 2020). As per the model, a 3-D model based on the ResNet50 and with the utilization of the layers of max pooling and fully connected layers recognizes the COVID-19 patients. Moreover, A DL-based model by Song Y (Song Y et al. 2020) for the 'CT scanned' image analysis of the COVID-19 patients manage 'lung CT' images gathered from the patients of COVID-19, pneumonia, and fit patients from two multi-facility healthcare organisations in china. The recommended model "Deep Pneumonia" claims an 'area under curve' metric (AUC) of 0.99 and a 'sensitivity' metric of 0.93.

Artificial Intelligence in Intensive Care Unit (ICU)

A critical patient suffering from COVID-19 on an ICU bed needs the utmost attention and constant monitoring care. Most advanced medical machines are designed to keep the patient alive and highly paid doctors who are taking their life at risk to monitoring the patient. Sovereign healthcare established at Hoboken City, New Jersey planned and assembled an AI system that can be implemented in an ICU to bid attentive watch, in the same way as a specialist on the patient's bedside all the time (Behnood Gholami et al. 2018). This system takes records steadily and watchfully regulates the machine consistently as per the patient's live reading. The oppressed staff of the critical care units could be supported by using an AI system, moreover, this would be beneficial as the patients can get out of the ICU speedily, moreover, it would help in cost-cut out of soaring expenses of the facilities in a healthcare department. In **Figure (4)**, a decision support system is shown (Behnood et al., 2018) using which the critically ill patient could be monitored using the automated system which would help in recommending the specialists to make adjustments as per the patients need. Penn Medicine (Epidemics 2020) also created a model 'CHIME' which stands for "COVID-19 Hospital Impact Model for Epidemics") that provides suggestions on the

Figure 1. Heat map for COVID-19 (Journal, 2020) (Lin Li et al., 2020)

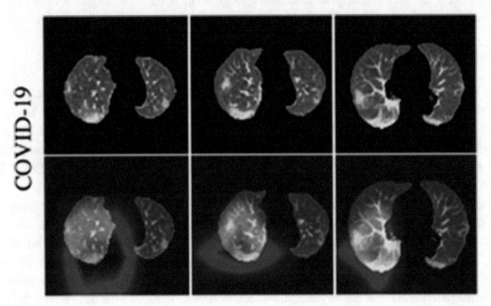

projection of the patients admitted in ICU and ventilated patients, respectively. A mathematical model based on the improvement measures such as social distancing, rate of hospitalization and detection likelihood has been employed in their approach. Furthermore, "Inception Migration Neuro Network" model based on convolutional neural networks (CNNs) proposed by (Wang S et al. 2020) built from the dataset from 2 medical associations in china suggested assessing the radiological features in volumetric chest photos of the patients. The goal of their work was to evaluate if the CT photos show the presence of COVID-19 or not. Model results (AUC and F1 metrics) proved cost-effective.

Figure 2. Heat map for community acquired pneumonia. (Journal, 2020), (Lin Li et al., 2020)

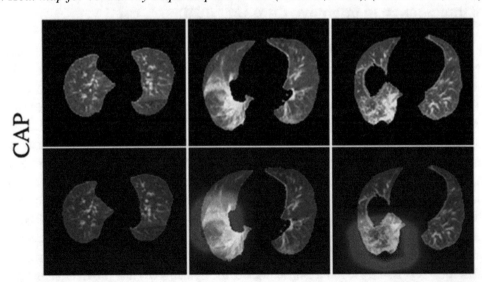

Figure 3. Heat map for non-pneumonia (Journal, 2020), (Lin Li et al., 2020)

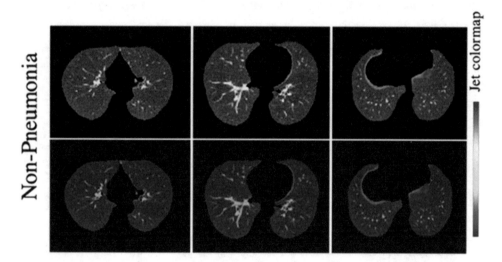

Mechanical Ventilators

An alarmingly unwell patient who has difficulty in breathing would be required to put on mechanical ventilators that rush air into the lungs, however, the pulse could escape accord with consistent patterns of breathing, and this would make the patient "battle the ventilator." An intelligent control system uses a machine-learning (ML) algorithm and inspects rushed air estimates, in addition, to identify numerous kinds of ventilator asynchrony with time. In an entirely self-ruling framework, a versatile controller constantly standardizes the flow of air to synchronize it with the patient. A decision support tool could be operated as a comparable framework in the ICU, giving ideas that breathing guides could use to plan (Behnood et al., 2018). **Figure 4**shows how the critically challenged patients who have trouble breathing could be placed on a mechanical ventilator machine, these devices push the oxygen to reach the lungs of the patient, however, these machines might go out of sync with the normal breathing response of the patient and thus, the necessity of an automated control system is extremely crucial for these purposes (1) To monitor the measurements of the airflow constantly (2) To obtain sorts of asynchronism in the ventilator (3) To make use in real-time using ML algorithms (4) To make constant adjustments using the adaptive controller.

To achieve the increasing need for intense clinical care, ICUs should build their ability just as their capacities. Preparing more experts is essential for the system—yet so is automation. AI frameworks could turn out to be the most essential for the healthcare crew, permitting medical experts and attendants to conduct their expertise when needed utmost (Behnood et al., 2018).

Length of Stay

Hospitals running out of beds even for critical patients of COVID-19 in both the private and government hospitals. Infected people requesting healthcare facilities are being directed to register on a waitlist as beds are unavailable in metro cities like Mumbai and Delhi in India. (The Indian Express, 2020). This is a very serious concern at this time of COVID-19 as a single minute is very crucial for critical patients.

Figure 4. Decision support system (Behnood et al., 2018). 1. Mechanical ventilator to help in breathing 2. To identify asynchronism types 3. Real-time usage with ML algorithm 4. Adaptive controller to adjust airflow as per the patient.

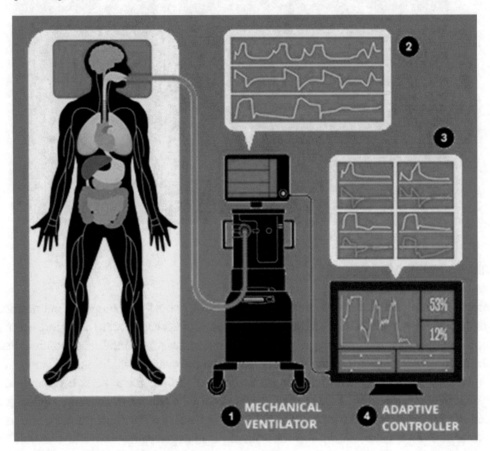

Researchers (Houthooft R et al., 2015) used ML by utilizing data of 14,480 patients to train a support vector machine (SVM) model on inference understanding endurance including patient's 'length of stay' in a healthcare unit (Gutierrez et al., 2020). 0.82 is the AUC for the respective prototype to anticipate the drawn-out length of stay for the patient. But according to the doctor's prediction as observed in the clinical report, the ICU length of stay was 53% which is a contradiction. To predict the 'length of stay' in the ISU, physiological estimations were noticed during the first two days of ICU admitted patients. This has been done using a hidden-markov (HMM) model framework. The aggregation and preprocessing techniques of the HMM framework is introduced for robustness and augmented learning concerning the metrics of the HMM framework. Accordingly, the time resolutions could be chosen to such an extent that each time window is probably going to have at least one new observation (Sotoodeh M et al., 2019). **Figure 5** demonstrates the non-overlapping and overlapping scheme for a single patient in the data set having time- resolution equals eight hours.

Using an algorithm based on an artificial neural network (ANN), implemented in the database of MIMIC-III stands for "medical information mart for intensive care III", the problem of ICU readmission was observed. This is a publicly accessible database created from a various patient who was treated in

Figure 5. Time windows with a time resolution of 8 hours (Sotoodeh M et al., 2019)

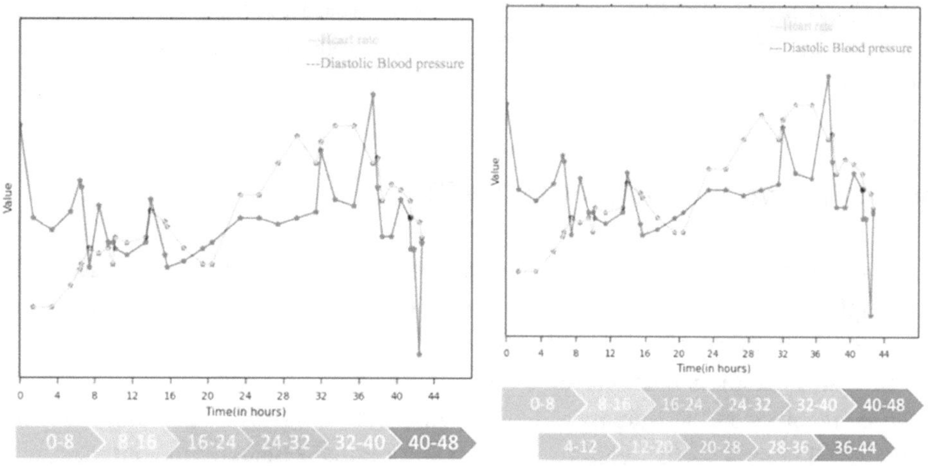

(a) Non-overlapping time windows   (b) Overlapping time windows

Beth Israel Deaconess Medical Centre's CCU. This database was created between 2001 and 2012 and had the preference to differentiate patients with the potential risk of ICU readmission with the AUC of 0.79 and sensitivity of 0.74 (Lin YW et al., 2019). Another ML model given by Sethy and Behera (Sethy PK et al. 2020) helped in the analysis of 'x-ray illustrations' built with the architecture of ResNet50 and SVM to detect the patients infected with COVID-19. Evaluation of the model showed the effectiveness and correctness in terms of quantitative metrics such as False-positive rate or FPR, Matthew's correlation coefficient or MCC, kappa and F1 score. By using the AI devised automated systems in medical techniques like radiology, radiography, and a decision support system in ICU, are not only giving the healthcare staff some relief but also providing maximum safety to the doctors and individuals coming to get other treatments in the hospital/clinic to not get infected, furthermore, timeliness and human error could be reduced. A doctor can use these artificial intelligent support systems to make the diagnosis and treatment very efficient and fast recovery could also be conceivable.

COMPUTER VISION FOR COVID-19

CV is an interdisciplinary subfield of AI and is defined as the understanding of visual environments and their contexts. It has enormous applications such as Face recognition, Image retrieval, surveillance cameras, smart cars, and many usages in healthcare (Le et al., 2019). CV has enlightened the recent triumph in resolving innumerable complex issues in healthcare and has the true potential to control the global crisis COVID-19.

CV has developed a huge extent of understanding in interpreting visual data such as images or videos and it has become the most enthusiastic research field, essentially with the power of DL, a sub-domain of ML (Megha Nain et al. 2021) (Anwaar Ulhaq et al., 2020). The CV techniques with the usage of deep learning in healthcare applications have vast potential that constitutes diagnosis, treatment, prediction of the disease, medical image processing and analysis, surgeries, and discoveries of the vaccines (Junfeng Gao et al., 2018).

Detecting objects accurately and proficiently in images is also a critical field in CV. This is on the grounds that to make useful inferences in images and video streams, computers need to accurately identify objects in them as an initial step (Yao et al., 2020). In sections (3.1, 3.2, 3.3), a demonstration of the CV for the detection purpose is provided. Afterwards, the contribution of CV in healthcare in the form of **Table 1** (3.4) has been given.

Face Mask Detection to Combat COVID-19

Adrian Rosebrock has trained a system to detect face mask on people with OpenCV, Keras/TensorFlow, and DL. This might be utilized to help guarantee our wellbeing and the security of others as well. Adrian has used a dataset of several people with and without a mask and trained the model in a way it automatically detects in case a person is not wearing a facial mask, even on a live video (Rosebrock, 2018). In **Figure 6,** Phases involved in the training and the implementation of the Face mask detector has been presented where ROI represents the region of interest and **Figure 7** displays the output after the training and implementation phase finishes.

Figure 6. Training and implementation phase (Rosebrock, 2018)

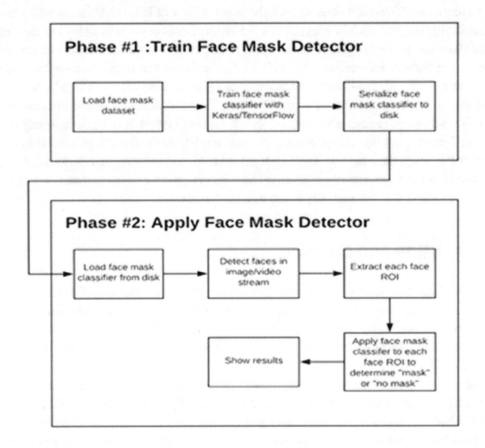

Figure 7. Output of face mask detector (Rosebrock, 2018)

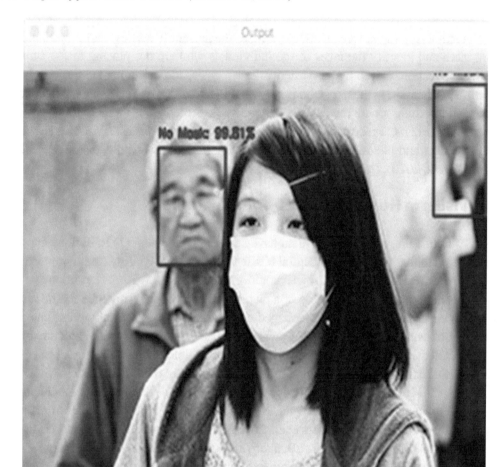

Covid Analytics and FebriEye for Covid-19

Vehant Technologies, which is a lead in the field of AI has given "COVID Analytics" and "FebriEye" which is an AI and CV based analytics software for the monitoring and detection of protective violations regarding the COVID-19 pandemic. Violations such as detection of face masks, social distance, and vehicle movement with the use of the Automatic Number Plate Recognition System (ANPR) can be checked and controlled with the assistance of these AI programs.

Construction sites, shops, traffic lights/junctions, manufacturing divisions, workplaces, airfields, and businesses can easily install these systems. On the other hand, apart from detecting the facemask and social distancing violations, FebriEye, a thermal Vision camera (Megha Nain et al. 2021), also do the task of checking the temperature. It has the system of generating alarms automatically in case of any violation (Mitra, 2020). By using such AI-driven software, we could control the infection to spread and thus serving the safety of everyone.

AppsStore.Ai for COVID-19

Face Mask Detection App (appsstore.ai, 2020) that uses the present IP address and surveillance cameras (CCTV) to search and identify the faces of the individuals who are not placing masks on their faces properly. This application, driven by an AI network, can easily identify a person not wearing a mask. The app sends a notification to the user who is not wearing a mask on a mobile phone, by recognizing a person's face and matching it with the dataset it already has. Moreover, if an induvial face is not recognized by the camera, then the report will be passed to the officer. This is a very useful application that can be used in offices and factories to maintain good hygiene, and this would ensure the safety during this pandemic (Hertz, 2020), (Megha Nain et al. 2021).

Computer Vision in Health Care for Diagnosis Purpose

The field of CV for the diagnosis of the patient have been explored using (1) Radiology approach, (CT Imaging) computed tomography and (2) Digital (CXR Imaging) Chest X-Ray Radiography as shown in **Table (1)** (Tao Ai et al., 2020). Chest CT scan comprises of 2 types, (i) High resolution and (ii) Spiral CT. The high-resolution provides an excess of a picture in just a single x-ray tube rotation, however, a table that moves consistently over a tunnel-shaped hole is included in a spiral kind of chest CT scan. The main benefit of using a spiral chest CT scan is that it uses a three-dimensional picture of the lungs (Website, 2020). On the other hand, CXR is the imaging methodology that utilizes a lower cost than CT Imaging and is more extensively accessible for the identification of chest diagnostics (Ming-Yen Ng et al., 2020). Hence, CXR becomes a very effective diagnostic method against the virus with the usage of automatic determination of the COVID-19 features (Anwaar Ulhaq et al., 2020). Apart from that, various diseases, such as osteoporosis (Paola Pisani et al., 2013), cancer (Mugahed A Al-antari et al., 2018) and cardiac diseases (Michael A Speidel et al., 2006) are also diagnosed with the CXR scans.

By using CV for the COVID-19 related violations, assurance of safety could be achieved. additionally, in healthcare, making use of the data set prepared from the patient's report of COVID-19 to apply CV techniques to increase the speed of treatment and to accomplish the recovery phase as early as possible to uphold the safety of one and all.

In **Table 1,** the author recognized various models with their corresponding dataset evidence and the accuracy achieved. CV plays a substantial role in diagnosing and treating patients and thereby, boosting the recovery rate. In terms of safety, CV could help in a tremendous way by managing the situation upon verifying a variety of parameters like face mask detection, monitoring of violations to curb virus spread (as discussed in 3.2, 3.2, 3.3).

DEEP LEARNING MODEL FOR COVID -19

A Hybrid AI Model was proposed by a group of researchers in China to control the COVID-19 pandemic. Initially, researchers proposed a conventional model ISI Model (Improved Susceptible Infected) to predict the variation in the infection rates. **Figure 8** describes the ISI Model, this ISI model treats people with an equal rate of infection and to overcome this issue, a hybrid AI model based on the DL concepts was built by integrating the NLP model and LSTM model (Long Short-Term Memory Network model) with the originally proposed traditional framework (ISI Model). The hybrid model has been used for accurate

Table 1. Study of diagnosis of patients based on CT scan and x-ray

Author Name	References	Description of the model used	Infected cases	Accuracy of the model
Cheng Jin et al	(Cheng Jin et al., 2020)	2-Dimensional-CNN based AI Model, Tested on 970 CT Imaging	496 confirmed cases with COVID-19	94.98% 97.91%: AUC
Chuansheng Zhengal.	(Michael A Speidel et al., 2006)	3D- Deep CNN to Detect COVID-19 using CT Imaging (DeCoVNet)	540 Patients were confirmed with COVID-19	95.90% 0.976: AUC
Linda Wang et al.	(Wong et al., 2020)	Deep CNN - COVID-Net, COVIDx dataset: 16,756 CXR images	More than 13,645 patients were confirmed with COVID-19	92.4%
Xiaowei Xu et al.	(Xu X et al., 2020)	3-Dimensional DNN model with 618 CT scans	110 patients were confirmed with COVID-19	86.7%
Ali Narin et al.	(Ali Narin et al., 2020)	ResNet50 Model	(open source) Git Hub Database and x-ray data (Pneumonia) (Refer: **Figure -1, 2 and 3**)	97%: (Inception V3) 87%: (Inception-ResNetV2)
Muhammad Farooq, Abdul Hafeez	(Hafeez et al., 2020)	ResNet-50 for the model enhancement	COVIDx dataset	96.23%

predictions for the coronavirus in China to control the infection spread. **Figure 9** shows the prediction procedure after combining LSTM and NLP models with the conventional model (Nanning Zheng et al., 2020). The measured metric MPEs (mean absolute percentage errors) with the proposed model have been 0.52%, 0.38%, 0.05%, 0.86% respectively for the 6 days in Wuhan, Beijing, Shanghai, and overall, China.

For making the epidemic model, the daily cases were observed under controlled conditions, those were generally due to the recently confirmed coronavirus cases, excluding the recovered and late cases of the COVID-19 as they would not have any role in the recently confirmed coronavirus patients and based on this observation, an ISI model was prepared which used a retrospective and Multiparameter approach (Hara et al., 2007) (N Imai et al., 2020).

$$I(t) = I(t-1) + {}^2{}_1(t,d)\sum_{i=1}^{d}\Delta I(t-i), d = 1,2,...,10 \tag{1}$$

Using equation (1) (Nanning Zheng et al., 2020), the rate of infection in the individuals were noted in numerous different areas and at diverse frames of time to detect whether the recently confirmed coronavirus cases were due to the cumulative number of confirmed coronavirus cases in the d days or not.

Here 't' represents each day, S(t): Susceptible persons on the day 't', I(t): cumulative confirmed cases on the day 't' and the recent confirmed cases on the day 't' can be determined using the formula, Δ I(t) = I(t) – I(t-1)

(I), $\hat{a}_1(t,k)$ .is to determine the stable relation between the Δ I(t) and $\sum\limits_{i=1}^{k} \Delta I(t-i)$. which implies to estimate the effects of cumulative confirmed cases in the 'k' past days against the recent confirmed cases on day 't'. (II) $\hat{a}_1^E(t,k)$ .can be obtained for each region and countrywide as per the equation (1) $L(t) = a \times e^{-bt}$., Exponential function, has been used to fit $\hat{\beta}_1(t,k)$ .for evaluation of the COVID-19 spread, where the parameters of the defined function are a and b, with a, b>0. As all the infected individuals could not be effectively quarantined, so they have a strong infection rate. Hence, $\hat{a}_1(t,k)$ .could be estimated by gradually increasing the value of k along with the new confirmed cases at a previous point in time is introduced into the model.

The rate of infection $\hat{a}_1(t,d)$ .s given by the equation (2) (Nanning Zheng et al., 2020).

$$ ^2{}_1(t,d) = \Delta I(t) / \sum_{i=1}^{d} \Delta I(t-i) \tag{2} $$

Figure 8. ISI model (Nanning Zheng et al., 2020)

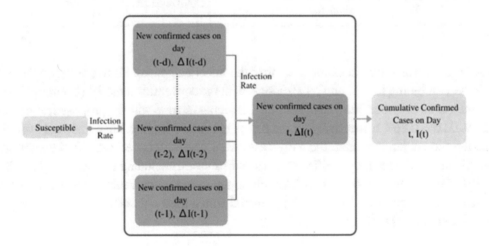

ISI model shown in **Figure 8** (Nanning Zheng et al., 2020) utilizes a retrospective and multiparameter approach and the notion behind this method is to apply the ratio of the latest confirmed cases (at a time 't') to the cumulative current verified cases across varying time scales (before time 't').

The requirement is to detect the time interval in which the possibility of the spread is maximum for understanding the effect of infected individuals on the successive infected person.

Thus, it is considered that the individual confirmed on the day 't' is affected by the confirmed individual between day 't-1' - day 't-10' and the in-depth analysis of the time laws of the rate of spread for the COVID-19 is necessary to determine for calculating the highest rate of infection spread. Most

Figure 9. Using ISI +NLP + LSTM (Nanning Zheng et al., 2020)

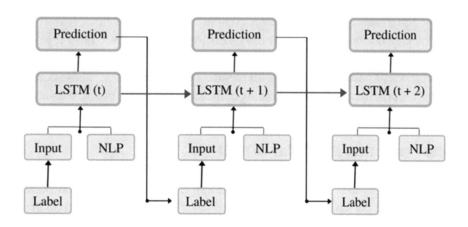

previous approaches are carried out based on stable days and considered the days of transmission as the past 'k' days.

NLP feature has been merged with the conventional model ISI and the LSTM network model to encrypt time-based information and hidden states for modelling the policies and news. Neural Network has been used for the bias prediction amongst the actual rate of infection and regressed rate of infection. $y(t) = {}^2(t) - {}^{2T}(t)$. here y(t) is taken as the bias prediction and therefore, LSTM network adds to the ISI Model.

The Mathematical Equation by Zheng (Nanning Zheng et al., 2020) gives a Standard "reproduction number" R_0 .implemented as an epidemiologic factor for checking an individual with infection of coronavirus, where R_0 .t) defines the average secondary cases of coronavirus given by the equation (3):

$$\beta_4\left(t+3\right)\Delta I\left(t\right), \beta_3\left(t+4\right)\Delta I\left(t\right), \ldots\ldots, \left(t+8\right)\Delta I\left(t\right) \tag{3}$$

Secondary coronavirus cases were given by a confirmed case at a given time t. Below is the mathematical expression (Nanning Zheng et al., 2020) for the Reproduction Number R_0 .t) at time t given in equation (4):

$$R_0\left(t\right) = \frac{\sum_{i=3}^{8} {}^2{}_4\left(t+i\right)\Delta I\left(t\right)}{\Delta I\left(t\right)} = \sum_{i=3}^{8} {}^2{}_4\left(t+i\right) \tag{4}$$

Wuhan recorded the larger values of R_0 and the hybrid AI model achieved success in tackling COVID-19 in China as per the data. Therefore, "ISI + NLP + LSTM" achieves the best predictions than any other models available. LSTM based approach was firstly introduced by Hochreiter and Schmidhuber (Hochreiter S et al. 1997). LSTM network model is a distinct form of recurrent neural networks (RNNs) having the capability to acquire dependencies for long-term. (Sayantani Basu et al. 2020) also recommended the LSTM based model for the prediction of the cumulative deaths and number of coronavirus cases. In comparison with Mathematical/statistical models which involve the comprehensive interpretation of the data as well as coefficient tuning for fitting the model for providing predictions, ML-based approaches enable the trained model to learn the complex features automatically from the data formed on the basis of the created model as well as the tuned hyperparameters. These types of methods are specifically useful for the time-series data such as COVID 19, where the cumulative curve of the virus spread, and the number of casualties varies with regards to time and place. These competencies of the LSTM network model provide a rich understanding of the aspect of future prediction and supports further in taking important health care decisions and measures (Sayantani Basu et al. 2020).

Mathematical Prediction Model for COVID-19

A diagnostic model given by the "King's College, London" and "health-science corporation, ZOE", for making predictions on the possibility for an individual to have COVID-19 based on the symptoms he/she gets. On data extraction from an app for the "COVID Symptom Study" and comparison of the individual's symptoms and results from the standard tests predicted the individuals who could have COVID 19 in future. A key symptom of the research was found to be "anosmia" —smell and taste loss. This key symptom of loss of taste and smell attributes to the infection more than any fever or cold symptoms. Age and sex were taken as the factors for the model prediction in addition to these 4 symptoms: exhaustion, appetite loss, taste and smell loss and plain/insistent cough to make the predictive mathematical model. This AI model tested on users from the United Kingdom and the United States, over 805,753 users in total got tested using a predictive mathematical model and those users confirmed that they are not tested for coronavirus. The result of the predictive model concluded that 140,312 users have a likelihood to catch the infection in the near future which is 17.42 percent. (International business, 2020) **Table 2** shows some of the AI models based on the concepts of ML and DL.

Based on the statistical evaluation, numerous research has been performed on the projections for the study on how the virus/infection is getting transmitted. SIR (Kermack W.O. et al. 1991) (Susceptible, Infected and Recovered) based model, statistical class of models for predicting the curve concerning the COVID-19 spread in future proposed by Neher RA et al. (Neher RA et al. 2020). According to their model, rate of infection, migration, and rates of community turnover are considered. A modern edition of the proposed model (Scenarios 2020) contemplates visualizing the projected clinical assets essential to aid a deadly disease like COVID-19.

Using the DL models, as discussed above (in section 4) hybrid model implementation, using such models specifically in china, has controlled the rate of infection spread enormously. So, using standard reproduction number for regulating infection, using key symptoms observed by the scientists and researchers along with some other parameters to make a future prediction for COVID-19 patients and models like these will ensure the safety of every individual.

In **Table (2)**, DL-based models are analyzed to check for the currently employed technologies and description of the same. DL Models are highly recommended to make predictions regarding the virus spread and managing the situation in a faster fashion with high precision. Using a similar type of LSTM methodologies, various aspects have been studied, for instance, patient's information, pandemic trends in China (Yang Z et al. 2020). Emphasis was on graphical analyses and prediction curve.

In addition to that LSTM network model provided by (Sayantani Basu et al. 2020) shows the quantitative analysis of the scale on which the mitigation practices are performing as per the predictions.

Table 2. AI models based mathematical models for COVID-19

Author Name	Model	Description	References
Li Yan et al.	Survival based Prediction Model	• Supervised ML algorithm • "XGBoost" classifier is used for prediction • Tested 375 cases • 90% accuracy	(Li Yan et al., 2020)
Nanning Zheng et al.	Hybrid AI Model	• Using DL model • LSTM and NLP along with ISI model • Introduced R0, reproduction number to control infection	(Nanning Zheng et al., 2020)
Tianqi Chen et al.	Tree Boosting System based on ML algorithm	• Using ML and DL for Scaling problems with scanty data • Using "XGboost" classifier (open source) Github link: [https://github.com/dmlc/xgboost]	(Tianqi Chen et al., 2016)
F Yu et al.	"Multi Scale context aggregation" using deep neural networks	• Deep Convolutional models • Image classification in dense prediction	(Yu F et al., 2016)
Qi1 X et al.	"Radiomics" model using ML	• ML based CT scans models for predicting the stay of an infected patient	(Qi1 X et al., 2016)

MACHINE LEARNING TECHNIQUES FOR COVID- 19

Contact Tracing is a significant instrument to minimize and stun the stretch of an outbreak like the novel coronavirus. It is providing us with the method of recognizing individuals who may have met a contaminated individual, and afterwards storing up additional data about the individuals who have been exposed to them (Kumar, 2020).

A contact tracing application named "Aarogya Setu" is launched by the government of India, this is available on all major mobile operating systems whether android or iPhone. This application will make calculations based on interactions with others, Bluetooth technology and AI. The Indian government has made the mandatory installation of this application for users who will travel by flights, to maintain the safety and tracking of passengers for any future threats using this AI application. Below **Figure 10** demonstrate the digital contact tracing. Singapore has also launched a channel named "SQREEM", this is an AI-based platform to digitally trace contact in real-time. This platform has a proximity sensor with inherent confidentiality specifications which does not require an application. This platform uses AI and ML (Kumar, 2020) algorithms to audit and analyses how many people might have contacted an infected person from a particular date until today. These platforms also detect digital patterns based on the previous detections by analyzing location and activities by user, this helps in predicting the next containment zone and ensure the safety of people living in that area.

A digital contact-tracing model arrangement for an area using GPS location. By this application, contacts of individual X (and all people utilizing the application) are followed utilizing GPS locations with the other users of the application, enhanced by examining quick response codes showed on large movement public places where global positioning system (GPS) is just extremely common. The X individual solicitations a SARS-COV-2 check (utilizing the Application) and on the other chance that their test outcome shows positive, at that point, it instantly actuates a warning alarm to people who were in close contact with the X person. The application prompts disengagement for the case (X person) and persons getting in touch with the X person (Ferretti, et al., 2020). Consequently, AI devised smart application/

Figure 10. Framework of digital contact-tracing (Ferretti, et al., 2020)

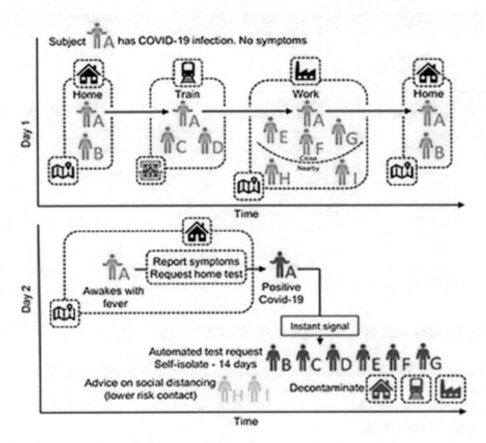

system is very effective for the safety of people and thus, helping in locating an infected individual in the very early stage to prevent any new transmission. In **Table 3** the author has shown the various contact tracing apps used worldwide to assist in safety.

In **Table 3,** the author cited all the presently implemented Contact tracing applications worldwide. Apart from that, the ML model given by (Hu Z et al. 2020) based on the stacked autoencoders is employed to estimate the cases of coronavirus in China built on historical facts and records. As per their model, regions/states were grouped in the form of clusters of the feature extraction from the recommended paradigm (Bandyopadhyay SK et al. 2020). To ensure a safer culture, pre-trained data applications based on ML are necessary to make sure that individuals are not entering any contaminated location or getting in contact with an infected person. ML-based algorithms would ensure our safety and aid in providing these advancements during the COVID-19 pandemics.

METHODS

The methodologies involve a comprehensive literature review, conducted for identifying the communications on existent applications of artificial intelligence in the domain of healthcare and pandemic management. Queries were run on to various databases of open journals such as Scopus, PubMed, Scien-

Table 3. List of contact tracing apps used worldwide

Country/ State	App Name	Description of Contact tracing app	References
South Korea	1. Corona 100m 2. Corona Map	1. Corona 100 m: for maintaining 100-meter distance (data collection: diagnosis date of the infected individual, nationality, age, gender, and location) 2. Corona map app plot the location of the infected patient 3. "Blue trace" system 4. surveillance cameras	(Tsang, 2020), (Yasheng Huang et al., 2020), (World, 2020), (Setzer, 2020), (Sommer., 2019), (Protocol, 2020), (Ketchell, 2020)
Australia	COVIDSafe app	1. Bluetooth-tracking 2. "Blue trace system" 3. Surveillance camera	
China	Close contact detector	1. GPS Tracking 2. Wi-Fi. 3. Database from railways, airline data and highway toll data	
Hawaii	Survey Method	Text messages and emails to build database to trace infected patients.	
Singapore	TraceTogether app	Tracing though Bluetooth	
Israel	HaMagen,	GPS Tracking: Individual location compared with confirmed cases within 14 days	
India	Aarogya Setu	1. Bluetooth 2. GPS Tracking 3. Data collection: name, birth date and biometric	

ceDirect and Google Scholar with the keyword search, AI or Artificial Intelligence, healthcare, machine learning, natural language processing, deep learning, computer vision and hybrid model along with the keyword COVID-19 pandemic or coronavirus. Up-to-date information regarding the COVID-19 and artificial intelligence has been examined for the management of the current pandemic as well as for any future outbreaks. Megha Nain et al. (Megha Nain et al. 2021) studied methods for the classification and localization of the objects in the digital images using various algorithms of ML, DL and CV including SVM, CNNs and RNNs and also YOLO (You Only Look Once), SSD (Single Shot Detector), Faster R-CNN, R-FCN (Region-based fully recurrent neural networks) which are highly essential in healthcare.

DISCUSSION

To present an in-depth analysis, the authors have shown **Table 4**for the various AI models in terms of their accuracy of the result. Higher the accuracy, more are the chances to implement the model for facilitating the actual practices for tackling the novel coronavirus.

Table 4 will be beneficial to have a quick view of the accuracy level of each model to make use of it in the true sense. These AI models are best suited for the development of the healthcare industry. Some observations are drawn as per the different sections contemplated in this chapter such as, In Section (2.1), it has been seen that (I) Sampling method produces satisfactory outcomes for the distribution of CAP subtypes (II) Transparency and interpretability were found to be lack in the DL methods (for example, it is not easy to pick the imaging features that could be chosen for concluding the output) (III) Overlapping comes in the demonstration of diseases inside the lung based on the parameters like age,

Table 4. List of tested AI models and their accuracy

Tested Model	Accuracy	References
2-D CNN based AI Model	94.98%	(Cheng Jin et al., 2020)
3-D Deep CNN Model (DeCoVNet)	95.90%	(Michael A Speidel et al., 2006)
Deep CNN Model (COVIDx)	92.40%	(Wong et al., 2020)
3-D Deep CNN Model	86.70%	(Xu X et al., 2020)
ResNet50 model with transfer learning (COVIDx)	97%: Inception V3 87%: Inception-ResNetV2)	(Ali Narin et al., 2020)
ResNet-50 architecture AI Model	96.23%	(Hafeez et al., 2020)
ML Prediction Model with "XGBoost" classifier	90%	(Li Yan et al., 2020)

immunity, drug reactivity etc. No solo method will help to distinguish all lung diseases, however, to separate COVID-19 from CAP, the usage of a ML method with a CNN would benefit (Lin Li et al., 2020). In Section (2.2), it has been perceived that, In ICU, a patient's level of fluid intake is recorded by an automated artificial intelligent framework like the pressure of blood and the blood volume variation at each pulse etc. An ML model is used to feed this information and continuously adjust the parameters as given by the prediction model (Behnood et al., 2018).

In section (4), It has been noted that the rate of the infection spread was found due to the recent confirmed COVID-19 cases which were due to the ones who do not get themselves quarantined and thus marked as the base for multiplying the rate of infection in the new confirmed COVID-19 cases and the rate of infection also varies with varying frames of time. (G. Chowell et al., 2004) (Gay et al., 2003) Several labs in china shared the information that the individual with COVID-19 have a high rate of infection from third to the eighth day after these individuals were found themselves infected with covid-19 which is quite large in comparison to the actual spread of the infection (S-L Yuang et al., 2001) (Fang et al., 2016). Also, the hybrid AI model significantly helped in controlling the situation in China based on the data. However, in this global outbreak of COVID-19, this model is valid for a short duration depending upon on how the disease spreads and being treated. Also, Models implemented and developed by China could not be applied in India due to the dissimilar country conditions and in the same way, a high-level country model might not work to make predictions locally. ML algorithms could be applied to the more detailed data and combine it with demographic information such as age, gender etc. from other sources to make out new inferences. For instance, (datarobot.com, 2020) DATA Robot (An Enterprise in Boston) made conclusions based on the preliminary data that the covid-19 virus will infect majorly the richest people first in comparison to the poor people as the rich people would be able to afford to travel extra unlike the poor people. In addition, NLP plays a great role in digging out valuable facts about the coronavirus, NLP could be utilized for understanding various things for the safety of people from virus, by studying the available literature such as understanding the structure of the protein, vaccination development, finding options and ways for the treatment, predicting the adverse effects from the coronavirus, determining the cure /dosage and so on. The regulatory body (government) is available to help us in giving news and updates regarding the virus using different platforms and that information could also be utilized to extract out several inferences. Also, individuals who use mobile apps, for example, a mobile application help user to find if they are infected with the COVID-19 virus by putting some data as input and getting their locations automatically to rate based on the degree of threat. In section (5), a situation wherein an infected individual's phone location is always open and whomever he got in contact with, the corresponding individual will be notified to stop the spread of infection. BERT is the most algorithm by Google to overcome the issues of NLP by carefully checking bi-directionally to each word and sentences to make inferences (Devlin, et al., 2018), (Jacob Devlin et al., 2019). The ML algorithms search for specific patterns with a given data set, using those patterns, classification and prediction on the data set could be achieved, clustering could possibly be done using the classification methods for an instance, location of coronavirus hotspot or ages of people who are more prone to coronavirus. On building the models for classification and prediction, 2 issues come into considerations such as, (I) The new data is constantly increasing; therefore, the model needs to consistently update and (II) Finding new attributes in the data will also call for rebuilding and retraining of the current model. For the prediction aspect, the LSTM model provides helpful information regarding how well the measures/decisions taken for monitoring the COVID-19 spread are running quantitatively in terms of spreads and deaths and accordingly the regulatory body (government) can plan to reopen the different locales. LSTM models can effectively be transferred for studying and understanding the disease aspects of any such future outbreaks (Sayantani Basu et al. 2020).

Some challenges have been observed, for instance, in section (4.1), Mathematical Prediction Model (International business, 2020) (I) The self-informing essence of the prediction model based application, both bogus negatives and positives, could be incorporated inside the data set devoid of any physiological evaluations.(II) As more reliable and accurate models are now available so the given model needs to be optimized, however, it is extremely important that if an individual is facing sudden symptoms of the loss of taste and smell, could be infected and they should do self-quarantine to prevent the spread any further. Likewise, in the section (5), Contact Tracing is incorporated with few interpretations. (Ferretti, et al., 2020) (I) Contact Tracing is one of the best safety measures against COVID-19 using AI devised mechanism, every nation has its own app and even organizations and states are to build their own app though this would invalidate the view of a worldwide online platform for cooperating the advanced healthcare services with individuals and private sectors for the betterment of outcome of the healthcare facilities. (II) Privacy is the second matter for every individual still moderately few people are okay with their data being on the server end after their identities are anonymized. Moreover, how to utilize the collected data as the massive extent of people must have been already out from the self-isolation for the control of the spread of infection to keep the safety of people in mind.

CONCLUSION

In this chapter, various technologies that explain how technology could be applied to tackle COVID-19 along with some challenges and scope for diverse Artificial Intelligence fields have been discussed. The rapid growth in AI technology has affected every industry with not just comfort in their work culture and but also to the level of satisfaction, safety, and easiness in their mundane and precarious tasks, still, a huge range of promising practices in the various fields of artificial intelligence call for development as well as enhancement covering the clinical and social challenges. The purpose of this chapter is to make an awareness about the current contribution of AI in this global crisis and anticipating AI to become more powerful and even better in future in terms of innovation and safety with the constant efforts of researchers and scientists in this perpetual field. Especially in the field of healthcare, AI takes control as an expert system to make fast diagnosis and treatment. The validated and systematic research in the domain of artificial intelligence, would yield an outstanding future and would assist in overcoming inevitable outbreaks with less human involvement.

REFERENCES

Ai, T., Yang, Z., Hou, H., Zhan, C., Chen, C., Wenzhi, L., Tao, Q., & Sun, Z. (2020). Correlation of chest ct and rt-pcr testing in coronavirus disease 2019 (covid-19) in China: A report. *Radiology*, *296*(2), E32–E40. Advance online publication. doi:10.1148/radiol.2020200642 PMID:32101510

Al-Antari, Al-Masni, Choi, Han, & Kim. (2018). (2018). A fully integrated computer-aided diagnosis system for digital x-ray mammograms via deep learning detection, segmentation, and classification. *International Journal of Medical Informatics*, *117*, 44-54.

Alvarez, F. E., Argente, D., & Lippi, F. (2020). *A simple planning problem for COVID-19 lockdown. Tech. Rep.* National Bureau of Economic Research. doi:10.3386/w26981

appsstore.ai. (2020). *Intelligent apps for any IP Cameras.* appsstore.ai.

Bandyopadhyay, S. K., & Dutta, S. (2020). Machine learning approach for confirmation of COVID-19 cases: positive, negative, death and release. doi:10.1101/2020.03.25.20043505

Basu & Campbell. (2020). Going by the numbers: Learning and modeling COVID-19 disease dynamics. 0960-0779/ doi:10.1016/j.chaos.2020.110140

Behnood, G. (2018). *North American.* https://spectrum.ieee.org/biomedical/devices/ai-could-provide-momentbymoment-nursing-for-a-hospitals-sickest-patients

Belfiore, Urraro, Grassi, Giacobbe, Patelli, Cappabianca, & Reginelli. (2020). *Artificial intelligence to codify lung CT in Covid-19 patients.*(doi:10.100711547-020-01195-x

Best, J., & the ZDNet News Website. (2020). *AI and the coronavirus fight: How artificial intelligence is taking on COVID-19.* https://www.zdnet.com/article/ai-and-the-coronavirus-fight-how-artificial-intelligence-is-taking-on-covid-19/

Broga, D. (2020). *How Taiwan used tech to fight COVID-19.* https://www.techuk.org/insights/news/item/17187-how-taiwan-used-techto-

Chen & Guestrin. (2016). *XGBoost: A Scalable Tree Boosting System KDD.*. doi:10.1145/2939672.2939785

Chowell, G., Castillo-Chavez, C., Fenimore, P. W., Kribs-Zaleta, C. M., Arriola, L., & Hyman, J. M. (2004). Model parameters and outbreak control for SARS. *Emerging Infectious Diseases*, *10*(7), 1258–1263. doi:10.3201/eid1007.030647 PMID:15324546

COVID-19 Projections. (2020). https://covid19.healthdata.org/united-states-of-america

Das, S., Ghosh, P., Sen, B., & Mukhopadhyay, I. (2020). *Critical community size for COVID- 19–a model based approach to provide a rationale behind the lockdown.* arXiv preprint arXiv: 200403126.

datarobot.com. (2020). *Enabling the AI-Driven Enterprise.* http://www.datarobot.com

Devlin, J., & Chang, M.-W. (2019). *Open Sourcing BERT: State-of-the-Art Pre-training for Natural Language Processing*. Google AI Blog.

Devlin, J., Chang, M.-W., Lee, K., & Toutanova, K. (2018). *BERT: Pre-training of Deep Bidirectional Transformers for Language Understanding*. arXiv:1810.04805v2

Epidemics, COVID-19 Hospital Impact Model for. (2020). https://penn-chime.phl.io

EstradaM. A. R. (2020). *The Uses of Drones in Case of Massive Epidemics*. doi:10.2139srn.3546547

Fang, T. (2006). A kind of epidemic model with infectious force in both latent period and infected period and nonlinear infection rate. *J. Biomath.*, *21*(3), 345–350.

Ferretti, L., Wymant, C., Kendall, M., Zhao, L., Nurtay, A., Abeler-Dörner, L., Parker, M., Bonsall, D., & Fraser, C. (2020). *Quantifying SARS-CoV-2 transmission suggests epidemic control with digital contact tracing*. doi:10.1126cience.abb6936

Gao, Yang, Lin, & Park. (2018). *Computer vision in healthcare applications*. doi:10.1155/2018/5157020

Gay, C. (2003). Dye and N., 2003. "Modeling the SARS epidemic. *Science*, *300*(5627), 1884–1885. PMID:12766208

GholamiB.HaddadW. M.BaileyJ. M. (2018). https://spectrum.ieee.org/biomedical/devices/ai-could-provide-momentbymoment-nursing-for-a-hospitals-sickest-patients

Global News. (2020). *Global news.* http://globalnews.ca

Gutierrez, G. (2020). *Artificial Intelligence in the Intensive Care Unit*. doi:10.118613054-020-2785-y

Hafeez, M. F. A. (2020). *Covid-resnet: A deep learning framework for screening of covid19 from radiographs*. arXiv preprint arXiv:2003.14395

Haleem, Ibrahim, & Abid. (2020). *Artificial Intelligence (AI) applications for COVID-19 pandemic*. doi:10.1016/j.dsx.2020.04.012

Hara, N. (2007). Global stability of a delayed SIR epidemic model with density dependent birth and death rates. *Journal of Computational and Applied Mathematics*, *201*(2), 339–347. doi:10.1016/j.cam.2005.12.034

Hertz, L. (2020). *Face Mask Detection System using Artificial Intelligence*. https://www.leewayhertz.com/face-mask-detection-system/

Hochreiter, S., & Schmidhuber, J. (1997). Long short-term memory. *Neural Comput.*

Houthooft, R., Ruyssinck, J., van der Herten, J., Stijven, S., Couckuyt, I., Gadeyne, B., Ongenae, F., Colpaert, K., Decruyenaere, J., Dhaene, T., & De Turck, F. (2015). Predictive modelling of survival and length of stay in critically ill patients using sequential organ failure scores. *Artificial Intelligence in Medicine*, *63*(3), 191–207. doi:10.1016/j.artmed.2014.12.009 PMID:25579436

Hu, Z., Ge, Q., Jin, L., & Xiong, M. (2020). *Artificial intelligence forecasting of COVID-19 in China*. arXiv preprint: 200207112.

Huang, Y., Sun, M., & Sui, Y. (2020). *How Digital Contact Tracing Slowed Covid-19 in East Asia.* https://hbr.org/2020/04/how-digital-contact-tracing-slowed-covid-19-in-east-asia

Imai, N. (2020). *Transmissibility of 2019-nCoV, WHO Collaborating Centre Infect. Dis. Model. MRC Centre Global Infect.Dis. Anal. J-IDEA, Imperial Coll.* doi:10.25561/77148

International Business, Times. (2020). *Scientists develop new AI model that can predict coronavirus without testing.* https://www.ibtimes.sg/scientists-develop-new-ai-model-that-can-predict-coronavirus-without-testing-44889

Jin, C., Chen, W., Cao, Y., Xu, Z., Zhang, X., Deng, L., Zheng, C., Zhou, J., Shi, H., & Feng, J. (2020). Development and evaluation of an ai system for covid-19 diagnosis. doi:10.1101/2020.03.20.20039834

Journal, R. (2020). *Radiology Journal.* https://pubs.rsna.org/journal/radiology

Kermack, W.O., & McKendrick, A.G. (1991). *Contributions to the mathematical theory of epidemics–I.* Academic Press.

Ketchell, M. (2020). *Why Singapore's coronavirus response worked – and what we can all learn.* https://theconversation.com/why-singapores-coronavirus-response-worked-and-what-we-can-all-learn-134024

Kumar, Gupta, & Srivastava. (2020). *A review of modern technologies for tackling COVID-19 pandemic.* doi:10.1016/j.dsx.2020.05.008

Kumar, V. (2020). *Tackling COVID-19: The Technology behind Contact Tracing.* https://www.mygreatlearning.com/blog/covid-contact-tracing/

Le, J. (2019). *The 5 Trends Dominating Computer Vision.* https://heartbeat.fritz.ai/the-5-trends-that-dominated-computer-vision-in-2018-de38fbb9bd86

Li, Qin, Xu, Yin, & Wang. (2020). *Artificial Intelligence Distinguishes COVID-19 from Community Acquired Pneumonia on Chest CT.* doi:10.1148/radiol.2020200905

Li, L., Qin, L., Xu, Z., Yin, Y., Wang, X., & Kong, B. (2020). Artificial intelligence distinguishes COVID-19 from community acquired pneumonia on chest CT. *Radiology, 296,* E65–E71. doi:10.1148/radiol.2020200905 PMID:32191588

Lin, Zhou, Faghri, Shaw, & Campbell. (2019). *Analysis and prediction of unplanned intensive care unit readmission using recurrent neural networks with long short term memory.* Academic Press.

Maghdid, H. S., Ghafoor, K. Z., Sadiq, A. S., Curran, K., & Rabie, K. (2020). A novel AI-enabled framework to diagnose coronavirus COVID 19 using smartphone embedded sensors: design study. doi:10.1109/IRI49571.2020.00033

Ming-Yen, N., & Elaine, Y. P. (2020). Imaging profile of the covid-19 infection: Radiologic findings and literature review. *Radiology. Cardiothoracic Imaging, 2*(1), e200034. doi:10.1148/ryct.2020200034 PMID:33778547

Mitra, G. (2020). *Vehant Technologies' Uses AI For Social Distancing, Face Mask And Vehicle Detection.* https://www.expresscomputer.in/indiaincfightscovid19/vehant-technologies-uses-ai-for-social-distancing-face-mask-and-vehicle-detection/55421/

Mooney, P. (2018). *Chest X-Ray.* https://www.kaggle.com/paultimothymooney/chest-xray-pneumonia

Nain, M., Sharma, S., & Chaurasia, S. (2021). Safety and Compliance Management System Using Computer Vision and Deep Learning. *IOP Conference Series: Materials Science and Engineering.*

Narin, A., Kaya, C., & Pamuk, Z. (2020). *Automatic detection of coronavirus disease (covid-19) using x-ray images and deep convolutional neural networks.* arXiv preprint arXiv:2003.10849

Nassar, A.P., Jr., & Caruso, P. (2016). *ICU physicians are unable to accurately predict length of stay at admission: a prospective study.* doi:10.1093/intqhc/mzv112

Neher, R. A., Dyrdak, R., Druelle, V., Hodcroft, E. B., & Albert, J. (2020). Potential impact of seasonal forcing on a SARS-CoV-2 pandemic. *Swiss Medical Weekly.* PMID:32176808

Nguyen, T.T., Waurn, G., & Campus, P. (2020). *Artificial intelligence in the battle against coronavirus (COVID-19): A survey and future research directions.* doi:10.13140/RG.2.2.36491.23846

Pisani, P., Renna, M. D., Conversano, F., Casciaro, E., Muratore, M., Quarta, E., Di Paola, M., & Casciaro, S. (2013). Screening and early diagnosis of osteoporosis through x-ray and ultrasound based techniques. *World Journal of Radiology*, *5*(11), 398. doi:10.4329/wjr.v5.i11.398 PMID:24349644

ProtocolB. T. (2020). https://bluetrace.io/

Qi, X., Jiang, Z., & Yu, Q. (2016). *Machine Learning based CT radiomics model for predicting hospital stay in patients with pneumonia associated with SARSCoV-2 infection: A multicentre study.* . doi:10.1016/S0031-3955(16)31867-3

Rosebrock, A. (2018). *OpenCV Face Recognition, PyImageSearch.* https://www.pyimagesearch.com/2018/09/24/opencv-face-recognition/

Scenarios, COVID-19. (2020). *COVID-19 Scenarios.* https://neherlab.org/covid19/

Sethy, P. K., & Behera, S. K. (2020). Detection of coronavirus disease (COVID-19) based on deep features. doi:10.20944/preprints202003.0300.v1

Setzer, E. (2020). *Contact-Tracing Apps in the United States.* https://www.lawfareblog.com/contact-tracing-apps-united-states

Sommer. (2019). *Israel Unveils Open Source App to Warn Users of Coronavirus Cases.* https://www.haaretz.com/israel-news/israel-unveils-app-that-uses-tracking-to-tell-users-if-they-were-near-virus-cases-1.8702055

Song, Y., Zheng, S., Li, L., Zhang, X., Zhang, X., & Huang, Z. (2020). Deep learning enables accurate diagnosis of novel coronavirus (COVID-19) with CT images. medRxiv.

Sotoodeh & Ho. (2019). *Improving length of stay prediction using a hidden Markov model.* Academic Press.

Speidel, Wilfley, Star-Lack, Heanue, & Van Lysel. (2006). Scanning-beam digital x-ray (sbdx) technology for interventional and diagnostic cardiac angiography. *Medical Physics*, *33*(8), 2714-2727.

The Indian Express. (2020). *Mumbai hospitals run out of beds for critical Covid patients.* https://indianexpress.com/article/cities/mumbai/mumbai-hospitals-run-out-of-beds-for-critical-covid-patients-6407221/

Tsang, S. (2020). *Contact tracing apps being deployed around the world.* https://iapp.org/news/a/here-are-the-contact-tracing-apps-being-employed-around-the-world/

Ulhaq, A., Khan, A., Gomes, D., & Paul, M. (2020). Computer vision for COVID-19 control. *Survey.* arXiv2004.09420

Wang, New, & Sun. (2020). *Response to COVID-19 in Taiwan big data analytics, new technology, and proactive testing.* doi:10.1001/jama.2020.3151

Wang, S., Kang, B., Ma, J., Zeng, X., Xiao, M., & Guo, J. (2020). A deep learning algorithm using CT images to screen for Corona Virus Disease (COVID-19). medRxiv. doi:10.1101/2020.02.14.20023028

Website. (2020). *Computed Tomography (CT) - Chest.* https://www.radiologyinfo.org/en/info

Wong & Wang. (2020). *Covid-net: A tailored deep convolutional neural network design for detection of covid-19 cases from chest radiography images.* arXiv preprint arXiv:2003.09871.

World Health. (2020). *Contact tracing apps: Which countries are doing what.* https://health.economictimes.indiatimes.com/news/diagnostics/contact-tracing-apps-which-countries-are-doing-what/75440095

World Health Organization. (2020). *WHO Coronavirus Disease (COVID-19) Dashboard.* https://covid19.who.int/

Xu, X., Jiang, X., & Ma, C. (2020). *Deep learning system to screen coronavirus disease 2019 pneumonia.* https://arxiv.org/abs/2002.09334

Yan, L., & Zhang, H.-T. (2020). A machine learning-based model for survival prediction in patients with severe COVID-19 infection. doi:10.1101/2020.02.27.20028027

Yang, Zeng, Wang, Wong, Liang, & Zanin. (2020). Modified SEIR and AI prediction of the epidemics trend of COVID-19 in China under public health interventions. *J Thorac Dis 2020, 12*(3), 165.

Yao & Leng. (2020). *Introduction to Computer Vision with Watson and OpenCV.* https://www.coursera.org/learn/introduction-computer-vision-watson-opencv/

Yu & Koltun. (2016). *Multi-scale context aggregation by dilated convolutions.* Academic Press.

Yuang, S.-L., Han, L. T., & Ma, Z. E. (2001). A kind of epidemic model having infectious force in both latent period and infected period. *J. Biomath., 16*(4), 392–398.

Zheng, Du, Wang, Zhang, Cui, Kang, Yang, Lou, Chi, Long, Ma, Yuan, Zhang, Zhang, Ye, & Xin. (2020). *Predicting COVID-19 in China Using Hybrid AI Model.* IEEE.). doi:10.1109/TCYB.2020.2990162

Chapter 8
Text Mining and Natural Language Processing for Health Informatics:
Recent Trends and the Way Forward

Anoop V. S.

Rajagiri College of Social Sciences (Autonomous), Kochi, Kerala, India

ABSTRACT

Health informatics deals with applying informatics to medicine and healthcare that aims to store, process, and retrieve large amounts of healthcare data to enable optimal collaboration between different stakeholders. This has several applications in the healthcare domain from extracting information from medical documents such as case reports and prescriptions to analyzing data from sensors available in wearable devices. Recent advancements in information and communication technologies fueled the need of devising intelligent technologies for analyzing such data – not only in various forms but also in large quantities. This has posed many challenges and opportunities to use techniques such as text mining, natural language processing (NLP), and deep learning to unearth the latent themes from the vast array of textual data. This chapter proposes some prominent works in health informatics that use text mining and NLP and also discusses some active research areas in these dimensions. This chapter will be useful to understand the recent advancements and future research dimensions.

INTRODUCTION

The recent developmental acceleration happens in the areas of intelligent computing, healthcare informatics is getting shifted to a new paradigm where advanced techniques such as deep learning and natural language processing are getting widely implemented in many areas. Since the major share of data accumulated and processed in healthcare are in the form of unstructured text, mining them to find latent patterns is an active research area with many open challenges. There are many innovative research reports in healthcare informatics for addressing these challenges, but there are still a lot of avenues where text

DOI: 10.4018/978-1-7998-7188-0.ch008

mining and natural language processing can be fully exploited for tackling the challenges. Compared with other areas of intelligent computing, health informatics is relatively new and attempts to use information technology capabilities to organize and analyze large quantities of unstructured text to unearth the patterns. Using computational techniques, health informatics attempts to leverage useful trends and information from humongous volumes of medical data that may support the healthcare decision-making process. This field has gotten significant attention in the very recent past due to the COVID-19 pandemic outbreak where millions of people got affected very adversely. The pandemic has affected the world unprepared and there were no clues among the healthcare workers and administrators on how to tackle the challenges posed by COVID-19. The manual way of fighting the pandemic with the activities such as case identification and contact tracing was proved inefficient in many situations and highlighted the need for using information technology-enabled approaches for dealing with the scenario in a better way. The government and public healthcare workers and officials are overwhelmed with the data - the most important tool for them to take decisions expedited and for planning, decision-making, and measuring effectiveness. This has again proved the need for automated techniques and tools to analyze this data effectively and the adoption of health informatics practices in better dealing with such situations.

Text mining and natural language processing attempts to analyze vast bodies of unstructured text documents and unearth the hidden patterns using processes such as information extraction, text classification, and topic modeling. Recent advancements in machine learning such as deep learning outperformed many state-of-the-art shallow machine learning approaches. From rule-based systems to machine learning to deep learning, this field has gone through many significant changes that improved the accuracy of many machine learning models. Healthcare domain generates large quantities of unstructured text in many forms such as patient generated data, social medical data, clinical narratives, discharge summaries, to name a few. So there exists a huge opportunity to analyze and unearth the patterns containing entities and relationships, that may find several applications in the healthcare industry. Health informatics which is a new but active research area that has got significant attention in the recent past which heavily makes use of text mining, natural language processing, and machine learning. There are several interesting research papers reported in the literature but there also exists many interesting research problems that need to be explored. In this connection, this chapter outlines some of the prominent state-of-the-art in health informatics and also future research trends and dimensions in this area.

The remainder of this chapter is organized as follows. Section 2 discusses some of the very recent and prominent works that were reported in the literature on healthcare informatics exploring the potentials of text mining and natural language processing techniques. Section 3 details the recent trends on adopting the intelligent computing paradigms to healthcare informatics and in Section 4, the future trends and further research dimensions are presented. Section 5 concludes this chapter.

STATE-OF-THE-ART IN HEALTH INFORMATICS USING NATURAL LANGUAGE PROCESSING AND TEXT MINING

This section discusses some of the prominent works in health informatics that uses techniques such as text mining, and natural language processing. The recently reported approaches which are closely related to the theme of this chapter have been presented for the readers to understand what is already in the literature. The applications of natural language processing for health-related text contents were discussed in detail by Dina Demner et. al. (Demner-Fushman et al., 2021) in a recent work reported in the health informatics literature. This work discusses some of the prominent approaches for health informatics using natural language processing such as language understanding, information retrieval, and cognitive virtual agents. Personal health informatics that comprises important components such as patient engagement and patient-generated health data was introduced by Robert M. Cronin et. al. (Shortliffe et al., 2021) in which they have discussed how the role of the person has evolved, and how personal health informatics broadly impacts both the person and the field of biomedical informatics. A systematic review has been conducted by Aziz Le Glaz et. al. on the applications of machine learning and natural language processing in mental health (Le Glaz et al., 2021). The authors have shown that machine learning and NLP techniques provide useful information from unexplored data such as patient's daily habits which are usually inaccessible for healthcare workers. The emerging trends of bioinformatics in health informatics and a detailed review on the same was reported in the recent literature and the work was carried out by Mahi Sharma et. al. (Sharma et al., n.d.). Big data technologies and their role in health informatics are also discussed by the authors. The key commercial platforms for healthcare data analytics and challenges along with prospects of bioinformatics in healthcare are also outlined in this work (Sharma et al., n.d.). Social media data is heavily mined for health informatics and the shared tasks that are organized in leading natural language processing conferences to show the significance of the same (Magge et al., 2021).

A qualitative and natural language processing analysis of spontaneously generated online patient experience is reported in the literature by Walsh et. al. (Walsh et al., 2021). The authors argue that the user-generated patient experience is a useful source for evaluating real-world effectiveness, identifying research gaps, and also for understanding patient perspectives. Another study of seven clinical natural language processing suites to check whether reproducibility can be improved in clinical natural language processing was conducted by Digan et. al. (Digan et al., 2021). The objective of their work was to study whether the workflow management systems heavily used in bioinformatics could impact the reproducibility of clinical NLP frameworks. The challenges and opportunities beyond structured data in the analysis of electronic health records were reported by Tayefi et. al. (Tayefi et al., 2021). For their advanced review, the authors have performed their search on two popular databases PubMed and Web of Science with sufficient queries. Their method showed and concluded that novel and innovative methods that can combine both unstructured and structured data are expected to be extremely important in future innovations (Tayefi et al., 2021). Jagadeesh and Rajendran showed different machine learning approaches for analysis in healthcare informatics (Jagadeesh & Rajendran, n.d.). With a focus on medical image processing, the authors showcased various machine learning modules used in the field of healthcare.

Reeves et. al. (Reeves et al., 2020) described how health informatics support outbreak management in an academic health system. The authors have outlined the design and the implementation of electronic health record-based rapid screening processes, clinical decision support, laboratory testing, reporting tools, etc. related to COVID-19 and stressed the importance of EHRin supporting the clinical needs of a health system for better dealing with the pandemic. Another recent work by Mantas showed the importance of health informatics in public health during the COVID-19 pandemic (Mantas, 2020). This work presented the challenges faced by health informatics in supporting healthcare professionals and public health authorities in the world (Mantas, 2020). Recently, Benson et. al. proposed an approach for leveraging clinical informatics to improve child mental healthcare (Benson et al., 2020). A study that was reported from Colorado by Lin et. al. (Lin et al., 2020) showed how clinical informatics accelerates health system adaptation to the COVID-19 pandemic. They have explained fourteen examples of innovative and effective informatics interventions in healthcare and showed how that would be helpful in dealing with the pandemic. An overview of health informatics and electronic health records to support clinical research in the COVID-19 pandemic (Dagliati et al., 2021) was reported in the healthcare informatics research by Dagliati et. al. This work gave special attention to collaborative data infrastructures to support COVID-19 research and on the open issues of data sharing and data governance that COVID-19 had made emerge (Dagliati et al., 2021). Barakati et. al. conducted an international survey on health informatics solutions in response to COVID-19 and the preliminary insights were reported (Barakati et al., 2020). Using the insights, the authors have concluded that the results are consistent with the claims made by the World Health Organization which has identified Health Information Technologies as "one of the most promising approaches to address this challenge in modern societies" (Barakati et al., 2020). Another interesting work by Sylvestre et. al. (Sylvestre et al., 2020) outlined how health informatics help supporting disease outbreak management and most interesting how to deal with it without an electronic health record. The works discussed above clearly shows the impact of informatics in healthcare to better deal with the disease outbreak and

From the literature analysis, it is highly evident that there are several pieces of literature that are being added to the repository that discusses the applications of artificial intelligence, specifically, natural language processing and text mining. An artificial intelligence-based approach that uses natural language processing applied to the electronic health record-based clinical research was reported very recently (Juhn & Liu, 2020). This work discussed the current literature on the secondary use of electronic health record data for clinical research concerning allergy, asthma, and immunology and highlights the potential, challenges, and implications of natural language processing techniques (Juhn & Liu, 2020). An interesting survey that discussed the applications of deep learning, the current hot topic in machine learning, in clinical natural language processing was reported by Wu et. al. (Wu, Roberts, Datta et al, 2020). This survey provides a quantitative analysis to answer research questions concerning methods, scope, and context of current research in deep learning for clinical research. Another prominent study that revealed the mental health support groups and heightened health anxiety on Reddit during COVID-19 was conducted by Low et. al. (Low et al., 2020). The aim of their study was to apply natural language processing techniques to identify the patterns and trends for mental support during the pandemic. Shoenbill et. al. applied natural language processing on lifestyle modification documentation to identify lifestyle modification details from electronic health records (Shoenbill et al., 2020). In this work, electronic health record notes from hypertension patients were analyzed using an open-source natural language processing tool to retrieve assessment and advice regarding lifestyle modification (Shoenbill et al., 2020). Another study on the use of natural language processing for the precise retrieval of key elements of health information technology evaluation studies was reported by Dornauer et. al. (Dornauer et al., 2020). They have applied four methods such as named entity recognition, bag-of-words, term frequency-inverse document frequency, and latent Dirichlet allocation topic modeling to health information technology evaluation studies. Their study has concluded that applying natural language processing and text mining would help retrieve hidden patterns in a speedy and effective manner (Dornauer et al., 2020).

An interesting piece of work on applying natural language processing for structuring clinical text data on depression was reported in the health and clinical informatics by Vaci et. al. (Vaci et al., 2020). The objective of their study was to apply natural language processing to capture real-world data on individuals with depression from the clinical record interactive search clinical text to foster the use of electronic healthcare data in mental health research. Their results showed a high degree of accuracy in the extraction of drug-related information (Vaci et al., 2020). Abbood et. al. developed a framework powered by natural language processing for event-based surveillance (Abbood et al., 2020). Their approach used named entity recognition and a naive bayes classifier for event-based surveillance and the authors claimed that this framework can be used for real-life applications. A natural language processing approach for extracting quantitative smoking status from clinical narratives was reported by Yang et. al. (Yang et al., 2020). The authors have annotated 200 clinical notes from patients who had low-dose CT imaging procedures for lung cancer screening and developed an NLP system using a two-layer rule-engine structure to implement their approach. They have reported that their system achieved the best F1 scores of 96.3% and 94.6% lenient and strict evaluation (Yang et al., 2020).

Mining large quantities of medical text, especially unstructured in nature, is an interesting and potential activity in health informatics. Advanced text mining approaches will help clinical practitioners and enthusiasts to leverage latent themes and patterns from medical text such as clinical narratives. BioBERT, a pre-trained biomedical language representation model for biomedical text mining was introduced by Lee et. al. (Lee et al., 2020). This domain-specific language representation model pre-trained on large-scale biomedical corpora is useful in many text mining and natural language processing tasks. Giummarra et. al. conducted a study on the evaluation of text mining approaches to reduce screening workload for injury-focused systematic reviews (Giummarra et al., 2020). The authors have examined the performance of text mining in supporting the second reviewer in a systematic review examining associations between fault attribution and health and work-related outcomes after transport injury (Giummarra et al., 2020). A text mining approach for automated detection of psychological risk factors was conducted by Uronen et. al. (Uronen et al., 2020). This study showed that it was possible to detect risk factors for sick leave, rehabilitation, and pension from free-text documentation of health checks (Uronen et al., 2020). Wu et. al. proposed a text mining technique to extract depressive symptoms and unearth the major depressive disorders from electronic health records (Wu, Kuo, Su et al, 2020). Their approach was aimed at improving the accuracy of the diagnostic codes for psychiatric disorders in NHIRD. A text mining approach for automated surgical term clustering from unstructured textual surgery descriptions was proposed by Khaleghi et. al. (Khaleghi et al., 2020). This work helps extract the most salient text features from the unstructured principal procedure and additional notes by effectively reducing the raw feature set dimension.

Text mining approaches for dealing with the ever growing and rapidly expanding literature on COVID-19 were presented by Wang and Lo (Wang & Lo, 2021). Automated text mining approaches such as searching, reading, and summarizations were discussed in this work. A text mining analysis that identifies addiction concerns on Twitter during the COVID-19 pandemic was reported by Glowacki et. al. (Glowacki et al., 2021). The authors have conducted their studies on 3,301 tweets captured between January 31 and April 23, 2020, and the study concluded that analyzing Twitter content enables health professionals to identify the public's concerns about addiction during the COVID-19 pandemic (Glowacki et al., 2021). There are several other approaches reported in health informatics literature that discuss the potential of deep natural language processing and deep text mining for enabling better accuracy in many areas of healthcare informatics.

NATURAL LANGUAGE PROCESSING AND TEXT MINING AS AN ENABLER FOR HEALTH INFORMATICS

The recent advancements in information communication and communication technologies have fueled the growth of generating large quantities of data, especially in the form of unstructured text. A recent study estimated that in 2020, around 2314 exabytes of data was accumulated from the healthcare domain and expected to be growing exponentially over the coming years. The major contributors of these data include electronic health records, the output of clinical research studies, data from patient wearable devices, patient's telehealth records including the data generated through chat applications, outpatient medical records, discharge summaries, etc. Manually analyzing these vast amounts of data to find out useful information for different stakeholders would be a very difficult task. Automated and intelligent algorithms can unearth interesting patterns from these data and these patterns would be highly useful for medical practitioners, medical enthusiasts, and researchers. Natural Language Processing and Text Mining techniques play a crucial role in leveraging those latent themes and interesting patterns and trends that would aid the clinical decision-making process. Some of the most prominent applications of Natural Language Processing and Text Mining are discussed in the subsequent parts of this section.

Named Entity Recognition (NER)

One of the most important applications of Natural Language Processing is identifying named entities from unstructured text documents. The medical text also contains different named entities such as the names of diseases, symptoms, reactions, drug names, medications, and dose. Manually annotating those entities is a time-consuming and difficult task thus natural language processing helps identify the named entities. Earlier approaches for named entity recognition were depending on a large set of rules handcrafted by domain experts and the accuracy, practicality, and maintenance of such rule-based systems were very less. Later, machine learning techniques came into the picture that could learn the patterns from the data in a supervised or unsupervised manner depending on the learning algorithm used. Again, the machine learning area underwent several upgrades and the current machine learning trend is on deep learning where the machine itself can learn without the human-crafted features. This has made significant improvements on the accuracy of machine learning techniques that use shallow learning-based approaches.

Relation Extraction (RE)

Relation extraction is the task of extracting the relationship between entities. In the biomedical field, there are many relations that need to be leveraged such as protein-protein relation, chemical reaction, and the drug-side effects that are very important to understand. Detection and classification of these types of semantic relationships will help healthcare practitioners understand the association with many biomedical entities. The earlier approaches were heavily dependent on rule-based approaches that could only classify only the highly relationships in a medical text, for example, a drug-drug interaction relationship. Later, several pre-trained models were introduced that could capture many types of relationships from the biomedical text and classify them with higher accuracy. Deep learning models that are trained using large quantities of data make use of these pre-trained models such as BioBERT (Lee et al., 2020) could yield better accuracy when compared with other machine learning models.

Text Summarization

Summarizing large bodies of text while preserving the meaning and context has many applications in real-world problems. This has also found applications in the biomedical domain where documents such as clinical notes, discharge summaries can be summarized that would significantly reduce the time required to understand the document. Text summarization techniques such as abstractive and extractive summarization can be applied for many applications such as healthcare news summarization and summarization of clinical research papers. With the advent of deep learning techniques and transformers, this area of natural language processing has also gotten significant attention in the recent past. Several techniques such as deep contextualized representations and semantic concepts-based summarization techniques have gained much momentum recently in the biomedical text mining field.

Knowledge Discovery

Natural Language Processing and text mining techniques are used in the biomedical field to discover latent themes from text data. There are a lot of patient-generated data that are getting added in the public domain which are goldmines containing useful patterns. Patterns such as risk factors, symptoms, reactions, disease outbreaks, and adverse drug events can be mined from such sources that could potentially help healthcare workers and medical practitioners to make intelligent decisions and also give necessary medical attention and aid to the needy.

Text Classification

Text classification refers to the process of automatically classifying text into predefined categories. There are many applications for text classification in the biomedical domain but that also imposes many challenges. Medical texts are very complicated and often contain abbreviations and other medical terminologies that are difficult to understand. For example, identification of a particular disease from free medical text and classifying that into a predefined ICD-10 code is an interesting area in healthcare that needs significant attention. Classifying the patient sentiments and classifying the severity of the symptoms and other medical conditions also remain open challenges in biomedical text classification.

Cognitive Virtual Agents

Cognitive Virtual Agents (CVA) are intelligent agents that can interact with humans in a natural way and this ability has many potential applications in healthcare. One of the most notable advantages of CVAs is that they can significantly reduce the workload of healthcare professionals as the virtual agents can converse with a patient as natural as humans. These virtual agents can be employed in many areas of healthcare such as monitoring the mental health of patients and pre-screening of medical conditions and other symptoms. There are several other applications for CVA in healthcare such as treatment and monitoring, healthcare services and support, and diagnosis. As the upcoming trend in healthcare is on providing personalized care, the cognitive virtual agent market will surely be growing exponentially in the future offering many innovative products and services for transforming the healthcare industry.

There are many other ways natural language processing can support healthcare applications such as improving the clinical documentation process, supporting clinical decisions, de-identification of personally identifiable information from medical texts, and clinical entity resolving. The cutting-edge deep learning models in the coming years will help to transform healthcare to the next level.

NLP AND TEXT MINING IN HEALTH INFORMATICS: FUTURE RESEARCH DIMENSIONS

This section details some future research dimensions of natural language processing and text mining in transforming health informatics. Recently the rate of adoption of electronic health records has grown significantly and that contributed to a massive clinical narrative data available electronically. The usage of social media in healthcare has increased and as a result, a large collection of medical text is available there. Mining these social network platforms is an interesting research area as this will explore many dimensions such as patient contact tracing, exploring patient connections, and social medical data mining. We have devised many techniques for identifying and extracting information such as entities from medical data such as clinical narratives and health records but there exists a huge gap in automatic inference of the relationship between these entities. This will help understand the context and associations in better ways and would aid the clinical decision making process efficiently. One of the most important challenges faced by health informatics researchers is the scarcity of annotated data for training machine learning and natural language processing models. There exist a lot of opportunities in creating such datasets and also techniques such as transfer learning should be exploited in its full swing for developing state-of-the-art systems. Temporal extraction is another interesting area in healthcare informatics as there is the temporal nature of the natural language text in the clinical domain. So focusing on temporal information extraction such as disease progression and clinical events which are recorded chronologically, with specific events being significant only in a particular temporal context is another interesting research dimension. De-Identification of personal and other sensitive data plays a major role in the current era and this demands more advanced data hiding and protection mechanisms. With the rapid developments in disruptive technologies such as Blockchain, Internet of Things, and Quantum Computing also have several applications in this complex field.

CONCLUSION

This chapter discussed the applications and recent trends of text mining and natural language processing in health informatics. Health informatics is a comparatively new and rapidly progressing area in healthcare that received significant attention in the recent past. The advancements in the digitization of medical data greatly demands innovative methods and mechanisms to unearth a large set of latent themes from the vast body of medical data. The innovations in text mining and natural language processing enables the ability of mining such datasets automatically with the aim of supporting clinical researchers and other medical practitioners. This chapter outlines some of those active research areas of text mining and natural language processing applied to health informatics. Some of the potential research dimensions of text mining and NLP is also discussed in this chapter. The author believes that this chapter would be highly useful for the health informatics researchers to widen their horizons and apply the innovative techniques in leveraging natural language processing in healthcare.

REFERENCES

Abbood, A., Ullrich, A., Busche, R., & Ghozzi, S. (2020). EventEpi-A natural language processing framework for event-based surveillance. *PLoS Computational Biology*, *16*(11), e1008277. doi:10.1371/journal.pcbi.1008277 PMID:33216746

Barakati, S. S., Topaz, M., Peltonen, L. M., Mitchell, J., Alhuwail, D., Risling, T., & Ronquillo, C. (2020). Health Informatics Solutions in Response to COVID-19: Preliminary Insights from an International Survey. *Studies in Health Technology and Informatics*, *275*, 222–223. doi:10.3233/SHTI200727 PMID:33227773

Benson, N. M., Edgcomb, J. B., Landman, A. B., & Zima, B. T. (2020). Leveraging Clinical Informatics to Improve Child Mental Health Care. *Journal of the American Academy of Child and Adolescent Psychiatry*, *59*(12), 1314–1317. doi:10.1016/j.jaac.2020.06.014 PMID:33248526

Cronin, R. M., Jimison, H., & Johnson, K. B. (2021). Personal Health Informatics. In E. H. Shortliffe & J. J. Cimino (Eds.), *Biomedical Informatics*. Springer. doi:10.1007/978-3-030-58721-5_11

Dagliati, A., Malovini, A., Tibollo, V., & Bellazzi, R. (2021). Health informatics and EHR to support clinical research in the COVID-19 pandemic: An overview. *Briefings in Bioinformatics*, *22*(2), 812–822. doi:10.1093/bib/bbaa418 PMID:33454728

Demner-Fushman, D., Elhadad, N., & Friedman, C. (2021). Natural language processing for health-related texts. In *Biomedical Informatics* (pp. 241–272). Springer. doi:10.1007/978-3-030-58721-5_8

Digan, W., Névéol, A., Neuraz, A., Wack, M., Baudoin, D., Burgun, A., & Rance, B. (2021). Can reproducibility be improved in clinical natural language processing? A study of 7 clinical NLP suites. *Journal of the American Medical Informatics Association: JAMIA*, *28*(3), 504–515. doi:10.1093/jamia/ocaa261 PMID:33319904

Dornauer, V., Jahn, F., Hoeffner, K., Winter, A., & Ammenwerth, E. (2020). Use of Natural Language Processing for Precise Retrieval of Key Elements of Health IT Evaluation Studies. *Studies in Health Technology and Informatics*, *272*, 95–98. doi:10.3233/SHTI200502 PMID:32604609

Giummarra, M. J., Lau, G., & Gabbe, B. J. (2020). Evaluation of text mining to reduce screening workload for injury-focused systematic reviews. *Injury Prevention, 26*(1), 55–60. doi:10.1136/injuryprev-2019-043247

Glowacki, E. M., Wilcox, G. B., & Glowacki, J. B. (2021). Identifying #addiction concerns on twitter during the COVID-19 pandemic: A text mining analysis. *Substance abuse*, *42*(1), 39–46. doi:10.1080/08897077.2020.1822489 PMID:32970973

Jagadeesh, K., & Rajendran, A. (n.d.). Machine Learning Approaches for Analysis in Healthcare Informatics. In Machine Learning and Analytics in Healthcare Systems (pp. 105-122). CRC Press.

Juhn, Y., & Liu, H. (2020). Artificial intelligence approaches using natural language processing to advance EHR-based clinical research. *The Journal of Allergy and Clinical Immunology*, *145*(2), 463–469. doi:10.1016/j.jaci.2019.12.897 PMID:31883846

Khaleghi, T., Murat, A., Arslanturk, S., & Davies, E. (2020). Automated Surgical Term Clustering: A Text Mining Approach for Unstructured Textual Surgery Descriptions. *IEEE Journal of Biomedical and Health Informatics, 24*(7), 2107–2118. doi:10.1109/JBHI.2019.2956973 PMID:31796420

Le Glaz, A., Haralambous, Y., Kim-Dufor, D. H., Lenca, P., Billot, R., Ryan, T. C., Marsh, J., DeVylder, J., Walter, M., Berrouiguet, S., & Lemey, C. (2021). Machine Learning and Natural Language Processing in Mental Health: Systematic Review. *Journal of Medical Internet Research, 23*(5), e15708. doi:10.2196/15708 PMID:33944788

Lee, J., Yoon, W., Kim, S., Kim, D., Kim, S., So, C. H., & Kang, J. (2020). BioBERT: A pre-trained biomedical language representation model for biomedical text mining. *Bioinformatics (Oxford, England), 36*(4), 1234–1240. doi:10.1093/bioinformatics/btz682 PMID:31501885

Lin, C. T., Bookman, K., Sieja, A., Markley, K., Altman, R. L., Sippel, J., Perica, K., Reece, L., Davis, C., Horowitz, E., Pisney, L., Sottile, P. D., Kao, D., Adrian, B., Szkil, M., Griffin, J., Youngwerth, J., Drew, B., & Pell, J. (2020). Clinical informatics accelerates health system adaptation to the COVID-19 pandemic: Examples from Colorado. *Journal of the American Medical Informatics Association: JAMIA, 27*(12), 1955–1963. doi:10.1093/jamia/ocaa171 PMID:32687152

Low, D. M., Rumker, L., Talkar, T., Torous, J., Cecchi, G., & Ghosh, S. S. (2020). Natural Language Processing Reveals Vulnerable Mental Health Support Groups and Heightened Health Anxiety on Reddit During COVID-19: Observational Study. *Journal of Medical Internet Research, 22*(10), e22635. doi:10.2196/22635 PMID:32936777

Magge, A., Klein, A., Miranda-Escalada, A., Al-Garadi, M. A., Alimova, I., Miftahutdinov, Z., . . . Gonzalez, G. (2021, June). *Proceedings of the Sixth Social Media Mining for Health (# SMM4H) Workshop and Shared Task.* Academic Press.

Mantas, J. (2020). The Importance of Health Informatics in Public Health During the COVID-19 Pandemic. *Studies in Health Technology and Informatics, 272,* 487–488. doi:10.3233/SHTI200602 PMID:32604709

Reeves, J. J., Hollandsworth, H. M., Torriani, F. J., Taplitz, R., Abeles, S., Tai-Seale, M., Millen, M., Clay, B. J., & Longhurst, C. A. (2020). Rapid response to COVID-19: Health informatics support for outbreak management in an academic health system. *Journal of the American Medical Informatics Association: JAMIA, 27*(6), 853–859. doi:10.1093/jamia/ocaa037 PMID:32208481

Sharma, M., Mondal, S., Bhattacharjee, S., & Jabalia, N. (n.d.). Emerging Trends of Bioinformatics in Health Informatics. *Computational Intelligence in Healthcare, 343.*

Shoenbill, K., Song, Y., Gress, L., Johnson, H., Smith, M., & Mendonca, E. A. (2020). Natural language processing of lifestyle modification documentation. *Health Informatics Journal, 26*(1), 388–405. doi:10.1177/1460458218824742 PMID:30791802

Sylvestre, E., Thuny, R. M., Cecilia-Joseph, E., Gueye, P., Chabartier, C., Brouste, Y., Mehdaoui, H., Najioullah, F., Pierre-François, S., Abel, S., Cabié, A., & Dramé, M. (2020). Health informatics support for outbreak management: How to respond without an electronic health record? *Journal of the American Medical Informatics Association: JAMIA, 27*(11), 1828–1829. doi:10.1093/jamia/ocaa183 PMID:32761100

Tayefi, M., Ngo, P., Chomutare, T., Dalianis, H., Salvi, E., Budrionis, A., & Godtliebsen, F. (2021). Challenges and opportunities beyond structured data in analysis of electronic health records. *Wiley Interdisciplinary Reviews: Computational Statistics*, 1549.

Uronen, L., Moen, H., Teperi, S., Martimo, K. P., Hartiala, J., & Salanterä, S. (2020). Towards automated detection of psychosocial risk factors with text mining. *Occupational Medicine (Oxford, England)*, *70*(3), 203–206. doi:10.1093/occmed/kqaa022 PMID:32086511

Vaci, N., Liu, Q., Kormilitzin, A., De Crescenzo, F., Kurtulmus, A., Harvey, J., O'Dell, B., Innocent, S., Tomlinson, A., Cipriani, A., & Nevado-Holgado, A. (2020). Natural language processing for structuring clinical text data on depression using UK-CRIS. *Evidence-Based Mental Health*, *23*(1), 21–26. doi:10.1136/ebmental-2019-300134 PMID:32046989

Walsh, J., Cave, J., & Griffiths, F. (2021). Spontaneously Generated Online Patient Experience of Modafinil: A Qualitative and NLP Analysis. *Frontiers in Digital Health*, *3*, 10. doi:10.3389/fdgth.2021.598431

Wang, L. L., & Lo, K. (2021). Text mining approaches for dealing with the rapidly expanding literature on COVID-19. *Briefings in Bioinformatics*, *22*(2), 781–799. doi:10.1093/bib/bbaa296 PMID:33279995

Wu, C. S., Kuo, C. J., Su, C. H., Wang, S. H., & Dai, H. J. (2020). Using text mining to extract depressive symptoms and to validate the diagnosis of major depressive disorder from electronic health records. *Journal of Affective Disorders*, *260*, 617–623. doi:10.1016/j.jad.2019.09.044 PMID:31541973

Wu, S., Roberts, K., Datta, S., Du, J., Ji, Z., Si, Y., Soni, S., Wang, Q., Wei, Q., Xiang, Y., Zhao, B., & Xu, H. (2020). Deep learning in clinical natural language processing: A methodical review. *Journal of the American Medical Informatics Association: JAMIA*, *27*(3), 457–470. doi:10.1093/jamia/ocz200 PMID:31794016

Yang, X., Yang, H., Lyu, T., Yang, S., Guo, Y., Bian, J., Xu, H., & Wu, Y. (2020). A Natural Language Processing Tool to Extract Quantitative Smoking Status from Clinical Narratives. medRxiv. doi:10.1101/2020.10.30.20223511

Chapter 9
Plant Disease Detection Using Machine Learning Approaches:
A Survey

Sukanta Ghosh

iD https://orcid.org/0000-0002-7715-7669

School of Computer Applications, Lovely Professional University, India

Shubhanshu Arya

School of Computer Application, Lovely Professional University, India

Amar Singh

School of Computer Application, Lovely Professional University, India

ABSTRACT

Agricultural production is one of the main factors affecting a country's domestic market situation. Many problems are the reasons for estimating crop yields, which vary in different parts of the world. Overuse of chemical fertilizers, uneven distribution of rainfall, and uneven soil fertility lead to plant diseases. This forces us to focus on effective methods for detecting plant diseases. It is important to find an effective plant disease detection technique. Plants need to be monitored from the beginning of their life cycle to avoid such diseases. Observation is a kind of visual observation, which is time-consuming, costly, and requires a lot of experience. For speeding up this process, it is necessary to automate the disease detection system. A lot of researchers have developed plant leaf detection systems based on various technologies. In this chapter, the authors discuss the potential of methods for detecting plant leaf diseases. It includes various steps such as image acquisition, image segmentation, feature extraction, and classification.

DOI: 10.4018/978-1-7998-7188-0.ch009

INTRODUCTION

India is a farming country. About 70% of the population depends on agriculture. Farmers can choose a variety of suitable crops and find suitable crop protection products. Plant disease refers to the study of visual observation patterns in plants. Plant health and disease control play an important role in successfully growing crops on the farm. In the past, the control and analysis of plant diseases were performed manually by experts in the field. This requires a lot of work and a long processing time. If plant diseases are detected, imaging tests can be used. In most cases, disease symptoms appear on leaves, stems and fruits. The leaves of plants are used to identify diseases by showing symptoms of diseases. This article describes imaging techniques used to detect plant diseases (Ghosh & Singh, 2020).

But agricultural production has also made a significant contribution to today's agricultural production. Significant changes have also taken place in agricultural production. With the increase of knowledge, technology has led to some modernizations in the field of agricultural production. Modern agronomy uses the best technical equipment and techniques. The use of modern tools has increased, making it easy to determine suitable conditions for increasing crop yields. Different types of fertilizers and pesticides are used for this. Even genetically modified seeds are being tested on a larger scale to increase the overall yield in each region.

Planting crops includes all activities aimed at increasing productivity at any time of the year. It includes a comprehensive analysis of the soil and the types of seeds used basically need nutrition. Especially the harvest and many others. The output of crops and other sources is not only used to meet the daily needs of farmers, but also to meet the daily needs of others, but because there are some problems in all fields, agriculture or crop production also faces serious problems in the agricultural field. As a plant disease, with the huge demand for food all over the world, it has become imperative to focus on plant production, the purpose of which is to protect the entire crop from loss before it goes to market. The earthquake and disease also explained the severe crop failure. In terms of quality or quality, the yield is reduced due to various types of plant diseases (Barbedo, 2016). These diseases will seriously affect crop production, and then affect the quality and quantity of the entire crop. Managing large crops requires multiple timely measures, such as disease surveillance, to reduce them to adverse events. This also includes seeking immediate solutions to various problems.

This disease affects the overall function of the plant. This can result in slower growth, decreased fruit yield, more leaves and many other diseases. Sometimes a disease can spread from one culture to another (Gavhale et al., 2014), or it can be spread through pathogens or other means. Sometimes they may be caused by fungi or bacteria, and sometimes viruses can even be carried from one place to another with the seeds.

The main cause of plant diseases is infection, such as pests, bacteria, fungi and viruses. These diseases are very common and can spread to any part of the plant, because any of the following can be found in stems, vegetables, fruits, etc.:

1. Define the affected area
2. Reconstruct the characteristics of the affected area
3. Identify and classify diseases

Agriculture is one of the important sources for India's economic development. India is a farming country, and about 70% of the population depends on agriculture. Farmers have a wide range of opportunities to choose from a variety of suitable crops and find suitable crop protection products. Plant diseases have caused a significant decline in the quality and quantity of crops product. Plant disease refers to the study of visual observation patterns in plants. Controlling plant health and disease plays an important role in successfully growing crops on the farm. In the past, the control and analysis of plant diseases were performed manually by experts in the field. This requires a lot of work and a long processing time. If plant diseases are detected, imaging tests can be used. In most cases, disease symptoms appear on leaves, stems, and fruits. The leaves of plants are used to identify diseases by showing symptoms of diseases. This article describes imaging techniques used to identify plant diseases.

LITERATURE SURVEY

M.Bhange et al. developed a web-based tool to detect fruit diseases by uploading fruit images to the system (Bhange et al., 2015). Use parameters such as color, shape, and CCV (color coherence vector) for feature extraction. Use k-means algorithm. SVM is used to classify infected and uninfected. In this work, the accuracy of the determination of pomegranate diseases was 82%.

Monica Jhuria et al used image processing for disease detection and fruit classification (Jhuria et al., 2013). They use artificial neural networks to detect diseases. They created two independent databases, one for training stored clinical pictures, and the other for image query. Backpropagation is used to adjust the weight of the training database. They consider three feature vectors, namely color, texture, and shape. They found that the morphological feature score was better than the other two.

J.D. Pujari et.al (2015) uses different types of crops, namely vegetables plants, fruit plants, commercial plants, and cereal plants, to identify fungal diseases on plant leaves. A different method is used for each plant species: (Pujari et al., 2015)

- For vegetable crops, the Chan-Vase method is used for segmentation, the local binary template is used for texture feature and SVM extraction, and the K-nearest neighbor algorithm is used for classification. The average overall accuracy rate reaches 87.825%.
- For fruit plants, k-means clustering is used as a segmentation method, and Artificial Neural Network and Nearest Neighbor Algorithm are used to focus and classify texture features. The average overall accuracy is 90.723%.
- Use grab-cut algorithm to segment commercial plants. Using wavelet-based feature extraction, Mahalnobis distance and PNN as the classifier, the overall average accuracy is 84.825%.
- Use k-means clustering and accurate boundary detector to cereal plants. Extract color, shape, texture, color texture and random transformation features. The overall average accuracy of SVM and nearest neighbor classifier is 83.72%.

It is proposed plant disease image recognition based on principal component analysis and neural network (Wang et al., 2012), which included 21 color features, 4 shape features and 25 texture features of wheat and grape disease images. These attributes are extracted using basic component neural networks, including Back Propagation Network (BP), Radial Basis Function Network (RBF), Generalized Regression Network (GRNN) and Probabilistic Neural Network (PNN), which are used as classifiers for disease detection of wheat and grapes.

Shantanu Phadikar and Jaya Sil used pattern recognition technology to identify rice diseases (Phadikar et al., 2008). This paper introduces a prototype of rice disease detection software based on rice infected images. Perform edge and stain detection to identify the infected part of the leaf.

The FPGA and DSP-based system was developed by ChunxiaZhang, Xiuqing Wang and Xudong Li to monitor and control plant diseases (Zhang et al., 2010). FPGA is used to obtain image or video data from the field system for monitoring and diagnosis. And encode the video or picture. Single chip radio 2.4 GHz nRF24L01The transmitter is used to transmit data. It has two data compressors and transmission methods to meet the needs of different users, and uses wireless multi-channel communication to reduce the overall system cost.

RGB images are used to identify diseases. After applying the k-means clustering technique, identify the green pixels, and then use the otsu method to obtain a variable threshold (Al-Hiary et al., 2011). The color symbiosis method is used for feature extraction. The image is converted to HSI translation. Calculate texture statistics, generate SGDM matrix, and use GLCM function to calculate features.

PROCESS FOR PLANT DISEASE DETECTION

The process of the plant disease detection system basically includes five steps, as shown in the figure. The first step is to use a digital camera and mobile phone or take pictures from the Internet. The second step is to use various pre-processing methods to remove noise or other objects in the image. The third step is to divide the image into several groups, and various techniques can be applied. Contains the method of extracting features, the last step is dedicated for Disease classification. All these concepts are visualized below in Figure 1.

Figure 1. Flowchart for plant disease detection

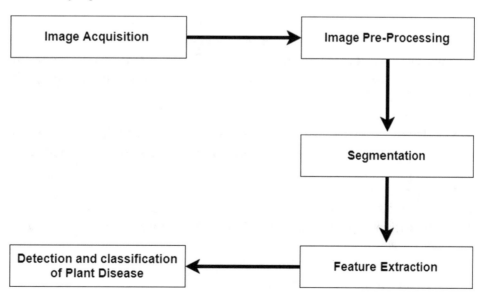

Image Acquisition

At this stage, images of plant leaves are collected using digital means, such as cameras, mobile phones, etc., with the required resolution and size. Images can also be obtained from the Internet. The creation of the image database is the sole responsibility of the application system developer. He is responsible for the best performance of the classifier in the final stage of the detection system (Al-Hiary et al., 2011). The images of plant leaves are taken by cameras. This image is in RGB format (red, green, and blue). Perform a color conversion structure on a single RGB image, and then perform a device-independent color space conversion on the color conversion suitable structure (Omrani et al., 2014).

Image Pre-Processing

When removing images or other objects, various pre-processing techniques are envisaged to remove noise. Crop the image i.e., Crop the image to get the image area you want. The image is smoothed using an anti-aliasing filter. Perform image enhancement to increase contrast.

According to equation (1), Color conversion from RGB image to grayscale image –

$$f(x)=0.2989*R + 0.5870*G + 0.114.*B \text{------------} \tag{1}$$

The histogram equalization is then applied to the image, which distributes the intensity of the image to enhance the image of plant diseases. The cumulative distribution function is used to distribute intensity values.

Image Segmentation

Segmentation refers to the segmentation of an image into several parts with the same attributes or some similarities. Various techniques can be used for segmentation, such as Otsu's method, K-Means grouping, converting RGB images to HIS models, etc.

1. Image Segmentation using Boundary and Spot Detection Algorithm:
    Convert RGB image to HIS model for segmentation. Edge detection and point detection help to find the infected part of the leaf, as described in (Phadikar et al., 2008). In order to determine the limit, the possibility of interconnecting 8 pixels is considered, and the algorithm for determining the limit is used.
2. K – Means Clustering –
    K-means clustering is used to classify objects into the number of K classes based on a set of features. Object classification is done by minimizing the sum of the squares of the distance between the object and the corresponding group.
    K –means Clustering Algorithm: -
    a. Choose the center of cluster K randomly or based on heuristics.
    b. Map each pixel in the image to a cluster that minimizes the distance between the pixel and the cluster center.
    c. Recalculate the cluster centers by averaging all pixels on the cluster. Repeat steps 2 and 3 until convergence is reached.

3. Otsu Threshold Algorithm: -

    The threshold method generates a binary image from a grayscale image by setting all pixels below a certain threshold to zero and all pixels above the threshold to 1. The Otsu algorithm defined in (Mrunalini et al., 2012) is as follows:

    a. Divide the pixels into two groups according to the threshold.
    b. Then calculate the average of each group.
    c. Square the difference between the averages.
    d. Multiply the number of pixels in one group by the number of pixels in the other group.

Infected leaf show symptoms of disease by discoloring the leaves. Therefore, the green color of the leaf can be used to identify the infected part of the leaf. Extract the R, G, and B components from the image. Calculate the threshold. According to Otsu Law, If the intensity of the green pixel is less than the calculated threshold, the green pixel will be masked and removed.

Feature Extraction in Image

Feature extraction plays an important role in object recognition. Many image Processing applications use feature extraction. Color, texture, shape, edge, etc. are the characteristics that can be used to detect plant diseases. In the article by Monica jhuria et al. uses color, texture, and shape as the characteristics for detecting diseases. It was found that the morphological results gave better results than other features. Texture refers to the distribution of colors in the picture, the roughness, and the hardness of the picture. It can also be used to identify infected areas of plants (Thangadurai et al., 2014).

After the segmentation, you are interested in the results obtained so far. Therefore, it is necessary to extract the features of this region of interest at this stage. These attributes are needed to determine the value of the sample image, Shape and texture (Dey et al., 2016). Recently, most researchers intend to use texture features to identify plant diseases. There are several feature extraction methods that can be used to design the system, such as gray-level co-occurrence matrix (GLLCM), color co-occurrence matrix, spatial gray-scale matrix and gray-scale extraction, based on the attributes of histograms. The GLCM method is a statistical texture classification technique.

Detection and Classification of Plant Disease

In the classification stage, it is determined whether the original image is healthy or sick. If an image is considered painful, it is divided into many diseases in some existing works. Classification requires a programming program written in MATLAB, also known as a series of classifiers, which has been used by researchers such as k nearest neighbours (KNN) in recent years. Support Vector Machine (SVM), Artificial Neural Network (ANN), Neural Back Propagation Network (BPNN), Decision Tree Classifier and Naive Bayes uses reliable technology (Gavhale et al., 2014).

1. Using ANN:

    After feature extraction, the images in the training database are classified using neural networks. These feature vectors are regarded as neurons in ANN. The neuron output is a function of the weighted sum of the inputs. SOM modified back-propagation algorithm; multiple types of reference vector machines can be used.

2.   Back Propagation:
      The BPNN algorithm is used to repeat the network. After the training is completed, the neural network weights are established, which can be used to calculate the output value of the new demand image that is not in the training database.

CHALLENGES

There are several challenges in detecting plant diseases using the following image processing techniques (Barbedo, 2016):

1.   **Dataset Collection:**
      The main requirement of image processing is to create an image database. To take photos of plant diseases, you need to travel to different places. Collecting data will be challenging because some farms may not have access to various plant diseases, and the diseases only occur at certain times of the year.
2.   **Background of Image:**
      Image segmentation is crucial section of photograph processing, wherein we separate maximum required a part of photograph. Leaf photograph segmentation can be a mission if background incorporates plants, leaves and a few different green elements.
3.   **Condition over Image Capturing:**
      If all the images are taken under the same conditions, the automatic plant disease detection system can provide consistent and effective results. Only in the laboratory can you take pictures under the same conditions. Due to the uncontrollable environment, it is difficult to take pictures under the same conditions in the wild.
4.   **Symptoms Segmentation:**
      Most plant disease symptoms have no clear boundaries and will slowly disappear on the plant, leading to incorrect segmentation, which affects the bottom line.
5.   **Symptoms Variations:**
      Symptoms depend on the environment, disease and plants. Each change of these elements will cause different symptoms. The task of identifying plant diseases with different symptoms.
6.   **Multiple simultaneous failures:**
      Many times, automatic plant disease detection systems may mistakenly believe that there is only one disease in the image. Pests and nutrient deficiencies can coexist because plants are more susceptible to other diseases after being infected.
7.   **Different diseases with similar symptoms**:
      Many plant diseases have similar symptoms, such as diseases, malnutrition, pests, phytotoxicity, cold or heat. It is not easy to distinguish and identify diseases using automatic plant disease detection methods.

CONCLUSION

Accurate detection and classification of plant diseases is very important for successful cultivation, which can be done through image processing. This article outlines and summarizes the various methods used by various researchers to detect plant diseases using image processing in the past few years. The main methods used are BPNN, SVM, K-Means clustering, Otsu's algorithm, CCM and SGDM. Determine whether the leaves are healthy or diseased. There were several problems in this process, including use complex images captured in street lights and harsh environments to automate the detection system. The conclusion of this review article is that these disease detection methods are very effective and accurate. In addition to some limitations, they can also run leaf disease detection systems. There is still a lot of work to be done in this area to improve the work that has already been done.

REFERENCES

Al-Hiary, Bani-Ahmad, Reyalat, Braik, & Al-Rahamneh. (2011). Fast and Accurate Detection and Classification of Plant Diseases. *International Journal of Computer Applications, 17*(1).

Badnakhe, M. R., & Deshmukh, P. R. (2012, March). Infected Leaf Analysis and Comparison by Otsu Threshold and k-Means Clustering. *International Journal of Advanced Research in Computer Science and Software Engineering, 2*(3).

Bhange, M., & Hingoliwala, H. A. (2015). Smart Farming: Pomegranate Disease Detection Using Image Processing. *Second International Symposium on Computer Vision and the Internet, 58,* 280-288. 10.1016/j.procs.2015.08.022

Dey, A. K., Sharma, M., & Meshram, M. R. (2016). Image Processing Based Leaf Rot Disease, Detection of Betel Vine (Piper BetleL.). *International Conference on Computational Modeling and Security,* 85, 748-754.

Garcia & Barbedo. (2016). *A review on the main challenges in automatic plant disease identification based on visible range images.* Science Direct, Biosystems Engineering.

Gavhale, K. R., & Gawande, U. (2014). An Overview of the Research on Plant Leaves Disease Detection using Image Processing Techniques. *IOSR Journal of Computer Engineering, 16*(1), 10–16.

Ghosh, S., & Singh, A. (2020). The scope of Artificial Intelligence in mankind: A detailed review. *Journal of Physics: Conference Series, 1531,* 012045.

Jhuria, M., Kumar, A., & Borse, R. (2013). Image Processing For Smart Farming: Detection Of Disease And Fruit Grading. *Proceedings of the 2013 IEEE Second International Conference on Image Information Processing (ICIIP-2013).* 10.1109/ICIIP.2013.6707647

Omrani, E., Khoshnevisan, B., Shamshirband, S., Saboohi, H., Anuar, N.B., & Nasir, M.H.N. (2014). Potential of radial basis function-based support vector regression for apple disease detection. *Journal of Measurement,* 233-252.

Phadikar, S., & Sil, J. (2008). Rice Disease Identification using Pattern Recognition. *Proceedings of 11th International Conference on Computer and Information Technology (ICCIT 2008)*.

Pujari, J. D., Yakkundimath, R., & Byadgi, A. S. (2015). Image Processing Based Detection of Fungal Diseases In Plants. *International Conference on Information and Communication Technologies*, 46, 1802-1808. 10.1016/j.procs.2015.02.137

Thangadurai & Padmavathi. (2014). Computer Visionimage Enhancement For Plant Leaves Disease Detection. *World Congress on Computing and Communication Technologies*.

Wang, H., Li, G., Ma, Z., & Li, X. (2012). Image Recognition of Plant Diseases Based on Principal Component Analysis and Neural Networks. In *8th International Conference on Natural Computation (ICNC 2012)* (pp. 246-251). IEEE.

Zhang, C., Wang, X., & Li, X. (2010). Design of Monitoring and Control Plant Disease System Based on DSP&FPGA. *Second International Conference on Networks Security, Wireless Communications and Trusted Computing*.

Chapter 10
Image Pre-Processing and Paddy Pests Detection Using Tensorflow

Rahul Sharma
Lovely Professional University, India

Amar Singh
Lovely Professional University, India

ABSTRACT

Agriculture is one of the important sources of earning worldwide. With the rapid expansion of the human population and food security for all, the agriculture sector needs to be boosted to increase the yield. Agriculture is the prime source of livelihood in India for more than 50% of the total population. As per Indian agriculture and allied industries industry report, agriculture is one of the major contributors in gross value. Agricultural crops suffer heavy losses due to insect damage and plant diseases. Worldwide, out of the crop losses, major losses are caused by plant pests. In this chapter, various image pre-processing methods and the need of pre-preprocessing are discussed in detail. For image classification, TensorFlow deep neural network is presented. Deep learning model is used for automatic and early detection of paddy pests. Early detection of the pests will aid farmers in adopting necessary preventive measures. Multiple ways to reduce overfitting during model training are also suggested.

INTRODUCTION

Computer vision has evolved over the years. Today with the availability of smartphones, tablets, etc raw digital lot of digital data is available. Different computer vision techniques can be used to extract hidden data patterns (O'Mahony et al., 2019) by processing images using machine learning techniques to draw meaningful information. Machine learning is being used for automating manual processes thereby increasing productivity.

DOI: 10.4018/978-1-7998-7188-0.ch010

Real-world images are collected using different types of devices having different device settings. So images collected from different sources may have a lot of variations. Image properties like resolution, aspect ratio, orientation, intensity level, contrast, sharpness, etc variations in the collected dataset must be handled properly before applying any machine learning algorithms (Sharma et al., 2020). No matter how good a machine learning model architecture is designed, it will not learn anything useful if the training data is invalid. A model trained on invalid data will give invalid results. Serious flaws in the data should be properly dealt with before starting the training phase of a machine learning model. The unwanted or invalid data can be disposed of during preprocessing.

IMAGE VARIATIONS AND PRE-PROCESSING METHODS

The image classification system must take into consideration the following variations in the images:

Viewpoint Variation: A single instance of an object can be photographed or viewed in many ways with different camera positions (Chu et al., 2019). The image of an object captured in different angles must be labeled to the same class.

Scale Variation: Images can have different sizes. During pre-processing, the images are resized for uniformity.

Deformation: Many objects of interest are not rigid bodies and can be deformed. Deformed object images must be labeled correctly.

Occlusion: The objects of interest can be hidden behind another type of object in the image and only a small portion of an object is visible.

Illumination Conditions: The effects of illumination are drastic on the pixel level. Image classification algorithm must be able to handle changes in illumination.

Background Clutter: When the object of interest and background of the image is similar. The objects of interest may blend into the background. This makes the image classification task hard.

Intra-Class Variation: When objects belonging to one category or class have variations. For example plant leaf images belonging to one type of disease has variation in symptoms.

Images acquired from different devices are not directly provided as input to a machine learning algorithm, instead, images are pre-processed to enhance the image dataset. Pre-processing involves noise reduction, brightness, and contrast enhancements. Thus the aim of image pre-processing is to remove noise or unwanted data and enhance the image features, the consistent physical geometry of the image, image resizing, image augmentation, etc (Elgendi et al., 2021). A consistent and enhanced image dataset will improve the accuracy of the model. Different image pre-processing techniques to enhance the pictorial information for interpretation and analysis are

1. **Resize Image**: Images captured from different devices may vary in size. Before inputting images to a machine learning algorithm, base size is defined for all the images. All the acquired images are resized accordingly.
2. **Uniform Aspect Ratio**
3. **Noise Removal by Image Filters**: Filter those images so that the noise present in the image can be removed and to enhance certain characteristics of the image like contrast enhancement. Acquired images may be blurred either due to the cammer's settings or the lens not properly focused. The other kind of blurred image maybe because of clicking the picture from a moving platform (mov-

ing car or train) due to which the image that you get is not clear but it is a blurred image. Another type of noise present in an image is speckle and salt and pepper noise. Different types of digital filters are mean filter, median filter, Gaussian smoothing, conservative smoothing, frequency filters, Crimmins Speckle Removal, etc. Salt and pepper noise can be removed by using conservative filters which use the intensity of the pixel. The Crimmins Speckle Removal method is used to remove speckle noise and smooth the edges of objects in an image. Image filters can be used to enhance the edges of the image for the precise and correct application of segmentation methods.

4. **Dimensionality Reduction and Color Model Conversion**: The number of input features or parameters or attributes determines the dimension of the dataset. Dimensionality reduction reduces the computation time of the image classifier, reduces noise in the dataset, avoiding overfitting, image compression, etc. Various dimensionality reduction techniques like Principal Component Analysis (PCA), Linear Discriminant Analysis (LDA), Factor Analysis (FA), Multidimensional Scaling (MDS), t-distributed Stochastic Neighbor Embedding (t-SNE), etc are very useful. RGB to Gray Scale model conversion may be considered for reducing the dimension of an image. Conversion of an image from the RGB space to the HSI space is very important as in many applications classification of the image is based on the intensity levels.

5. **Normalization of Image**: Normalization is done to change the intensity of image pixels to a standard interval. After Image normalization means is set so that it is the midpoint of the standard interval and variance is set to one. Machine vision can be used for identifying objects. Different images of the same object under different lighting conditions should be classified into the same class.

6. **Image Augmentation**: Another common pre-processing technique is augmentation. Different operations like rotation, flip, crop, scaling, brighten, darken, and other affine transformations. Image augmentation supports the training of the machine learning algorithm by exposing it to a wide variety of variations.

STEPS FOR LABELING IMAGES

In addition to image pre-processing steps as shown in Fig. 1 are used for labeling images.

Segmentation is the process of extracting the region of interest(ROI)(Wang et al., 2020). Thus the process of segmentation can be referred to as the process of grouping the pixels of an image to form meaningful regions. Segmentation techniques such as Clustering methods, FCM, Thresholding based, histogram methods, edge detection, region growing, watershed, etc (Kaur et al., 2021) methods are used to select the regions of interest or diseases. Thresholding is a simple technique that is used for the separation of foreground and background regions in an image. The edge detection method is used to trace the boundary of the object in an image. Canny edge detection produces better results. There are two types of segmentation semantic and instance segmentation.

Image mining techniques can be used for unique feature extraction in the form of color information, texture information, and spatial frequency information. Feature extraction is an important part of image classification. Different methods like LBP, HOG, SURF, GLCM, MSER, Histogram features, wavelets, canny edge detection (Patel et al., 2021; Toennies, 2017), etc are applied for feature extraction. Nature-inspired optimization techniques like Ant Colony Optimization, Genetic Optimization, Three parent genetic optimization, parallel three parent genetic optimization, Big Bang Big Crunch, Parallel Big Bang

Figure 1. Steps for image classification

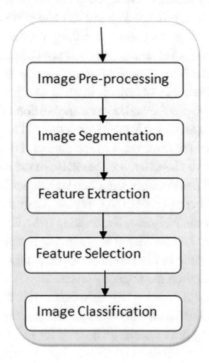

Big Crunch, Artificial Bee Colony Optimization (Kumar et al., 2018; Singh et al., 2015; Singh, 2020; Singh et al., 2019) etc can be used for optimal feature selection.

Image classification is a process of labeling the images as per their type. For the classification task, the computer allots confidence scores for each class. The class with the highest confidence score is the resulting prediction. Image classification analyzes the numerical properties of various image features and organizes the data into different categories. Identifying the objects of interest in an image is an interesting computer vision problem.

Image classification for which different machine learning algorithms like SVM, Naïve Bayes, Decision Tree, KNN, Random Forest, AdaBoost, Nural Networks, Fuzzy classifiers, CNN, etc are used. CNN represents a huge breakthrough in image recognition. They're most commonly used to analyze visual imagery and are frequently working behind the scenes in image classification. A CNN has Convolutional layers ReLU layers, Pooling layers, a Fully connected layer. Convolution is using a 'kernel' to extract certain 'features' from an input image. A kernel is a matrix, which is slid across the image and multiplied with the input such that the output is enhanced in a certain desirable manner. Instead of using manually made kernels for feature extraction, through Deep CNNs, we can learn these kernel values which can extract latent features. Performance measures such as sensitivity, specificity, accuracy, error rate, ROC curve, AUC, F-score create confidence in the image classification (Dhingra et al., 2018; Flach, 2016).

IMAGE CLASSIFICATION USING TENSORFLOW

TensorFlow is a free, open-source mathematical computation library developed by Google for training and building machine learning and deep learning model using simple to use high-level APIs(Abu et al., 2019). In this section, we will study how to train a CNN model to classify images using TensorFlow. We will identify the overfitting and suggest techniques to reduce generalization errors.

For a demonstration of image classification, we will use two-class "Paddy Pests Datasets" Kaggle Dataset. This classifier can be used for the early prediction of paddy pests so that farmers can adopt effective preventives measures. The dataset has total of 648 images belonging to two types i.e.

1. Paddy with pests (135 images)
2. Paddy without pests (513 images)

Now we will learn how to classify these images. TensorFlow library provides rich set of API's. TensorFlow's image_dataset_from_directory utility is used for loading image data efficiently from the

Figure 2. Paddy pests dataset sample images

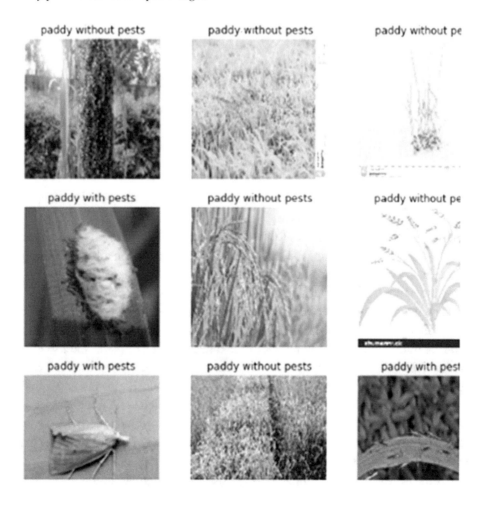

Figure 3. CNN model training graphs

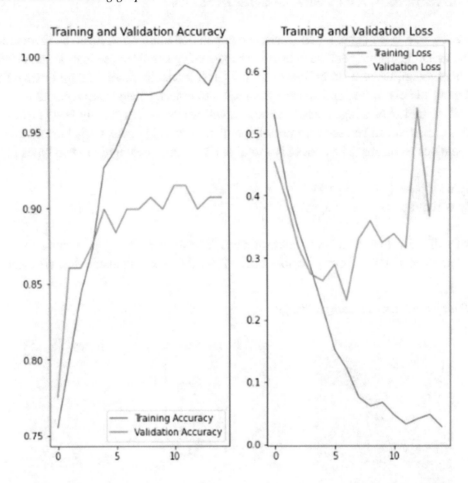

directory. Dataset is split using 80-20% split configuration. So 80% of images (519) are used for training and 20% images (129) are used for validation.

RGB images are used for classification. RGB values are in (0-255) range. Normalization of images is done to obtain standardize values in (0-1) range. CNN model with convolution layer, pooling layer and fully connected layers with 'adam' optimizer is trained for 15 epochs.

The training and validation accuracy of the trained model are shown below

As you can see there is a difference in the training and validation accuracy. This difference in accuracy will result in overfitting. Overfitting may be due to small dataset(Thanapol et al., 2020), noise in the dataset. During training the CNN model learns the unwanted data or noise and use it for prediction. Overfitting is not desirable and can be reduced by data augmentation, dropout (Park & Kwak, 2016) etc. Data augmentation is done by applying different transformations like zoom, flip, rotation, blurring etc. As shown in the Fig. 4 random transformations are being applied to an image.

Data augmentation helps in reducing the generalization error. Drop out is another technique for reducing overfitting (Perez & Wang, 2017). Dropout drops randomly selected neurons during training pause. Dropout layer of tensorflow accepts decimal number (less than 1) as input where .2 means randomly dropping 20% of the neurons. This technique is very effective for regularization.

Figure 4. Data augmentation applied to same image.

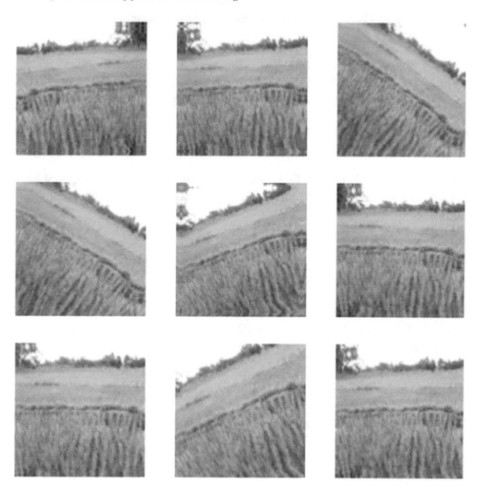

Overfitting reduces the model test accuracy. If the training dataset has noise, the trained model will learn the data points which do not contribute for labeling of the class. Using unnecessary attributes for training will result in overfitting and testing error will be high. Regularization is a technique used in machine learning to reduce the error by fitting a simple function and discourages learning of a complex function. Cross validation can also be used for avoiding overfitting.

REFERENCES

Abu, M. A., Indra, N. H., Abd Rahman, A. H., Sapiee, N. A., & Ahmad, I. (2019). A study on Image Classification based on Deep Learning and Tensorflow. *International Journal of Engineering Research & Technology (Ahmedabad)*, *12*(4), 563–569.

Chu, R., Sun, Y., Li, Y., Liu, Z., Zhang, C., & Wei, Y. (2019). Vehicle re-identification with viewpoint-aware metric learning. In *Proceedings of the IEEE/CVF International Conference on Computer Vision* (pp. 8282-8291). IEEE.

Dhingra, G., Kumar, V., & Joshi, H. D. (2018). Study of digital image processing techniques for leaf disease detection and classification. *Multimedia Tools and Applications*, *77*(15), 19951–20000. doi:10.100711042-017-5445-8

Elgendi, M., Nasir, M. U., Tang, Q., Smith, D., Grenier, J. P., Batte, C., ... Nicolaou, S. (2021). The effectiveness of image augmentation in deep learning networks for detecting COVID-19: A geometric transformation perspective. *Frontiers in Medicine*, 8. PMID:33732718

Flach, P. A. (2016). ROC analysis. In *Encyclopedia of Machine Learning and Data Mining* (pp. 1–8). Springer.

Kaur, A., Kaur, L., & Singh, A. (2021). State-of-the-art segmentation techniques and future directions for multiple sclerosis brain lesions. *Archives of Computational Methods in Engineering*, *28*(3), 951–977. doi:10.100711831-020-09403-7

Kumar, S., Singh, A., & Walia, S. S. (2018). Parallel Big Bang - Big Crunch Global Optimization Algorithm: Performance and its Applications to routing in WMNs. *Wireless Personal Communications, Springer*, *100*(4), 1601–1618. doi:10.100711277-018-5656-y

O'Mahony, N., Campbell, S., Carvalho, A., Harapanahalli, S., Hernandez, G. V., Krpalkova, L., ... Walsh, J. (2019, April). Deep learning vs. traditional computer vision. In *Science and Information Conference* (pp. 128-144). Springer.

Park, S., & Kwak, N. (2016, November). Analysis on the dropout effect in convolutional neural networks. In *Asian conference on computer vision* (pp. 189-204). Springer.

Patel, A., Swaminarayan, P., & Patel, M. (2021). Identification of Nutrition's Deficiency in Plant and Prediction of Nutrition Requirement Using Image Processing. In *Proceedings of the Second International Conference on Information Management and Machine Intelligence* (pp. 463-469). Springer. 10.1007/978-981-15-9689-6_50

Perez, L., & Wang, J. (2017). The effectiveness of data augmentation in image classification using deep learning. arXiv preprint arXiv:1712.04621.

Sharma, P., Hans, P., & Gupta, S. C. (2020, January). Classification Of Plant Leaf Diseases Using Machine Learning And Image Preprocessing Techniques. In *2020 10th International Conference on Cloud Computing, Data Science & Engineering (Confluence)* (pp. 480-484). IEEE. 10.1109/Confluence47617.2020.9057889

Sharma, R., & Singh, A. (2019). Overview of different machine learning techniques for plant disease detection. *Journal of the Gujarat Research Society*, *21*(6), 416–425.

Sharma, R., Singh, A., & Sharma, V. (2018). Potato Leaf Diseases Identification using CNN. *Journal of Emerging Technologies and Innovative Research*, *5*(12), 519–527.

Singh, Kumar, Walia, & Chakravorty. (2015). Face Recognition: A Combined Parallel BB-BC & PCA Approach to Feature Selection. *International Journal of Computer Science & Information Technology*, *2*(2), 1-5.

Singh, A. (2020). *Parallel 3-Parent Genetic Algorithm with Application to Routing in Wireless Mesh Networks, Implementations and Applications of Machine Learning.* Springer.

Singh, A., Kumar, S., Singh, A., & Walia, S. S. (2019). Three-parent GA: A Global Optimization Algorithm. *Journal of Multiple-Valued Logic and Soft Computing, 32,* 407–423.

Thanapol, P., Lavangnananda, K., Bouvry, P., Pinel, F., & Leprévost, F. (2020, October). Reducing Overfitting and Improving Generalization in Training Convolutional Neural Network (CNN) under Limited Sample Sizes in Image Recognition. In *2020-5th International Conference on Information Technology (InCIT)* (pp. 300-305). IEEE.

Toennies, K. D. (2017). Feature Detection. In *Guide to Medical Image Analysis* (pp. 173–207). Springer. doi:10.1007/978-1-4471-7320-5_5

Wang, E. K., Chen, C. M., Hassan, M. M., & Almogren, A. (2020). A deep learning based medical image segmentation technique in Internet-of-Medical-Things domain. *Future Generation Computer Systems, 108,* 135–144. doi:10.1016/j.future.2020.02.054

Chapter 11
Deep Learning Models for Detection and Diagnosis of Alzheimer's Disease

Gowhar Mohiuddin Dar
Lovely Professional University, India

Ashok Sharma
University of Jammu, India

Parveen Singh
Government SPMR College of Commerce, Jammu, India

ABSTRACT

The chapter explores the implications of deep learning in medical sciences, focusing on deep learning concerning natural language processing, computer vision, reinforcement learning, big data, and blockchain influence on some areas of medicine and construction of end-to-end systems with the help of these computational techniques. The deliberation of computer vision in the study is mainly concerned with medical imaging and further usage of natural language processing to spheres such as electronic wellbeing record data. Application of deep learning in genetic mapping and DNA sequencing termed as genomics and implications of reinforcement learning about surgeries assisted by robots are also overviewed.

INTRODUCTION

Deep learning (LeCun et al., 2015) is a subpart of a machine learning family and has very high computational power. The sudden and extreme growth of deep learning is because of its very high computational power and the availability of huge datasets. The dramatic advancement in the field of deep learning is the manipulation capability of machines especially speech (Hinton et al., 2012), images (Russakovsky et al., 2015), and languages (Hirschberg & Manning, 2015). Deep learning models can manipulate large datasets with the requirement of high computing hardware and will improve gradually with the increas-

DOI: 10.4018/978-1-7998-7188-0.ch011

ing size of data and thus enhancing its capability to do better than many traditional machine learning approaches. The striking feature of deep learning is to accept many data types as input which specifies its aspect of specific pertinence for different health care data. The figure below depicts a simple, multilayer deep neural network that takes input data from two different classes of data, with two different colors, and separates them in a linear fashion linearly by recursively changing the data as it flows from one layer to next layer. The classification is done by last output layer and generates the possible output from any one of the class. This illustration explains the straightforward perception implemented by huge scale networks.

ALZHEIMER'S DISEASES

From the medical point of perspective, the illness is not a complete scientific concept, as an additional health concern. Every person possesses remembrance or distinctive awareness of the long-standing disease and one of the most important anthropological apprehensions (Armstrong & Hilton, 2014). De facto definition of any disease in medical sciences is the general ailment of the normal functioning of the body with specific signs and indications. (Armstrong & Hilton, 2014; Scully, 2004). The ailment is an amalgam of visible signs and indications that doctors must understand properly. Analysis and treatment have guided this course of action. The Disease diagnosis in healthcare is a complicated and difficult process, that is why doctors find several reasons and conditions for medical signs at the same time (Leaman et al., 2013). Disease prediction in healthcare situations have no specified definition, but addresses the assessment building process in overall healthcare, which helps in understanding complex health issues of a patient (Committee on Diagnostic Error in Health Care, 2015). Evaluation of the disease is central in the formation of clinical judgment, which includes various individual and unprejudiced factors. A prompt and crystal-clear diagnosis, therefore, has the dynamic role in critical diseases or disorders. That is why, the recovery plan can't be determined until an absolute diagnosis is regulated (Scheuermann et al., 2009). The main objective of present medical science projects with the

Figure 1.

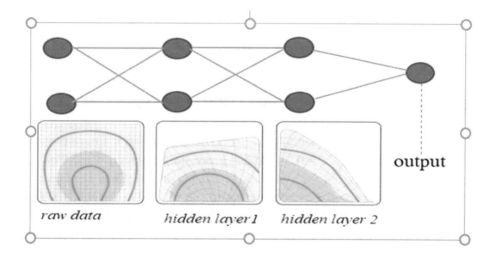

Figure 2. Feature learning from variety of data types by deep learning

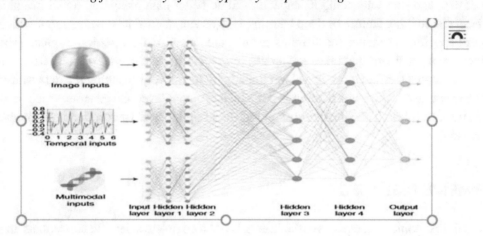

ensemble of artificial intelligence is to attain accurate results, thereby helping consultants to control the disease at its early stage. (Croft et al., 2015; Malmir et al., 2017; Nashi et al., 2018; Nilashi et al., 2017). So globally researchers are exploring different neural network implications in the prediction of some dreadful diseases. Scholars explain the cycle of health science in various formats to overcome the elusiveness of an examination of ailment It is incredibly challenging to explain all the evidence of real-world in terms of crusty values, innovative technology must be developed to model this imprecise. Few persuaded algorithms are implemented by deep learning, even though veiled intuitions can begin from statistics, here machine training is not done, but DL's recurrent learning procedure permits technologies to hurriedly acclimate their systems and outcomes, according to new environments and information. The indispensable aspiration of the paper is to investigate diverse studies in deep learning concerning Alzheimer's disease prediction (A permanent challenging illness categorized by brain degeneration, followed by several symptoms like unable to recognize, malnutrition, dehydration, and infection in late stages which finally leads to death) through a systematic review. Around 5.8 million people in America have Alzheimer's disease in 2019.After analyzing the data from the past eight years, it is evident that people above the age of 65 years are having diagnosed or have chances to get affected by this disorder. 5.6 million people falling in the age group of 65(Nashi et al., 2017) and 2 million individuals fall in the age group below 65, though, the accurate estimate regarding the young generation is yet to emphasized properly. Population living with Alzheimer's is roughly 8.5 million and 81 percent among them are falling in the age group of 75 or over (Hebert et al., 2013).

RECURRENT NEURAL NETWORKS AND IMAGE PROCESSING

The remarkable success of Recurrent Neural Networks (RNNs) is found in image captioning (Vinyals et al., 2015), machine translation (Wu, 2016), and text generation (Kannan, 2016). The contribution of natural language processing in the field of healthcare is found in the domain of electronic health records (EHRs). EHRs are becoming pervasive at very fast speed (The Office of the National Coordinator for Health Information Technology, 2017). The capability of EHR is to procure the transactions of a medical organization up to the ten million patients throughout the progression of a decade. Thus, the appliance of deep learning technology in the field of electronic health data (EHRs) is briskly expanding (Rajkomar et al., 2018; Shickel et al., 2017). The whole procedure involved in the formation of deep learning systems for EHRs are shown in figure 3.

Figure 3. Steps involved in building deep learning systems for EHRs.

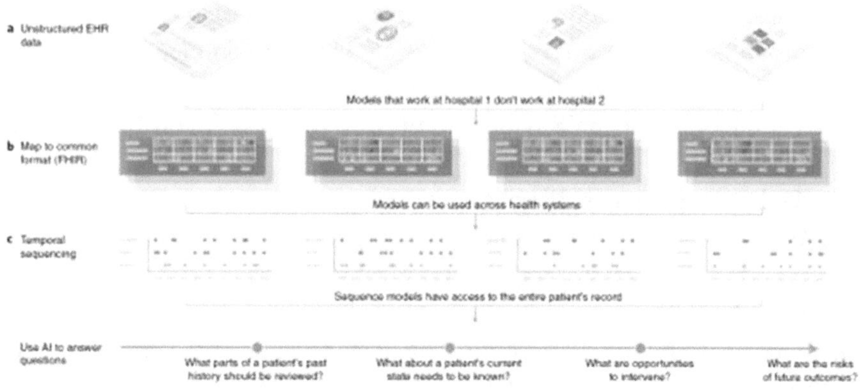

COMPUTER VISION AND IMAGE PROCESSING

There is a distinction between image processing and computer vision. The basic definition of image processing is to draw out a new image from an existing image. This whole procedure is usually done by enhancing or simplifying the content of image in one or other way. The procedure followed in image processing is summarized as:

1. Photometric proprieties of the image are normalized like brightness or color.
2. Image cropping, such as centered alignment of the objects in the image is done.
3. unwanted digital noise is removed from the image.

CNN AND MEDICAL SCIENCES

Diagnosis and detection of diseases based on images is very successful by implementing CNN based methods. The main reason behind the success of CNN is because it has acquired performance up to the level of humans in case of object classification assignments [Alzheimer's Association, 2006] where CNN learns classification procedure of objects present within images. Satisfactory results out of these similar CNN networks are acquired in case of transfer learning (Richard, 2010). We train CNN's initially on large datasets in case of transfer learning. Dataset is not however related to the specified task, for example ImageNet (Yosinski et al., 2014) a dataset comprising of millions of some common objects. Same CNN is further fine-tuned on some other small dataset which is as per target requirement (medical images). The preliminary work of algorithm is to clout huge amount of data to learn basic information present in images e.g., curves, straight lines etc. higher layers of the algorithm are then trained again to make clear distinction between different diagnosis cases. Same procedure is then followed in image segmentation and object detection algorithms to identify those parts of images which correspond to specific objects.

The Convolutional neural networks have outstanding results in the field of medical science. The brief description of some remarkable performance is outlined below:

1. Identification of a tiny, pigmented spot called the mole in case of skin cancer, which is called melanoma in medical terminology.
2. Diabetic retinopathy: it is a complication that affects the eyes. The main cause of diabetic retinopathy is the damage of blood vessels present in the retina. The main problem is because of uncontrolled blood sugar level. The occurrence of this disease is very rare and cannot be cured completely. It can last for years or lifelong. The main symptoms of these diseases are difficulty in observing colors, blurriness, and blindness.
3. Cardiovascular risk: it is the condition that creates a problem to heart like diseased vessels, blood clots, and other structural problems. Some broad types of cardiovascular diseases are as under:
    a. Coronary artery disease: it is a condition in which damage occurs to major blood vessels of the heart.
    b. High blood pressure: the force of blood against the walls of the artery is very up.
    c. Cardiac arrest: an abrupt, unforeseen loss of heart function, breathing and consciousness

TRANSFER LEARNING AND MEDICAL SCIENCE

Transfer learning is a process where a certain model trained on one problem is reused in some way on a second problem that is linked to it. Transfer learning can reduce the training time for a neural network model while also lowering the error rate.

How to Use Pre-Trained Models

The only limit to using a pre-trained model is your imagination. A model, for example, might be downloaded and used in its current form, such as incorporating it into an application and then using it to categorize fresh images. Models can be downloaded and used as feature extraction models as well. The output of a layer anterior to the model's output layer is used as input to a new classifier mode in this case. The pre-trained model can be used as a standalone feature extraction programme, in which case the model or a component of the model can pre-process each input image to produce an output (e.g., a vector of numbers) that may subsequently be utilized as input for training a new model. We can summarize some of these usage patterns as follows:

Classifier: To classify new images, the pre-trained model is used directly.
Standalone Feature Extractor: Image pre-processing or feature extraction is done by applying pre-trained model or portion of that model.
Integrated Feature Extractor: The pre-trained model, or some portion of the model, is integrated into a new model, but layers of the pre-trained model are frozen during training.
Weight Initialization: The pre-trained model, or some portion of the model, is integrated into a new model, and the layers of the pre-trained model are trained in concert with the new model.

Models for Transfer Learning

There are probably a few or more high-performing image recognition models available for download and use as the foundation for image recognition and other computer vision tasks. The following are three of the most well-known models:

- GoogLeNet (e.g., InceptionV3).
- VGG (e.g., VGG16 or VGG19).
- Residual Network (e.g., ResNet50).

Almost all these models are widely utilized for transfer learning, not only because of their performance, but also because they were examples of architectural advances, such as consistent and repetitive structures (VGG), inception modules (GoogLeNet), and residual modules (GoogLeNet) (ResNet).

GoogleNet: The accuracy of GoogleNet is very high however it requires high computational power since the order of computations is very high. At the last connected layer fully, connected layer is replaced by average pooling layer to minimize the parameters (Szegedy et al., 2017; Szegedy, Liu, Jia, Sermanet, Reed, Anguelov, & Rabinovich, 2015).

ResNet: Increasing the network depth has resulted in an increase in accuracy. However, with ResNet (He et al., 2016a), there are several issues associated with network depth. However, with ResNet (He et al., 2016a), there are several issues associated with network depth. Because of the increased depth, which necessitated adjusting the weights, the prediction becomes modest at the first layers. Another issue is the large amount of parameter space it necessitated. To avoid these issues, leftover modules were created. To prevent these problems residual modules are came into picture. ResNet50 and ResNet152 are example networks of ResNet.

VGG (e.g., VGG16 or VGG19): VGG (Scully, 2004) stands for Visual Geometry Group in its entire form. VGG16 and VGG19 are usually found in the VGG network. The large size kernels are substituted by the small size kernels in this network. By the virtue of the features are extracted at low cost

Transfer Learning in DCNN

Deep CNNs, also known as DCNNs, typically require large, annotated image datasets to achieve a high level of classification accuracy. Nonetheless, in several sectors, obtaining such an image dataset is difficult, and annotating it is costly In the face of such challenges, the use of "off-the-shelf" attributes of well-known DCNNs like Alexnet (Russakovsky et al., 2015), GoogLeNet (Szegedy, Liu, Jia, Sermanet, Reed, Anguelov, Erhan et al, 2015), ResNet50 (He et al., 2016b), ResNet101 (Simonyan & Zisserman, 2014), Vgg-16 (Szegedy et al., 2016), Vgg-19 (Szegedy et al., 2016), Inceptionv3 (), and Inception-ResNetV2 (Szegedy et al., 2017) pre-trained on huge datasets (like ImageNet) have established to be valuable for solving cross-domain image classification problems by means of transfer learning (Hoo-Chang et al., 2016). The structure of transfer learning employing any of the above-examined models is briefly depicted in Figure 4.

Figure 4. Description of transfer learning

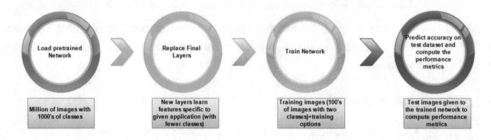

BLOCKCHAIN AND MEDICAL SCIENCE

Blockchain technology offers multifold advantages to the medical sciences. There are multiple domains in medical technology where Blockchain technology can make advancements in the future. These areas are summarized as:

1. Monitoring configuration
2. Administrative management.
3. Reduction in processing time at clinics by collecting complete data at a time, once a patient gets enrolled due to the availability of distributed ledger.

Big Data and Medical Sciences

To analyze pictorial information so that medical diagnosis, monitoring, and therapy through imaging is an effective tool for every working professional in multiple domains like radiography, medical imaging, etc.[16] Big data is a focus center in the present era and has become very crucial for big companies like Microsoft, Google, IBM, etc. Big data is consociated with the concept of "4 V's" and is based upon the concept of Moor's law.

V=Volume: Quantity of Big data in healthcare means Volume, which is appraised to sudden and extreme increase until the order of Zettabytes (1021by 2020). The report published by Stanford Medicine 2017, the Volume of healthcare data is increasing at an astronomical rate approx. 153 Exabytes where 1 Exabyte=1 billion gigabytes were produced in 2013 and 2314 Exabytes are going to be produced in 2020.

V=Variety is defined as a heterogeneous type of healthcare big data collection including their different characteristics and structured and unstructured nature.

CONCLUSION

Deep learning has got remarkable breakthrough in the area of research fields notably in medical sciences. This chapter has outlined some broad areas and especially the Alzheimer's diseases where the deep learning is applicable. Author is presently working on the development of deep learning framework for early prediction of Alzheimer's diseases.

REFERENCES

Alzheimer's Association. (2006). *Early-Onset Dementia: A National Challenge, a Future Crisis.* Alzheimer's Association.

Armstrong, N., & Hilton, P. (2014). doing diagnosis: Whether and how clinicians use a diagnostic tool of uncertain clinical utility. *Social Science & Medicine, 120,* 208–214. doi:10.1016/j.socscimed.2014.09.032 PMID:25259659

Committee on Diagnostic Error in Health Care. (2015). *Board on Health Care Services, Institute of Medicine, T.N.A.o, Sciences, Improving Diagnosis in Health Care.* The National Academies Press.

Croft, P., Altman, D. G., Deeks, J. J., Dunn, K. M., Hay, A. D., Hemingway, H., LeResche, L., Peat, G., Perel, P., Petersen, S. E., Riley, R. D., Roberts, I., Sharpe, M., Stevens, R. J., Van Der Windt, D. A., Von Korff, M., & Timmis, A. (2015). The science of clinical practice: Disease diagnosis or patient prognosis? Evidence about "what is likely to happen" should shape clinical practice. *BMC Medicine, 13*(1), 20. doi:10.118612916-014-0265-4 PMID:25637245

He, K., Zhang, X., Ren, S., & Sun, J. (2016a). Deep residual learning for image recognition. In *Proceedings of the IEEE conference on computer vision and pattern recognition.* IEEE. 10.1109/CVPR.2016.90

He, K., Zhang, X., Ren, S., & Sun, J. (2016b). Deep residual learning for image recognition. *Proceedings of the IEEE conference on computer vision and pattern recognition,* 770–778.

Hebert, L. E., Weuve, J., Scherr, P. A., & Evans, D. A. (2013). Alzheimer disease in the United States (2010-2050) estimated using the 2010 Census. *Neurology, 80*(19), 1778–1783. doi:10.1212/WNL.0b013e31828726f5 PMID:23390181

Hinton, G., Deng, L., Yu, D., Dahl, G., Mohamed, A., Jaitly, N., Senior, A., Vanhoucke, V., Nguyen, P., Sainath, T., & Kingsbury, B. (2012). Deep neural networks for acoustic modeling in speech recognition: The shared views of four research groups. *IEEE Signal Processing Magazine, 29*(6), 82–97. doi:10.1109/MSP.2012.2205597

Hirschberg, J., & Manning, C. D. (2015). Advances in natural language processing. *Science, 349*(6245), 261–266. doi:10.1126cience.aaa8685 PMID:26185244

Hoo-Chang, S., Roth, H. R., Gao, M., Lu, L., Xu, Z., Nogues, I., Yao, J., Mollura, D., & Summers, R. M. (2016). Deep convolutional neural networks for computer-aided detection: CNN architectures, dataset characteristics and transfer learning. *IEEE Transactions on Medical Imaging, 35*(5), 1285–1298. doi:10.1109/TMI.2016.2528162 PMID:26886976

Kannan, A. (2016). Smart reply: automated response suggestion for email. In *Proceedings of the 22nd ACM SIGKDD International Conference on Knowledge Discovery and Data Mining.* ACM. 10.1145/2939672.2939801

Krizhevsky, A., Sutskever, I., & Hinton, G. E. (2012). Imagenet classification with deep convolutional neural networks. Advances in neural information processing systems, 1097–1105.

Leaman, R., Islamaj Do ˘gan, R., & Lu, Z. (2013). DNorm: Disease name normalization with pairwise learning to rank. *Bioinformatics (Oxford, England)*, *29*(22), 2909–2917. doi:10.1093/bioinformatics/btt474 PMID:23969135

LeCun, Y., Bengio, Y., & Hinton, G. (2015). Deep learning. *Nature*, *521*(7553), 436–444. doi:10.1038/nature14539 PMID:26017442

Malmir, B., Amini, M., & Chang, S. I. (2017). A medical decision support system for dis- ease diagnosis under uncertainty. *Expert Systems with Applications*, *88*, 95–108. doi:10.1016/j.eswa.2017.06.031

Nashi, M., Ahmadi, H., Shahmoradi, L., Mardani, A., & Ibrahim, O. (2017). E. Yade- garidehkordi, Knowledge discovery and diseases prediction: A comparative study of machine learning techniques. *J. Soft Comput. Decis. Support Syst.*, *4*, 8–16.

Nashi, M., Ibrahim, O., Ahmadi, H., Shahmoradi, L., & Farahmand, M. (2018). A hybrid intelligent system for the prediction of Parkinson's disease progression using machine learning techniques. *Biocybernetics and Biomedical Engineering*, *38*(1), 1–15. doi:10.1016/j.bbe.2017.09.002

Nilashi, M., Ibrahim, O., Ahmadi, H., & Shahmoradi, L. (2017). O. bin Ibrahim, H. Ahmadi, L. Shahmoradi, An analytical method for diseases prediction using machine learning techniques. *Computers & Chemical Engineering*, *106*(106), 212–223. doi:10.1016/j.compchemeng.2017.06.011

Rajkomar, A., Oren, E., Chen, K., Dai, A. M., Hajaj, N., Hardt, M., Liu, P. J., Liu, X., Marcus, J., Sun, M., Sundberg, P., Yee, H., Zhang, K., Zhang, Y., Flores, G., Duggan, G. E., Irvine, J., Le, Q., Litsch, K., ... Dean, J. (2018). Scalable and accurate deep learning with electronic health records. *NPJ Digital Medicine*, *1*(1), 18. doi:10.103841746-018-0029-1 PMID:31304302

Richard. (2010). *Computer Vision: Algorithm and Application*. Academic Press.

Russakovsky, O., Deng, J., Su, H., Krause, J., Satheesh, S., Ma, S., Huang, Z., Karpathy, A., Khosla, A., Bernstein, M., Berg, A. C., & Fei-Fei, L. (2015). Imagenet large scale visual recognition challenge. *International Journal of Computer Vision*, *115*(3), 211–252. doi:10.100711263-015-0816-y

Scheuermann, R. H., Ceusters, W., & Smith, B. (2009). Toward an ontological treatment of disease and diagnosis. *Summit on Translational Bioinformatics*, *2009*, 116–120. PMID:21347182

Scully, J. L. (2004). what is a disease? *EMBO Reports*, *5*(7), 650–653. doi:10.1038j.embor.7400195 PMID:15229637

Shickel, B., Tighe, P. J., Bihorac, A., & Rashidi, P. (2017). Deep EHR: A survey of recent advances in deep learning techniques for electronic health record (EHR) analysis. *IEEE Journal of Biomedical and Health Informatics*, *22*(5), 1589–1604. doi:10.1109/JBHI.2017.2767063 PMID:29989977

Simonyan, K., & Zisserman, A. (2014). Very deep convolutional networks for large-scale image recognition. arXiv Prepr. arXiv:1409.1556.

Szegedy, C., Ioffe, S., Vanhoucke, V., & Alemi, A. A. (2017). Inception-v4, inception-resnet and the impact of residual connections on learning. Association for the Advancement of Artificial Intelligence (AAAI), 4.

Szegedy, C., Liu, W., Jia, Y., Sermanet, P., Reed, S., Anguelov, D., Erhan, D., Vanhoucke, V., & Rabinovich, A. (2015). Going deeper with convolutions. *Proceedings of the IEEE conference on computer vision and pattern recognition*, 1–9.

Szegedy, C., Liu, W., Jia, Y., Sermanet, P., Reed, S., Anguelov, D., & Rabinovich, A. (2015). Going deeper with convolutions. In *Proceedings of the IEEE conference on computer vision and pattern recognition*. IEEE. 10.1109/CVPR.2015.7298594

Szegedy, C., Vanhoucke, V., Ioffe, S., Shlens, J., & Wojna, Z. (2016). Rethinking the inception architecture for computer vision. *Proceedings of the IEEE conference on computer vision and pattern recognition*, 2818–2826. 10.1109/CVPR.2016.308

The Office of the National Coordinator for Health Information Technology. (2017). *Quick stats: health IT dashboard*. https://dashboard.healthit.gov/quickstats/ quickstats.php

Vinyals, O., Toshev, A., Bengio, S., & Erhan, D. (2015). Show and tell: a neural image caption generator. *Proceedings of the IEEE Conference on Computer Vision and Pattern Recognition, 3156*–3164. 10.1109/CVPR.2015.7298935

Wu, Y. (2016). Google's neural machine translation system: bridging the gap between human and machine translation. Preprint at https://arxiv.org/ abs/1609.08144

Yosinski, J., Clune, J., Bengio, Y., & Lipson, L. (2014). How transferable are features in deep neural networks? Advances in Neural Information Processing Systems, 3320–3328.

Chapter 12
Data Analytics to Predict, Detect, and Monitor Chronic Autoimmune Diseases Using Machine Learning Algorithms:
Preventing Diseases With the Power of Machine Learning

Jayashree M. Kudari

iD https://orcid.org/0000-0003-2720-8250

Jain University, India

ABSTRACT

Developments in machine learning techniques for classification and regression exposed the access of detecting sophisticated patterns from various domain-penetrating data. In biomedical applications, enormous amounts of medical data are produced and collected to predict disease type and stage of the disease. Detection and prediction of diseases, such as diabetes, lung cancer, brain cancer, heart disease, and liver diseases, requires huge tests and that increases the size of patient medical data. Robust prediction of a patient's disease from the huge data set is an important agenda in in this chapter. The challenge of applying a machine learning method is to select the best algorithm within the disease prediction framework. This chapter opts for robust machine learning algorithms for various diseases by using case studies. This usually analyzes each dimension of disease, independently checking the identified value between the limits to monitor the condition of the disease.

DOI: 10.4018/978-1-7998-7188-0.ch012

INTRODUCTION

Over the past few decades Machine Learning has grown into one of the supports of information technology, a rather central, albeit usually hidden, part of our life. With the ever increasing amounts of data becoming available there is good reason to believe that smart data analysis will become even more pervasive as a necessary ingredient for technological progress. (2020, Infographics)

One of the main ambitions why we develop (computer) programs to computerize various kinds of processes. Originally developed as a subfield of Artificial Intelligence (AI), one of the goals behind machine learning was to replace the need for developing computer programs "manually." Considering that programs are being developed to automate processes, we can think of machine learning as the process of "automating automation." In other words, machine learning lets computers "create" programs (often, the intent for developing these programs is making predictions) themselves. In other words, machine learning is the process of turning data into programs. It is said that the term machine learning was first coined by Arthur Lee Samuel, a pioneer in the AI field, in 19591. (Mike Thomas, 2020) says the quote that almost every introductory machine learning resource cites is the following, which summarizes the concept behind machine learning nicely and concisely:

In the last decade, machine learning techniques have been used comprehensively for a varied range of tasks comprising of various algorithms. These algorithms used in a variety of application areas such as bioinformatics, speech recognition, spam detection, computer vision and fraud detection, health care to detect disease and managing disease. The algorithms and techniques usage come from many various domains including statistics, mathematics, neuroscience, and computer science.

This chapter deals with the Machine learning algorithm for prediction of disease, diagnostics of disease, and monitoring disease by using suitable case study. This chapter is to opt for robust machine learning algorithms for various diseases by using case studies. This chapter is to monitoring disease, this usually analyzes each dimension of disease independently checking the identified value between the limits to monitor the condition of the disease.

BACKGROUND

What is Learning?

"Learning makes someone Intelligent and perform a task better"

- Learning is the process of acquiring new understanding, knowledge, behaviors, or skills through study, experience or being taught.
- The ability to learn is possessed by humans, birds and animals, even certain plants – Natural Learning.
- Now, computers/ machines are able to learn- Artificial Learning/ Machine Learning.
- Computers can learn and act like humans do, and improve their learning over time in autonomous fashion, by taking input data in the form of observations and real-world interactions.

What is Machine Learning?

Learning is the process of acquiring new understanding, knowledge, behaviors, or skills through study, experience or being taught. The ability to learn is possessed by humans, birds and animals, even certain plants – Natural Learning. Now, computers/ machines are able to learn- Artificial Learning/ Machine Learning. Computers can learn and act like humans, and improve their learning over time in independent mode by taking input data in the form of observations and real-world interactions.

The Real-World Benefits of Machine Learning in Healthcare

Digitalization disturbing every field, including healthcare, the ability to capture, share and deliver data is becoming a high priority. Machine learning, big data and artificial intelligence (AI) can help address the challenges that vast amounts of data pose. (Infographics, 2020)

Machine learning has become essential and mandatory applications in the healthcare industry. It is assisting to map and treat contagious diseases and personalize medical treatments. Mike Thomas (2020).

According to LISA M. KRIEGER (March 3, 2017) Machine learning in medicine is playing vital role, and google has made headlines. Google has developed a machine learning algorithm to help in identify cancerous tumors on mammograms. Google research teams say that; team is surrounded throughout to handle complex problems. So Machine learning and Artificial Intelligence have confronted related challenges.

And (google computer) team witnessed in this work, the whole bunch of people worked on applying deep learning to create an algorithm for automated detection, by ECG, scanning photos, of retinal damage in patients with diabetes etc. "To confirm the best clinical outcome for patients, the various algorithms need to be incorporated in a way that complements the pathologist's workflow.

According to (Taylor Kubota, 2017), Stanford university is implemented a deep learning technique to identify skin cancer.

According (Jonathan Waring,2020) the usage of machine learning techniques have proven the possibilities to improve health results, reduce the costs of medical and to advance medical research. Jonathan Waring and team says, automated machine learning (AutoML) has emerged in order to make machine learning techniques simpler to apply and to reduce the burden of a doctor. This spontaneously select, comprise, and parametrized machine learning model to achieve finest performance by using given dataset.

One of the articles like JAMA article, it has conveyed the results of a deep learning algorithm was able to detect diabetic retinopathy in retinal images. This is how the machine learning creates its demand in the field of clinical decision making. (JAMA, 2016)

Vembandasamy K, Sasipriya, R. and Deepa, E. (2015) is used Naive Bayes algorithm to identify the heart disease. Therefore, Naive Bayes algorithm has powerful independence hypothesis capabilities. The dataset is collected from one of the prominent diabetic research institute in Chennai. Data set contains of 500 patients. Weka tool is used and executes classification technique for splitting 70% of data. In this, researcher achieved Naive Bayes offers 86.419% of accuracy in identifying the heart disease

(Corbet, 2017) perceives that, medical should take significant move to machine learning techniques as a innovative concept to deploy in this current era. Corbet says, we must find specific use cases in which machine learning's proficiencies provide the value from a specific technological application like Google and Stanford.

(O'Brien J, 2014) observes that, Hidden Markov Models and Spark were used to mine ECG data, coalescing accurate Hidden Markov Model (HMM) techniques with Apache Spark to improve the speed of ECG analysis. The paper has proven that there is potential for developing a fast classifier for heartbeats classification.

This chapter attempting to deal with the various prediction algorithms used to detect, predict and managing the disease.

MACHINE LEARNING ALGORITHMS

Machine Learning has several techniques such as Supervised Learning, Unsupervised Learning and Reinforced Learning

Machine learning techniques are categorized in to three types.

Figure 1. source: http://www.cognub.com/index.php/cognitive-platform/

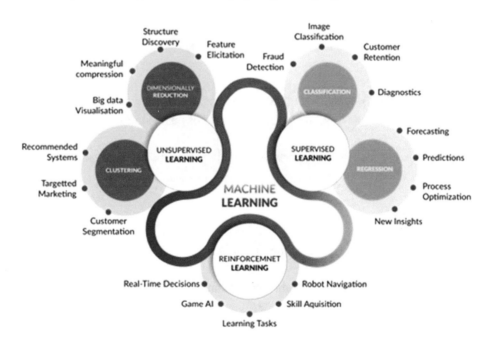

1. Supervised Learning technique deals with training data, data has to be labelled with the correct answers, for example yes or no or some other label. Significant common types of supervised learning are Classification and regression. Classification is results the outputs in discrete labels, as in spam filtering and second one is Regression which has the results are real-valued.

2. Unsupervised learning technique deals with unlabelled data set. Here required to analyse dataset and discover patterns out of it. The two important examples of unsupervised learning are dimension reduction and clustering.

Figure 2. Source: https://www.javatpoint.com/machine-learning

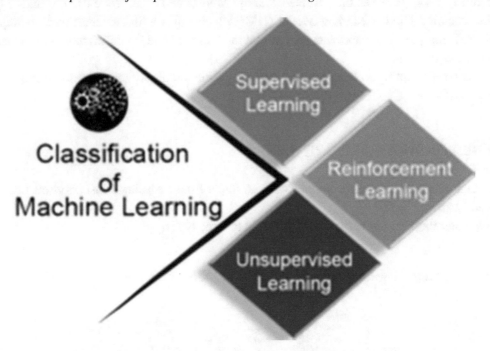

3.   Reinforcement learning is a technique deals with an agent, agent may be robot or controller which try to learn the ideal actions to go for right the results of past actions.

   This chapter completely focuses on supervised learning. Various types of supervised learning used in medical field.

Supervised Learning

The objectives of supervised machine learning are to build a model that decides the prediction based on the available data set with uncertain data. A supervised learning algorithm takes a well-known set of input data and known responses to the data (output) and trains a model to generate rational predictions for the response to new data. Supervised learning uses classification and regression techniques to develop predictive models.

Types of Supervised Learning

Classification: Classification is predictive model; class labels are predicted for given set of input data. makes to group the output inside a class. If the algorithm attempting to label input into two different classes, this is called binary classification. Choosing between more than two classes is called as multi-class classification. For example, determining whether or not someone will be a defaulter of the loan.

Figure 3. Types of supervised learning
Source: *(Supervised Machine Learning: What is, Algorithms with Examples, n.d.)*

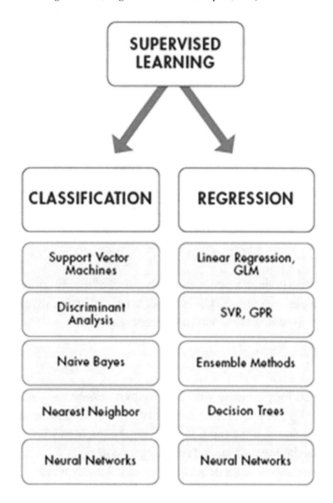

Types of Classification Algorithm

Naïve Bayes Classifiers

Naïve Bayesian classifiers are collection classification based on Naïve Bayes theorem. It is a family of algorithm shares common principle is class independence assumption.

Decision Trees

Decisions trees performs classification of the instance by sorting data based on the feature value. In this method, each kind is the feature of an instance. It should be classified, and every branch represents a value which the node can assume. It is a widely used technique for classification. In this method, classification is a tree which is known as a decision tree. It helps you to predict real values (cost of purchasing a car, number of calls, total monthly sales, etc.).

Nearest Neighbor

The nearest neighbour is a type of classifiers uses some or all the patterns available in the training set to classify a test pattern. These classifiers essentially involve finding the similarity between the test pattern and every pattern in the training set.

Support Vector Machine

Support vector machine (SVM) is a popular machine learning algorithm or classification, Basically Support Vectors are normally the co-ordinates of individual observation. For example, (33,210) is a support vector which corresponds to a female. Support Vector Machine is a boundary values which segregates the Male from the Females. In this case, the two classes are well separated from each other, hence it is easier to find a SVM.

Neural Network

Neural Network by the human brain, a neural network consists of highly connected networks of neurons that relate the inputs to the desired outputs. The network is trained by iteratively modifying the strengths of the connections so that given inputs map to the correct response.

Logistic Regression:

Regression models are used for problems where the output variable is a real value such as a unique number, dollars, salary, weight or pressure. It is most often used to predict numerical values based on previous data observations. Some of the more familiar regression algorithms include linear regression, logistic regression, polynomial regression, and ridge regression.

Regression is a method of modelling a dependent variable based on independent variables known as predictors. The anticipated output is continuous. This method is mostly used for forecasting and finding out cause and effect relationship between variables. Regression techniques mostly differ based on the number of independent variables and the type of relationship between the independent and dependent variables. Regression is used to predict the house price from training data. The input variables will be locality, size of a house, etc.

Supervised Machine Learning in Medical

The health care industries collect huge amounts of data that contain some hidden information, which is useful for making effective decisions. For providing appropriate results and making effective decisions on data, some advanced data mining techniques are used. This chapter attempting to apply various machine algorithm in the health care industry.

Machine learning can also assist healthcare organizations reach developing medical demands, improvise the operations and lower the expense. At the outset, machine learning innovation assist healthcare doctors to predict, detect and monitor disease more proficiently and with more accuracy and personalized care. (Infographics, 2020).

This chapter focuses on few diseases like heart, liver, diabetes, dengue, Hepatitis diagnosis and prediction.

Diagnosis of Diseases by using Different Machine Learning Algorithms

Many authors have been working on various machine learning algorithms for disease diagnosis. Currently authors have been witnessed in acknowledging machine-learning algorithms in in health care industry successfully. Authors says that machine learning algorithms blend well in diagnosis of various diseases.

Figure 4. Diseases diagnosed by machine learning technique.
(Source- Survey of Machine Learning Algorithms for Disease Diagnostic, Meherwar Fatima1, Maruf Pasha 2, JILSA Vol.9 No.1, February 2017)

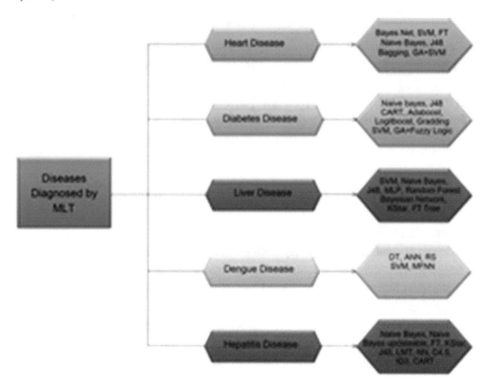

LITERATURE REVIEW

(Ma'sum M. A et al H,2016), Enhanced huge works related to ECG classification implanted with big data tools and without big data when dataset is small. Authors implemented several studies that depend on big data techniques. Since Indonesia has high mortality rate due to heart disease, researchers attempted to decrease the mortality rate, in order to deal with big data, a tele-ecg system was built for heart diseases early detection and monitoring using Hadoop framework. The system can classify the ECG data using decision tree and random forest, it was the first real system for heartbeats classification using big data tools. The system was built on cluster computer with 4 nodes. The server was able to handle 60 requests at the same time. The accuracy was 97.14% and 98,92% for decision tree and random forest respectively. In (Dalvi RdF et al, 2016), uses of Neural networks and dimensionality reduction technique and tested on the Massachusetts Institute of Technology arrhythmia database. The classification performance on a test set of only 18 ECG records of 30 min each achieved an accuracy of 96.97%.

In, many types of heartbeat were extracted and used for classification, classification method is used to classify independent type (3 records for each type); each type of heartbeats has its own model (model to classify normal heartbeats, model to classify type 1 of heartbeats and so forth). Neural network and SVM were applied and the accuracy of results was high good (more than 90%), but there was not unified model to classify all multi-types together at once. In (Ince T et al,2009), Feed-forward and fully connected artificial neural networks aided by particle swarm optimization technique are employed to recognize two patterns of heartbeats. Tuning parameters of proposed method has improved accuracy of classification to 96% comparing to the same method with default value of parameters. Not all features were used (only morphological and temporal) and a total of 83,648 beats were selected for training and testing.

In (Ince T et al, 2009), Hidden Markov Models and Spark were used to mine ECG data, combining accurate Hidden Markov Model (HMM) techniques with Apache Spark to improve the speed of ECG analysis. The paper has proven that there is potential for developing a fast classifier for heartbeats classification.

In (Celesti F, et al,2017), DNN (Deep Neural Network) has been used for deep learning to classify heartbeats. The author has compared results with many studies, accuracy of classifying has reached 99%, but the classification was only two types (Normal and Abnormal) and dataset size was almost 85,000 records.

Case Study on Heart Attack Risk Prediction using Machine Learning

Source-(Amayomordecai, 2020)

Heart disease can be managed effectively with a combination of lifestyle changes, medicine and, in some cases, surgery. With the right treatment, the symptoms of heart disease can be reduced and the functioning of the heart improved. The predicted results can be used to prevent and thus reduce cost for surgical treatment and other expensive.

The overall objective of my work will be to predict accurately with few tests and attributes the presence of heart disease. Attributes considered form the primary basis for tests and give accurate results more or less. Many more input attributes can be taken but our goal is to predict with few attributes and faster efficiency the risk of having heart disease. Data mining holds great potential for the healthcare industry to enable health systems to systematically use data and analytics to identify inefficiencies and best practices that improve care and reduce costs.

The dataset is publically available on the Kaggle website, and it is from an ongoing cardiovascular study on residents of the town of Framingham, Massachusetts. The classification goal is to predict whether the patient has 10-year risk of future coronary heart disease (CHD). The dataset provides the patients' information. It includes over 4,000 records and 15 attributes. Variables Each attribute is a potential risk factor. There are both demographic, behavioural and medical risk factors.

Attributes used for Prediction

Demographic

Sex: Male or female(Nominal)

Age: Age of the patient;(Continuous - Although the recorded ages have been truncated to whole numbers, the concept of age is continuous)

Education: No Further Information Provided

Behavioral

Current Smoker: Whether or not the patient is a current smoker (Nominal)

Cigs Per Day: The number of cigarettes that the person smoked on average in one day.(can be considered continuous as one can have any number of cigarettes, even half a cigarette.)

Information on Medical History

BP Meds: Whether or not the patient was on blood pressure medication (Nominal)

Prevalent Stroke: Whether or not the patient had previously had a stroke (Nominal)

Prevalent Hyp: Whether or not the patient was hypertensive (Nominal)

Diabetes: Whether or not the patient had diabetes (Nominal)

Information on Current Medical Condition

Tot Chol: Total cholesterol level (Continuous)

Sys BP: Systolic blood pressure (Continuous)

Dia BP: Diastolic blood pressure (Continuous)

BMI: Body Mass Index (Continuous)

Heart Rate: Heart rate (Continuous - In medical research, variables such as heart rate though in fact discrete, yet are considered continuous because of large number of possible values.)

Glucose: Glucose level (Continuous)

Target Variable to Predict

10 year risk of coronary heart disease (CHD) coronary heart disease - (binary: "1", means "Yes", "0" means "No")

Data Cleaning and Pre-Processing

Here, dealt with missing and duplicate values from the used data set as these can totally affect the performance of different machine learning algorithms.

Exploratory Data Analysis

To understand the significant statistical perceptions from the data. This chapter deals with the scatterings of the various attributes, correlations of the factors with each other and the target variable, calculated probabilities and sizes for the categorical attributes.

Feature Selection

If dataset has irrelevant features that could be decreased to get the accuracy of the model, here the Boruta Feature Selection technique to select the most important features for future selection of the different model.

Model Development and Comparison

In this, four classification models are used, i.e., Logistic Regression, K-Nearest Neighbors, Decision Trees and Support Vector Machine, then later stage compared the performance of the of algorithms using their accuracy and F1 scores to decide best fit algorithm.

Load Data

```
#Loading Dataset
#load the data
data = pd.read_csv('data/framingham.csv')
data.drop(['education'],axis=1,inplace=True)
data.head()
```

In this demo, dropped the education column since it has not involved in correlation with heart disease.

Data Cleansing

Then the data has been taken to the further main process which is 'DATA CLEANING' which means to find all the null and missing values. The data is being cleansed by Python code.

```
#total percentage of missing data
missing_data = data.isnull().sum()
total_percentage = (missing_data.sum()/data.shape[0]) * 100
print(f'The total percentage of missing data is {round(total_percentage,2)}%')
```

In the complete dataset the total percentage of missing data is 12.74%

```
# percentage of missing data per category
total = data.isnull().sum().sort_values(ascending=False)
percent_total = (data.isnull().sum()/data.isnull().count()).sort_
values(ascending=False)*100
missing = pd.concat([total, percent_total], axis=1, keys=["Total", "Percent-
age"])
missing_data = missing[missing['Total']>0]
missing_data
```

Table 1. Attribute wise missing data

Attribute	Total	Percentage
glucose	388	9.150943
BPMeds	53	1.25
totChol	50	1.179245
cigsPerDay	29	0.683962
BMI	19	0.448113
heartRate	1	0.023585

The blood glucose column would be dropped since because it has the highest percentage of missing data i.e 9.15%. Since missing entries account for only 12% of the total data that could be dropped.

Exploratory Data Analysis

To understand the significant statistical perceptions from the data. This chapter deals with the scatterings of the various attributes, correlations of the factors with each other and the target variable, calculated probabilities and sizes for the categorical attributes.

This analysis is required to understand the distribution different attributes. The data is not distributed on the on the stroke, diabetes, and blood pressure.

```
#Heart disease case count
sns.countplot(x='TenYearCHD',data=data)
plt.show()
cases = data.TenYearCHD.value_counts()
print(f"There are {cases[0]} patients without heart disease and {cases[1]} pa-
tients with the disease")
```

Case Count

Result: There are 3179 patients without heart disease and 572 patients with the disease

Correlation Heat Map

Correlation matrices are needed tool of exploratory data analysis. Correlation heat maps contain the information visually which is appealing and meaningful.

```
plt.figure(figsize=(15,8))
sns.heatmap(data.corr(), annot = True)
plt.show()
```

Figure 5. Histogram plot for exploratory analysis of disease with all attributes

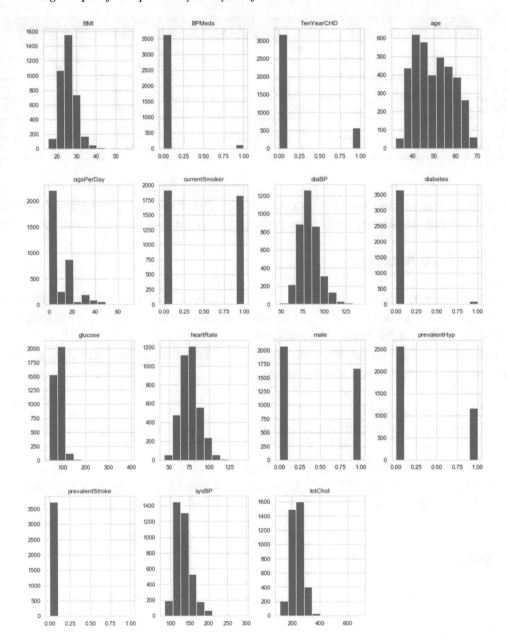

Findings

According to heat map, there is no feature having more than 0.5 correlation coefficient value with the 10-year risk of developing CHD and this demonstration that the attributes are poor predictors.

Since there are only couple of attributes highly correlated with each other but implementation of machine learning is highly not affordable to predict the disease. Therefore, it is important to carry out feature selection to pick the best features

Figure 6. Histogram plot to count hear disease case out of the sample

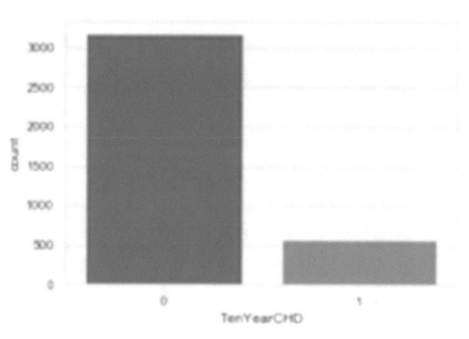

Feature Selection

Here, Boruta algorithm used due to a wrapper built around the random forest classification algorithm. And it tries to capture all the significant attributes in a data set with respect to an outcome variable.

Step 1:   It adds randomness to the given data set by creating shuffled copies of all features.

Step 2:   Then, it trains a random forest classifier on the extended data set and applies a feature importance to evaluate the importance of each feature where higher means more important.

```
from sklearn.ensemble import RandomForestClassifier
from boruta import BorutaPy
In [16]:
#define the features
X = data.iloc[:,:-1].values
y = data.iloc[:,-1].values
forest=RandomForestClassifier(n_estimators=1000,n_jobs=-1, class_
weight='balanced')
# define Boruta feature selection method
feat_selector = BorutaPy(forest, n_estimators='auto', verbose=2)
# find all relevant features
feat_selector.fit(X, y)
```

Figure 7. Heat-Map shows no features with more than 0.5 correlation with the Ten-year risk of developing CHD and this shows that the features a poor predictor.

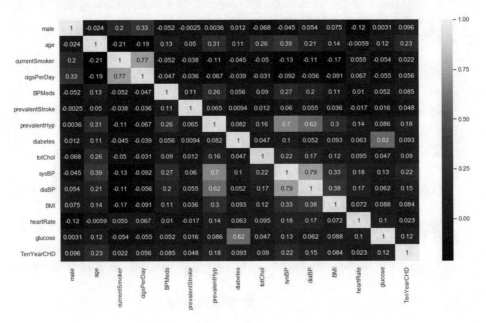

Step 3: At every iteration, it checks whether a real feature has a higher importance than the best of its shadow features (i.e. whether the feature has a higher Z-score than the maximum Z-score of its shadow features) and constantly removes features which are deemed highly unimportant.

Step 4: Finally, the algorithm stops either when all features get confirmed or rejected or it reaches a specified limit of random forest runs.

BorutaPy finished running.

Iteration: 100 / 100
Confirmed: 2
Tentative: 1

```
BorutaPy(alpha=0.05,
         estimator=RandomForestClassifier(bootstrap=True,
                                           class_weight='balanced',
                                           criterion='gini', max_depth=None,
                                           max_features='auto',
                                           max_leaf_nodes=None,
                                           min_impurity_decrease=0.0,
                                           min_impurity_split=None,
                                           min_samples_leaf=1,
                                           min_samples_split=2,
                                           min_weight_fraction_leaf=0.0,
```

```
                                        n_estimators=28, n_jobs=-1,
                                        oob_score=False,
                                        random_state=<mtrand.RandomState ob-
ject at 0x000001E839B74828>,

                                        verbose=0, warm_start=False),
        max_iter=100, n_estimators='auto', perc=100,
        random_state=<mtrand.RandomState object at 0x000001E839B74828>,
        two_step=True, verbose=2)
# show the most important features
most_important = data.columns[:-1][feat_selector.support_].tolist()
most_important
```

Rejected: 10

Here, the age and the systolic blood pressures are selected as the most important features for predicting

```
# select the top 6 features
top_features = data.columns[:-1][feat_selector.ranking_ <=6].tolist()
top_features
the Ten-year risk of developing CHD. Those are ['age', 'sysBP']
```

The top features are:

1. Age
2. Total cholesterol
3. Systolic blood pressure
4. Diastolic blood pressure
5. BMI
6. Heart rate
7. Blood glucose

```
import statsmodels.api as sm
X_top = data[top_features]
y = data['TenYearCHD']
res = sm.Logit(y,X_top).fit()
res.summary()
```

```
params = res.params
conf = res.conf_int()
conf['Odds Ratio'] = params
conf.columns = ['5%', '95%', 'Odds Ratio']
print(np.exp(conf))
```

Table 2. Logit regression results, descriptive summary about the regression results.

Dep. Variable:	TenYearCHD	No. Observations:	3751
Model:	Logit	Df Residuals:	3744
Method:	MLE	Df Model:	6
Date:	Sat, 25 Apr 2020	Pseudo R-squ.:	0.02354
Time:	22:16:47	Log-Likelihood:	-1564
converged:	TRUE	LL-Null:	-1601.7
Covariance Type:	nonrobust	LLR p-value:	3.17E-14

Plotting all other features constant, the odds of getting diagnosed with heart disease increases with about 2% for every increase in age systolic blood pressure. Rest factors show no significant change in the result.

Table 3. Odds ratio is a measure of association between an exposure and an outcome.

5% 95% Odds Ratio
age 1.011381 1.033813 1.022536
totChol 0.994963 0.999184 0.997071
sysBP 1.018236 1.031493 1.024843
diaBP 0.962258 0.984627 0.973378
BMI 0.929304 0.973798 0.951291
heartRate 0.963690 0.977730 0.970685
glucose 1.001074 1.007518 1.004291

Models: In this chapter other algorithms are implemented and done the model comparison
Logistic Regression:
The objective of logistic regression is to find the best fitting model to describe the relationship between dependent variable and response or outcome variable and a set of independent (predictor or explanatory) variables. Logistic regression produces the coefficients and its standard errors and significance levels of a formula to predict a logit transformation of the probability of presence of the characteristic of interest:

Logistics Regression Implemented using Sklearn Library

```
from sklearn.linear_model import LogisticRegression
from sklearn.model_selection import GridSearchCV
from sklearn.metrics import confusion_matrix
from sklearn.metrics import accuracy_score
from sklearn.metrics import f1_score
from sklearn.metrics import classification_report
```

```
from sklearn.metrics import recall_score,precision_score,classification_
report,roc_auc_score,roc_curve
# search for optimun parameters using gridsearch
params = {'penalty':['l1','l2'],'C':[0.01,0.1,1,10,100],
         'class_weight':['balanced',None]}
logistic_clf = GridSearchCV(LogisticRegression(),param_grid=params,cv=10)
#train the classifier
logistic_clf.fit(X_train,y_train)
logistic_clf.best_params
#make predictions
logistic_predict = logistic_clf.predict(X_test)
log_accuracy = accuracy_score(y_test,logistic_predict)
print(f"Using logistic regression we get an accuracy of {round(log_accura-
cy*100,2)}%")
```

Here, using Using logistic regression got an accuracy of 67.6%

```
Implecm=confusion_matrix(y_test,logistic_predict)
conf_matrix=pd.DataFrame(data=cm,columns=['Predicted:0','Predicted:1'],index=[
'Actual:0','Actual:1'])
plt.figure(figsize = (8,5))
sns.heatmap(conf_matrix, annot=True,fmt='d',cmap="YlGnBu")mentation of Confu-
sion Matrix and Plot
```

Figure 8. Logistic regression using confusion matrix

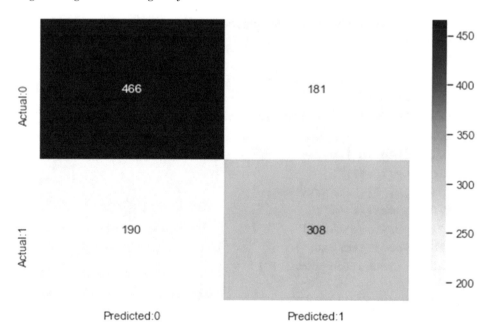

```
print(classification_report(y_test,logistic_predict))
```

Table 4. F1 score of logistic regression

precision recall f1-score support
0 0.71 0.72 0.72 647
1 0.63 0.62 0.62 498
accuracy 0.68 1145
macro avg 0.67 0.67 0.67 1145
weighted avg 0.68 0.68 0.68 1145

```
logistic_f1 = f1_score(y_test, .logistic_predict)
print(f'The f1 score for logistic regression is {round(logistic_f1*100,2)}%')
```

Result: F1 Score for Logistic Regression is 62.41%

ROC AND AUC

Receiver Operating Characteristic curve is a plot shows the performance of a classification

```
# ROC curve and AUC
probs = logistic_clf.predict_proba(X_test)
# keep probabilities for the positive outcome only
probs = probs[:, 1]
# calculate AUC
log_auc = roc_auc_score(y_test, probs)
# calculate roc curve
fpr, tpr, thresholds = roc_curve(y_test, probs)
# plot curve
sns.set_style('whitegrid')
plt.figure(figsize=(10,6))
plt.plot([0, 1], [0, 1], linestyle='--')
plt.plot(fpr, tpr, marker='.')
plt.ylabel('True positive rate')
plt.xlabel('False positive rate')
plt.title(f"AUC = {round(log_auc,3)}")
plt.show()
```

model at all classification edges. This curve plots two parameters: True Positive Rate and False Positive Rate Area under the UC: AUC is used for "Area under the ROC Curve." That is, AUC measures the entire two-dimensional area below the entire ROC curve (think integral calculus) from (0,0) to (1,1).

Figure 9. ROC and accuracy plot shows inclined toward false positive rate in logistic regression

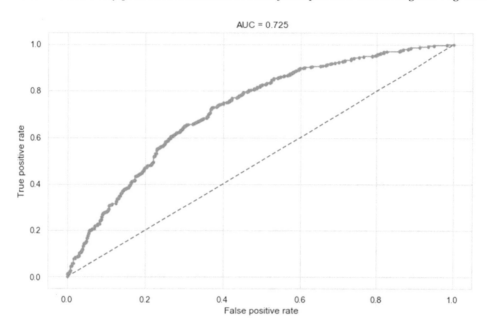

K-Nearest Neighbors

It tries to define the group a data point is in by observing at the data points around it

```
from sklearn.neighbors import KNeighborsClassifier
# search for optimun parameters using gridsearch
params= {'n_neighbors': np.arange(1, 10)}
grid_search = GridSearchCV(estimator = KNeighborsClassifier(),
param_grid = params, scoring = 'accuracy', cv = 10, n_jobs = -1)
knn_clf = GridSearchCV(KNeighborsClassifier(),params,cv=3, n_jobs=-1)
# train the model
knn_clf.fit(X_train,y_train)
knn_clf.best_params_
{'n_neighbors': 1}
# predictions
knn_predict = knn_clf.predict(X_test)
#accuracy
knn_accuracy = accuracy_score(y_test,knn_predict)
```

```
print(f"Using k-nearest neighbours we get an accuracy of {round(knn_accura-
cy*100,2)}%")
```

OUTPOUT: Using k-nearest neighbors we get an accuracy of 82.53%

Confusion Matrix Applying on K-Nearest Neighbor

```
m=confusion_matrix(y_test,knn_predict)
conf_matrix=pd.DataFrame(data=cm,columns=['Predicted:0','Predicted:1'],index=[
'Actual:0','Actual:1'])
plt.figure(figsize = (8,5))
sns.heatmap(conf_matrix, annot=True,fmt='d',cmap="YlGnBu")
```

Figure 10. Confusion matrix for KNN

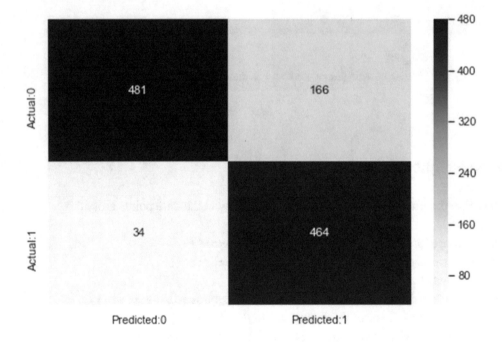

The **confusion matrix** is a table that is used to show the number of correct and incorrect predictions on a classification problem when the real values of the Test Set are known

```
print(classification_report(y_test,knn_predict))
```

Table 5. F1 score of k-nearest neighbour

	precision recall f1-score support
0 0.93 0.74 0.83 647	
1 0.74 0.93 0.82 498	
accuracy 0.83 1145	
macro avg 0.84 0.84 0.83 1145	
weighted avg 0.85 0.83 0.83 1145	

```
knn_f1 = f1_score(y_test, knn_predict)
print(f'The f1 score for K nearest neignbours is {round(knn_f1*100,2)}%')
```

The f1 score for K nearest neighbors is 82.27%

ROC Curve and AUC for KNN

```
# ROC curve and AUC
probs = knn_clf.predict_proba(X_test)
# keep probabilities for the positive outcome only
probs = probs[:, 1]
# calculate AUC
knn_auc = roc_auc_score(y_test, probs)
# calculate roc curve
fpr, tpr, thresholds = roc_curve(y_test, probs)
# plot curve
sns.set_style('whitegrid')
plt.figure(figsize=(10,6))
plt.plot([0, 1], [0, 1], linestyle='--')
plt.plot(fpr, tpr, marker='.')
plt.ylabel('True positive rate')
plt.xlabel('False positive rate')
plt.title(f"AUC = {round(knn_auc,3)}")
plt.show()
```

Decision Trees

```
from sklearn.tree import DecisionTreeClassifier
dtree= DecisionTreeClassifier(random_state=7)
# grid search for optimum parameters
params = {'max_features': ['auto', 'sqrt', 'log2'],
```

Figure 11. ROC and accuracy applying on KNN

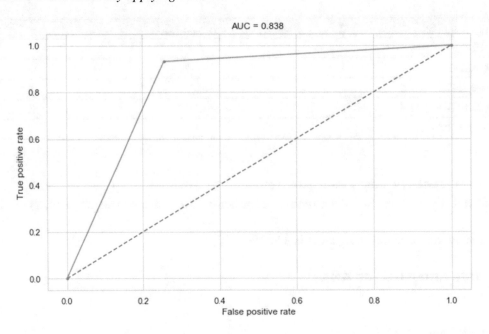

```
              'min_samples_split': [2,3,4,5,6,7,8,9,10,11,12,13,14,15],
              'min_samples_leaf':[1,2,3,4,5,6,7,8,9,10,11]}
tree_clf = GridSearchCV(dtree, param_grid=params, n_jobs=-1)
# train the model
tree_clf.fit(X_train,y_train)
tree_clf.best_params_
# predictions
tree_predict = tree_clf.predict(X_test)
#accuracy
tree_accuracy = accuracy_score(y_test,tree_predict)
print(f"Using Decision Trees we get an accuracy of {round(tree_accura-
cy*100,2)}%")
```

It is a tree-like graph with nodes signifying an attribute and ask a question; edges indicate the answers, and leaves represent the actual output. Decision trees classify the data by sorting them down the tree from the root to some leaf node, with the leaf node providing the classification. Each node in the tree acts as a test case for some attribute, and each edge descending from that node corresponds to one of the possible answers to the test case. This process is recursive in nature and is repeated for every sub-tree rooted at the new nodes.

Using Decision Trees we get an accuracy of 72.4%

```
cm=confusion_matrix(y_test,tree_predict)
conf_matrix=pd.DataFrame(data=cm,columns=['Predicted:0','Predicted:1'],index=[
'Actual:0','Actual:1'])
```

```
plt.figure(figsize = (8,5))
sns.heatmap(conf_matrix, annot=True,fmt='d',cmap="YlGnBu")
```

Apply Confusion Matrix

```
print(classification_report(y_test,tree_predict))
```

Figure 12. Confusion matrix for decision tree

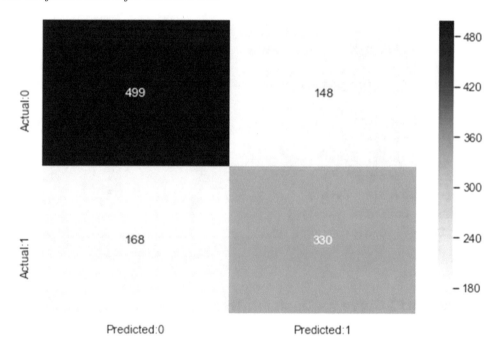

```
tree_f1 = f1_score(y_test, tree_predict)
print(f'The f1 score Descision trees is {round(tree_f1*100,2)}%')
```

The f1 score Decision trees is 67.62%

ROC Curve and AUC Applying on Decision Tree

```
# ROC curve and AUC
probs = tree_clf.predict_proba(X_test)
# keep probabilities for the positive outcome only
probs = probs[:, 1]
```

Table 6. f1 score of Decision Tree

	precision recall f1-score support
0 0.75 0.77 0.76 647	
1 0.69 0.66 0.68 498	
accuracy 0.72 1145	
macro avg 0.72 0.72 0.72 1145	
weighted avg 0.72 0.72 0.72 1145	

```
# calculate AUC
tree_auc = roc_auc_score(y_test, probs)
# calculate roc curve
fpr, tpr, thresholds = roc_curve(y_test, probs)
# plot curve
sns.set_style('whitegrid')
plt.figure(figsize=(10,6))
plt.plot([0, 1], [0, 1], linestyle='--')
plt.plot(fpr, tpr, marker='.')
plt.ylabel('True positive rate')
plt.xlabel('False positive rate')
plt.title(f"AUC = {round(tree_auc,3)}")
plt.show()
```

ROC Curve and AUC Curve for Decision Tree

Support Vector Machine

Support vector machine (SVM) is a popular machine learning algorithm or classification, Basically Support Vectors are normally the co-ordinates of individual observation. For example, (33,210) is a support vector which corresponds to a female. Support Vector Machine is a boundary values which segregates the Male from the Females. In this case, the two classes are well separated from each other, hence it is easier to find a SVM.

```
cm=confusion_matrix(y_test,svm_predict)
conf_matrix=pd.DataFrame(data=cm,columns=['Predicted:0','Predicted:1'],index=[
'Actual:0','Actual:1'])
plt.figure(figsize = (8,5))
sns.heatmap(conf_matrix, annot=True,fmt='d',cmap="YlGnBu")
from sklearn.svm import SVC
```

Figure 13. ROC And AUC for decision tree

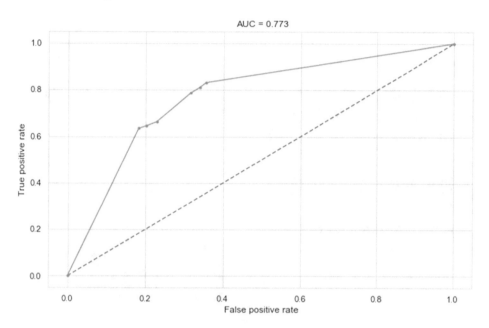

```
In [62]:
#grid search for optimum parameters
Cs = [0.001, 0.01, 0.1, 1, 10]
gammas = [0.001, 0.01, 0.1, 1]
param_grid = {'C': Cs, 'gamma': gammas}
svm_clf = GridSearchCV(SVC(kernel='rbf', probability=True), param_grid, cv=10)
In [63]:
# train the model
svm_clf.fit(X_train,y_train)
svm_clf.best_params_
Out[63]:
{'C': 10, 'gamma': 1}
In [64]:
# predictions
svm_predict = svm_clf.predict(X_test)
In [65]:
#accuracy
svm_accuracy = accuracy_score(y_test,svm_predict)
print(f"Using SVM we get an accuracy of {round(svm_accuracy*100,2)}%")
Using SVM we get an accuracy of 86.46%
```

Confusion Matrix for SVM

Figure 14. Confusion matrix for SVM

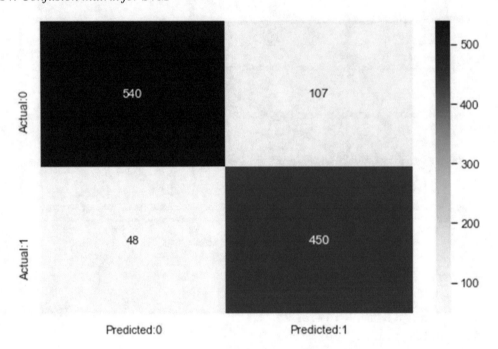

```
print(classification_report(y_test,svm_predict))
```

Table 7. F1 score of SVM

	precision recall f1-score support
0 0.92 0.83 0.87 647
1 0.81 0.90 0.85 498
accuracy 0.86 1145
macro avg 0.86 0.87 0.86 1145
weighted avg 0.87 0.86 0.87 1145

```
svm_f1 = f1_scor(y_test, svm_predict)
print(f'The f1 score for SVM is {round(svm_f1*100,2)}%')
```

The f1 score for SVM is 85.31%

```
# ROC curve and AUC
probs = svm_clf.predict_proba(X_test)
# keep probabilities for the positive outcome only
probs = probs[:, 1]
# calculate AUC
svm_auc = roc_auc_score(y_test, probs)
# calculate roc curve
fpr, tpr, thresholds = roc_curve(y_test, probs)
# plot curve
sns.set_style('whitegrid')
plt.figure(figsize=(10,6))
plt.plot([0, 1], [0, 1], linestyle='--')
plt.plot(fpr, tpr, marker='.')
plt.ylabel('True positive rate')
plt.xlabel('False positive rate')
plt.title(f"AUC = {round(svm_auc,3)}")
plt.show()
```

ROC Curve and AUC Applying on SVM

Figure 15. ROC And AUC for SVM

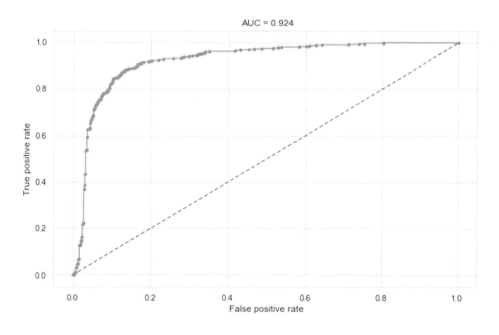

```
comparison = pd.DataFrame{
    "Logistic regression":{'Accuracy':log_accuracy, 'AUC':log_auc, 'F1
```

```
score':logistic_f1},
    "K-nearest neighbours":{'Accuracy':knn_accuracy, 'AUC':knn_auc, 'F1
score':knn_f1},
    "Decision trees":{'Accuracy':tree_accuracy, 'AUC':tree_auc, 'F1
score':tree_f1},
    "Support vector machine":{'Accuracy':svm_accuracy, 'AUC':svm_auc, 'F1
score':svm_f1}
}).T
Comparison
```

Model Comparison

Comparison of Models

Table 8. Comparison of models used with AUC, accuracy and f1 score

	AUC	Accuracy	F1 score
Logistic regression	0.725005	0.675983	0.624113
K-nearest neighbors	0.837579	0.825328	0.822695
Decision trees	0.773151	0.724017	0.67623
Support vector machine	0.92362	0.864629	0.853081

Plot of All Models with Respect to AUC, Accuracy and F1 Score

```
fig = plt.gcf()
fig.set_size_inches(15, 15)
titles = ['AUC','Accuracy','F1 score']
for title,label in enumerate(comparison.columns):
    plt.subplot(2,2,title+1)
    sns.barplot(x=comparison.index, y = comparison[label], data=comparison)
    plt.xticks(fontsize=10)
    plt.title(titles[title])
plt.show()
```

Comparison of all Four Models

Figure 16. Comparison of models

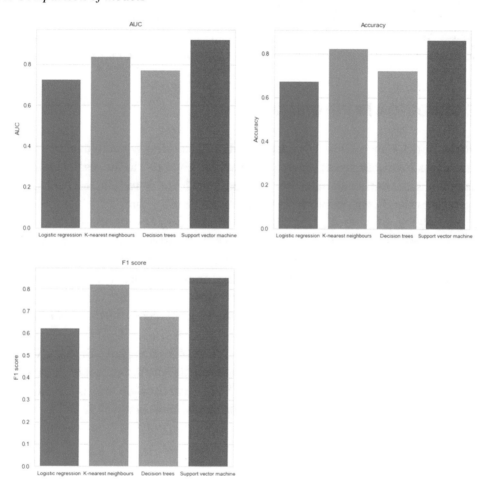

CONCLUSION OF THE CASE STUDY

The most important features in predicting the ten-year risk of developing coronary heart disease (CHD) were age and systolic blood pressure. The Support vector machine is the best model for performing in terms of accuracy and the F1 score. High value of AUC and shows high true positive rate. Balancing the dataset by using the SMOTE technique helped in improving the models sensitivity, with more data (especially that of the minority class) better models can be built.

FUTURE SCOPE

The health care industry is wide field, this chapter can be extended for more disease and to detect and control medical anomalies after treatment. Engaging machine learning algorithms to observe diseased environments simplifies model-building and provides multiple. Machine learning can absolutely

Impact on maintain and care of patient. For an instance, it would assist in identifying and diagnosing treatable disease. Machine Learning Applications in healthcare can also modernize healthcare industry and improve treatment, operation planning, preparation planning and execution planning.

DISEASE CONDITION MONITORING

According to (Dr Patrick Bangert, 2018) Disease Condition Monitoring typically analyzes each dimension separately and check for imbalance of the dimensions. This gives rise to the results in false alarms and unhealthy conditions that are not alarmed. By using machine learning techniques, the big data gathered to analyze to take up significant decisions about its present health status.

According (S. Nashif, M. R. et al,2018) initial detection of cardiac diseases and frequent monitoring of patients can decrease the mortality rate, doctor can monitor heart disease patients by sensing real-time parameters such as BP, body temperature, heartbeat etc. (S. Nashif et al, 2018) So from this, the doctors can visualize the patient's real-time sensor data by using the application and auto start live video for the doctor, if there is any immediate treatment needed. One more feature authors have anticipated that notification would reach to doctor real-time parameter of the patient exceeds the threshold and immediately notified to assigned doctor over GSM technology.

According to (Wan Nor Liyana, et al, 2019), authors have compared Naive Bayes method for prediction. They have done prediction accuracies of Bayesian technique with three machine learning algorithms K-nearest neighbor (K-NN), support vector machine (SVM), and decision tree (DT). The results proved that the best performance was from the Bayesian algorithm with accuracy of 97.281%.

CONCLUSION

This chapter demonstrated CHD by comparing four models to concludes best model for prediction.

This chapter recommends SVM as best fit model prediction of heart disease risk. This might assist Doctor to understand the parameters involved in the heart disease risk. Prevention could be suggested through the prediction predicted the algorithm. Here the concentration was only on CHD risk prediction, but this can be expanding for various diseases.

REFERENCES

Amayomordecai. (2020, April 26). *Heart disease risk prediction machine learning*. Kaggle. https://www. kaggle.com/amayomordecai/heart-disease-risk-prediction-machine-learning

Bangert. (2018). *Smart Condition Monitoring Using Machine Learning*. Algorithmica technologies GmbH.

Celesti, F., Celesti, A., Carnevale, L., Galletta, A., Campo, S., Romano, A., Bramanti, P., & Villari, M. (2017). *Big data analytics in genomics: the point on deep learning solutions. IEEE symposium on computers and communications (ISCC).* IEEE.

Corbett. (2017, April 25). The Real-World Benefits of Machine Learning in Healthcare. *The Medical Officer.*

Dalvi Rd, F., Zago, G. T., & Andreão, R. V. (2016). Heartbeat classification system based on neural networks and dimensionality reduction. *Research on Biomedical Engineering, 32*(4), 318–326. doi:10.1590/2446-4740.05815

Fatima & Pasha. (2014). Survey of Machine Learning Algorithms for Disease Diagnostic. *JILSA, 9*(1).

Gulshan, Peng, & Coram. (2016). *Development and Validation of a Deep Learning Algorithm for Detection of Diabetic Retinopathy in Retinal Fundus Photographs.* doi:10.1001/jama.2016.17216 PMID:27898976

Ince, T., Kiranyaz, S., & Gabbouj, M. A. (2009). generic and robust system for automated patient-specific classification of ECG signals. *IEEE Transactions on Biomedical Engineering, 56*(5), 1415–1426. doi:10.1109/TBME.2009.2013934 PMID:19203885

Infographics. (2020). *Machine Learning in Healthcare: Examples, Tips & Resources for Implementing into Your Care Practice.* Author.

Krieger. (2017). *Google computers trained to detect cancer.* Bay Area News Group.

Kubota. (2017). *Stanford researchers have trained an algorithm to diagnose skin cancer.* Academic Press.

Liyana, Ibeni, Salikon, & Salleh. (2019). Comparative analysis on bayesian classification for breast cancer problem. *Computer Science, Bulletin of Electrical Engineering and Informatics.*

Ma'sum, M. A., Jatmiko, W., & Suhartanto, H. (2016). Enhanced tele ECG system using hadoop framework to deal with big data processing. In *International workshop on Big Data and information security (IWBIS).* New York: IEEE. 10.1109/IWBIS.2016.7872900

Nashif, S., Raihan, M. R., & Imam, M. H. (2019). *Heart Disease Detection by Using Machine Learning Algorithms and a Real-Time Cardiovascular Health Monitoring System. World Journal of Engineering and Technology.*

O'Brien, J. (2014). *Using hidden Markov models and spark to mine ECG data.* Academic Press.

Supervised Machine Learning. (n.d.). *What is, Algorithms with Examples.* Guru99. https://www.guru99.com/supervised-machine-learning.html

Thomas. (2020). *15 examples of machine learning in healthcare that are revolutionizing medicine.* Academic Press.

Vembandasamy, K., Sasipriya, R., & Deepa, E. (2015). Heart Diseases Detection Using Naive Bayes Algorithm. IJISET-International Journal of Innovative Science. *Engineering & Technology, 2,* 441–444.

Waringa, Lindvallc, & Umeton. (2020). *Automated machine learning.* Academic Press.

KEY TERMS AND DEFINITIONS

AI: Artificial intelligence.
AUC: Area under the curve.
BN: Bayesian networks (BN).
CHD: Coronary heart disease.
DT: Decision Tree.
ECG: Electrocardiogram.
KNN: K-nearest neighbor.
PCA: Principal component analysis.
ROC: Receiver operating characteristic.
SVM: Support vector machine.

Chapter 13

Criticality of E-Privacy and Data Leakage Amid the Pandemic:
Privacy-Preserving Techniques and Frameworks

Gaurav Roy

EC Council University, India

ABSTRACT

The global pandemic has led to an undeniable surge in using digital technologies due to the social distancing norms and nationwide lockdowns. Firms and organizations are conforming to the new culture of work and life. The use of internet services, digital devices, and cloud systems has seen surges in usage from 40% to 100%, compared to pre-lockdown levels. With the rapid growth of this technological use, people are exposing their digital assets, presence, and behavior out to the binary world where AI-driven data analysis algorithms, data-gathering systems, and spyware are continuously monitoring their behavior. These subconsciously exposed data are then carried forward for delivering customized ads and recommend features.

INTRODUCTION

In today's digital epoch, data has become an asset for every organization and is valued more than gold. Every organization thinks of preserving the organization's data + the client's data or consumer's data. Recent advances and trends in technology like sensors & IoT systems, cloud, data analytics, databases, Smart devices, etc., are plausible to collect data effectively and pervasively. Organizations are taking data through static apps, cloud-connected apps, web apps, websites, online services, ads, and other malicious content. This chapter will primarily focus on the impact of e-privacy caused during the pandemic.

DOI: 10.4018/978-1-7998-7188-0.ch013

THE DATA FLOW

The use of internet services, digital devices, and cloud systems have seen surges in usage from 40 percent to 100 percent, compared to pre-lockdown levels (De, 2020). With the rapid growth of this technological use, people are exposing their digital assets, presence, and e-behavior out to the binary world. AI-driven data analysis algorithms, data-collecting systems, and spyware continuously monitor user behavior. These subconsciously exposed data are then carried forward for delivering customized ads and recommend features. But people are not consciously aware of it.

According to some reports, due to lockdown and increase in remote working culture, people's credentials are experiencing data breach due to remote work, organization's data are getting compromised because of the employee's negligence. 76% of participants realized that remote work increases the time to identify and contain a data breach (IBM, 2021). Healthcare systems went digital due to the increase in the number of patients during this pandemic. Weak systems with lesser security tests led to the data breach. Cybercriminals are attacking healthcare systems - stealing patient records and selling them on the dark web against monetary benefits.

Even though people are working promptly on data security and privacy for the last 25 years, we are still facing difficulty in data security and privacy challenges (Tawalbeh, p. 2020). It is the attack surface that is spreading wider every day - because of the deployments of new data collection & processing devices like IoT systems, data monitoring apps, cloud, online services, web apps, websites, etc. In the subsequent sections, you will get to know the different data breach and e-behavior leakage mechanisms taking place behind our back. Also, we will stretch further to how cybercriminals and legitimate organizations are selling our data to the dark web. Next, we will discuss how surveillance in individual e-privacy is becoming a concern. Lastly, we will cover the prevention mechanisms and comprehensive solutions organizations are using for preserving data privacy. Let us now peep into each topic in detail.

DATA BREACH AND E-BEHAVIOR LEAKAGE

A data breach is a form of cyber-attack that might change the course of your life or change the revenue graph of any business. Yes, it's the most vulnerable and attractive attack that intentionally and unintentionally makes an attacker release private or sensitive credentials to any untrusted digital ecosystem. Through this process, the cybercriminal gains monetary and other benefits by leaking the sensitive credentials of the victim. You might have heard about sensitive data disclosure, unintentional information disclosure, massive data leak, info leak, delicate data spill, and terms like this. Yes, all of them belong to the data breach. Most organized crimes also leverage the use of data breaches. During this attack process, cybercriminals extract the protected and sensitive data such as credit card information, personal health information (PHI), financial records, Personal Identifiable Information (PII), trade secrets, bank details, project plans, stat reports, behavioral analysis data, and other vulnerable unstructured data, files, or documents.

More than 3.5 billion people parts with their personal and sensitive data compromised in the top 2 breaches of the 21st century. Many other data breaches were untold. Did you know, Covid-19 had also brought cyber pandemics. Since so many trades, communication, and sensitive synergies went online without significant blackouts or business repercussions has unknowingly invited cyber-terror. Digitizing everything and remotely managing it from home has enabled you to make mistakes more. It is allowing nation-state cybercriminals the ability to find flaws in plenty. The World Health Organization (WHO) reported a fivefold increase in cyberattacks in April 2020 (WHO, 2020). *Wired* magazine also posted "Internet Freedom Has Taken a Hit During the COVID-19 Pandemic where everything right from Surveillance to arrests, governments were using the coronavirus as a camouflage for a breakdown/seize on digital liberty.

Governments & private firms of many countries started mass surveillance on user's online behavior, also known as e-behavior. E-behavior is the interpersonal, intrapersonal, and functional behaviors of people while they use the internet. Right from marketing behavior, scrolling social media, subscribing, following, visiting websites of interest or need are all monitored and recorded for further analysis. Think of a situation where someone is monitoring your every online action. Such a situation arises in one of the two cases - either you have done some national or international-level crime, or you are the source of constant profit production. Here we will talk about the latter one. Large companies and government organizations are developing new products and services, launching them into the market, and targeting user behavior to analyze whether the user is interested in a particular product or not. Furthermore, companies stitched various ads beside your search page that allows navigating more options. But subconsciously, you are triggering and providing your interest as input to the autonomous algorithm running behind such apps. Every user has a unique representation in their semi-structured or unstructured database. Data analysis uses those cleaned data to further analyze the needs and requirements of the user. Future item recommendations and choices are also predicted through such algorithms.

Another side of the coin is where ISPs and other apps take our location data, what services we are using, our movement, IP address, MAC address, screen resolution, size, other PC data, etc. Modern apps are equipped with scroll behavior analysis. It secretly records the amount of time we spent on each post or section of a web page on social media, blog, service, etc. These data help in identifying which user is inclined more in what topics. Accordingly, automated-running AI algorithms prepare a recipe for what to serve the next day and so on. Hence, ISPs and search engines serve many websites and product-based ads with high bandwidth; search engine searches become customized; smart-crawlers became aware of the user preferences & present to us only what the company wants to sell. It dramatically reduces net neutrality, and every user is under the trap of such illicit privacy violations. With the increase in the use of digital assets during this pandemic era, people are drowning more in such a digital trap.

There are various organizations and social media brands who not only take user data for their benefit but also sell them to third-party firms, organizations, or dark web for monetary benefits. Imagine a situation, your wife is looking for precautions to medical complications because she is pregnant. Unfortunately, if she searches the medicine on any popular search engine like Google or Bing, that engine will use that search data & analyze it to suggest similar products. The search system sold your data in real-time to any other pharmaceutical company, which is not only allowing the ad company to show custom ads but also pushing emails with the latest product of that medical complications.

There are many other case studies showing eCommerce companies showing ads based on your previous preferences and collecting your online habits at bulk. Ask yourself, who is storing these data? Are you actually aware of it? Organizations are not only taking our online habits, choices, preferences, and details but also our live locations, movement, distance traveled, system data, etc. We are facing this deadly pandemic. The future might be full of such bio attacks that will be more data-driven.

A question might come to your mind, why hackers choose the darknet to sell the data extracted from a data breach or data leak? A simple answer is, sellers and buyers here at darknet are anonymous, which makes the selling of such illicit entities easy. That is why cybercriminals and black hat hackers prefer this platform.

DATA PRIVACY PREVENTION TECHNIQUES

Keeping all the online credentials, financial records, and personal information safe from outside intruders has always been a priority for enterprises and organizations. But it is more decisive for users to have proper data protection habits and practice sound methods to manage all sensitive personal information safely and securely. Modern companies store a broad spectrum of data about their users. These data include your phone number, credit card details, address, computer information, etc. Here are some essential techniques you can use to protect your data from any data breach or stealing your sensitive data.

1. Encryption: With the advent of the pandemic, more data went online. Protection of the data at rest (on the server) & the data-in-transit (data getting used frequently) in real-time becomes arduous to perform. Therefore, it is better to use data encryption to encrypt data, emails, files, and other sensitive information flowing outside the organization or from your browser. Modern cloud storage uses encryption for both structured and unstructured data.

2. Anti-malware: Malware is one of the sophisticated tools cybercriminals use to target their victim. The pandemic triggered a 72% rise in malware growth, (Security, 2020) carrying 77 new ransomware campaigns with the arrival of the first few months of the pandemic (Lohrmann, 2020). The world has also witnessed a 50% increase in malware-oriented mobile attacks during this short span. Among the mentioned ransomware and malware count, nearly 75% of them targeted healthcare organizations due to the increase in data traffic. Therefore, it is essential for organizations to install anti-malware programs for better data safety.

3. Less is more: You might use apps like Dominos, Zomato, UberEats to order meals online, Air India, Indigo, and other flights to travel. Likewise, every one of us performs some online actions on a daily basis. It is a good practice not to share all the information. We can share the bare minimum information and leave those fields that are not mandatory (*). Also, try not to share that phone number (on those online apps) with which your credit card is linked. The less you share, the more you can protect your data from getting misused.

4. Less is more because, recently, Air India faced a data breach losing data of about 4.5 million passengers since 2011. Payments giant MobiKwik said in late March that they investigated claims of a data breach that exposed the private information of nearly 100 million users. Domino's India has fallen victim to a significant data leak where cybercriminals hacked their database, leaking worth 13 TB (terabytes) data on the Dark Web . This breach includes 180,000,000 order details holding names, phone numbers, emails, addresses, payment details, and a whopping 1,000,000 credit cards.

5. Install Updates: It is a mandatory action to update apps and OS as and when demands. Although leveraging this gigantic pain for users, this is a necessary evil. Failing to install these updates means your computer is at risk. Updates contain radical programs with bug fixes that help protect your system from further breaches. Patching an app reduces attacks and mitigates vulnerabilities of a system. It's best to set your operating system to update automatically. Updates and patches also protect your data leak from recently discovered threats.

6. Backup and security: From the organization's perspective, a public data breach means damage reputation, costing millions, and a possibility of altering millions of data if you don't have a data backup. Enterprises can address the first two using strong encryption, firewall, anti-malware, and other means. But, one of the most elementary yet often overlooked data assurance tips is to back up the data. Duplicating a copy of your data saves a lot of effort when your system data gets stolen or compromised. Backing up your data periodically; saves you from losing your important information.

7. Use VPN: VPN renders your online privacy & anonymity by forming a private network from a public internet connection. VPN has the ability to mask your IP address so that your online actions become untraceable and virtual. VPNs also deliver services by establishing a secure and encrypted connection for providing greater privacy. Every website stores your history, data location, computer information (OS you are using, IP, geolocation, latitude & longitude, monitor resolution, size, other hardware attached, and sometimes MAC address). Using VPN can help you protect yourself from letting others steal your data. Also, VPNs make it harder for companies and cybercriminals to track your e-behavior while you are doing online activities. Make sure your VPN includes IKEv2, OpenVPN, and L2TP/IPsec to keep your data safe. Also, make sure whether your VPN has a no-user data storage policy or not.

8. Passwords and paraphrases: Account users and employees should use paraphrases rather than passwords. Paraphrases are nothing but random words or sentences that may or may not have appropriate meaning and contain numbers, spaces, special characters, symbols, etc. Also, experts recommend keeping these paraphrases meaningless so that cybercriminals and illicit hackers do not get the sense or use social engineering on your paraphrases.

9. Data masking: It is an exciting concept that ensures the security of data. Data masking helps in data obfuscation. This process involves hiding the initial/sensitive data with codes, raw data, and other random characters. It is the most popular data security technique or situation that can help organizations and enterprises secure classified information. Data masking also have the ability to mask data in such a way that the database admins or the internal management employees will find it difficult to extract user data and private detailing from it easily. This way, enterprises can be certain that only internal employees knowing the data's details, masking algorithms, & randomization mechanism can understand the data.

10. Row-level Security: This particular way of protecting confidential or sensitive data helps restricting access to the data for specific users. If you are familiar with Microsoft's Power BI tool, you'd know - it allows you to add restrictive filters to the company's dashboards, data sets, and reports using Row Level Security. Through this, different users in a company can achieve access; and can manage sensitive data accessibility that requires adequate attention. Row-level security is exceptionally suitable when dealing with Business Intelligence (BI) or data warehousing.

11. Vendors and partners' Data protection standards: Enterprises and organizations these days take the cloud and other data-related services from different vendors and partners. They should keep in mind that the vendors or partners they got associated with should maintain high data protection standards. When working with other companies that can handle your customer data, make sure that they must possess adequate systems for protecting the data.

ANONYMITY IN DATA PUBLISHING AND MINING

In the previous section, we have learned the various ways to preserve our data from getting into the wrong hands. In this section, we will go through some anonymous data publishing and mining techniques that we can place to secure the data. Data security for privacy protection should go in such a way that even if cyber criminals steal our data, they won't be able to extract the meaning out of it or analyze it meaningfully. In this section, we will understand some deeper techniques that can use to protect data in this pandemic. There are two ways to anonymize data.

- Anonymity by Randomization: Various data privacy researchers and firms use the latest randomization methods to modify data to preserve the privacy of sensitive information. This method was earlier meant for statistical disclosure control. But now, enterprises and data security and privacy development engineers and professionals use it in privacy-preserving and data mining implementations. In the randomization technique, data gets blended with reliable random noise to perturb the data. By doing this, even the internal employees won't be able to steal those sensitive data because random noise data gets added in such a way that it becomes difficult to extract the original value out of it. But the randomization algorithms attached to it can fetch back the original data from the perturbed data. There are two sub-techniques of anonymizing data with random distorted data merging. These are

  - Data distortion by Additive Randomization: During the last two years, especially during the excitation state of this COVID, adding noise to the data and distorting its originality to preserve the sensitive data and its privacy became a general approach for enterprises. Let suppose, O = {O1, O2, O3, ..., On} is an original dataset that requires anonymity using randomization for better privacy-preserving. A new distorted dataset D = {D1, D2, D3, ..., Dn} will be added to it as noise. The value of this distorted dataset will be randomly picked and using a probability distribution, a noise amount n_i will be added to each record of the distorted dataset. The final output will be P (Privacy-preserved dataset) = O (Original dataset) + D (Distorted dataset)

  - Data distortion by Multiplicative Random Perturbation: This is popular in data-mining security and privacy. This technique leverages two different multiplicative noises. The first technique uses the logarithmic transformation of data for generating random noise. Then the second technique uses multivariate normal distribution. Finally, the antilog of the noise data is accepted and multiplied with the original dataset.

- Anonymity by Indistinguishability: The randomization technique becomes effective if the randomization input is very dynamic and real-time user-driven. Also, the randomization technique that uses hashing is much more beneficial. But many enterprises use other random data generation techniques that might fall apart. Randomization with these weak techniques might not be beneficial for expert privacy-breakers if they have prior knowledge of the algorithms and randomization process. That is where anonymity by indistinguishability comes into action. This technique helps better in reducing the probability of record identification from any public or stored dataset. It uses the suppression technique, where the algorithm will suppress some of the data values while keeping other data intact. This technique of anonymity by indistinguishability is known as k-anonymity. Unfortunately, k-anonymity might go fragile if the attacker performs homogeneity attacks or background knowledge attacks on the suppressed dataset. That is where the l-diversity framework got proposed. It another form of anonymity by indistinguishability technique that takes care of maintaining a diversity of sensitive data attributes so that background knowledge, guess and figure out attacks, and homogeneity attacks won't impact stealing the data.

Organizations and enterprises should opt these measures to protect their data privacy and leakage for better service to customers.

CONCLUSION

An enormous set of sensitive data are getting produced daily. Nurturing them with care & privacy-preserving interest should be a concern - especially in this global pandemic situation, where everything from learning to office work went digital. Also, companies are harvesting big data for business insight, customer behavioral insights, and understanding their products better from the users' perspective. All these raise a deafening privacy concern, and hence this chapter focuses on data privacy and the impact it could cause from a slight mistake. Enterprises & organizations involved in data mining, storage, and analysis should implement proper measures to use these data privacy-preserving techniques to anonymize and protect the true essence of users' data.

REFERENCES

COVID-19 Pandemic Sparks 72% Ransomware Growth, Mobile Vulnerabilities Grow 50%, Skybox Security. (2021). https://www.prnewswire.com/in/news-releases/covid-19-pandemic-sparks-72-ransomware-growth-mobile-vulnerabilities-grow-50--817268901.html

Domino's India data hacked? 1 million credit card details, phone numbers allegedly leaked. (2021). *Business Today.* https://www.businesstoday.in/latest/corporate/story/omg-dominos-india-hacked-1-million-credit-card-details-names-phone-numbers-leaked-293943-2021-04-20

During, R. (2020). *COVID-19.* https://www.govtech.com/blogs/lohrmann-on-cybersecurity/ransomware-during-covid-19.html

Impact of digital surge during Covid-19 pandemic: A viewpoint on research and practice. (2020). https://www.ncbi.nlm.nih.gov/pmc/articles/PMC7280123/

IoT Privacy and Security. Challenges and Solutions. (2020). https://www.mdpi.com/2076-3417/10/12/4102/pdf

Must-Know Data Breach Statistics for 2021. (n.d.). *IBM.* https://www.varonis.com/blog/data-breach-statistics/

WHO reports fivefold increase in cyber attacks, urges vigilance. (2020). *WHO.* https://www.who.int/news/item/23-04-2020-who-reports-fivefold-increase-in-cyber-attacks-urges-vigilance

Chapter 14
Designing a Real–Time Dashboard for Pandemic Management:
COVID–19 Using Qlik Sense

Rahul Rai
Indira Gandhi National Open University, India

ABSTRACT

COVID-19 is very dynamic in nature, and it is varying drastically with time, and this requires continuous monitoring of the situation for better resource management during the pandemic such as medical facilities and daily necessities. The situation needs to be evaluated on a regular interval by all the stakeholders such as all the government officials for making strategic decisions such as lockdown or lifting lockdown in a phase-wise manner. In order to manage pandemics such as COVID-19, the administration needs to know statistical information, trends, forecasting, and overall aggregated real-time information, and this can be achieved through a well-designed dashboard. A dashboard is used for efficient monitoring of continuously evolving situations, and it provides an overall picture in addition to historical information. This chapter proposes a real-time dashboard design for COVID-19, and it will provide insight about different elements such as design and application of the dashboard in pandemic management.

COVID -19 OUTBREAK

Covid-19 stands for Coronavirus diseases. "Co" stands for Corona, "Vi" stands for virus, "d" stands for diseases and "19" stands for 2019 because the first case was confirmed in 2019. Talking of the first case, it was identified in Wuhan, Hubei, China in December 2019. Initially also referred to as "Wuhan Coronavirus". SARS-Cov-2 (Severe accurate respiratory syndrome coronavirus 2) was the official name given by WHO (World Health Organization) on February 11, 2020. It is believed to be an animal origin disease. The first identified patient was named as "Patient Zero".

DOI: 10.4018/978-1-7998-7188-0.ch014

From China it travelled to several countries and reached India on January 30 through a student from Wuhan in Kerala. The first three cases identified in India were all through students who returned from Wuhan and all the three cases were in Kerala only. The fourth case was identified in Delhi and the patient had returned from Italy. Similarly, the fifth case was identified in Hyderabad with a travelling history from UAE (United Arab Emirates). The sixth and the seventh both cases were identified in Jaipur, Rajasthan and both were with a travelling history from Italy. And from there it started spreading all across the nation.

SARS-CoV-2 originated in bats and is also responsible for MERS (Middle East respiratory syndrome) and SARS (Severe accurate respiratory syndrome). Coronavirus was first identified in humans in 1965. It was named Coronavirus after its crown-like appearance. SARS first emerged in Southern China in 2002 and MERS started in Saudi Arabia in 2012 According to "COVID-19 pandemic in India"(2021).

Coronavirus has mutated over time. Alpha was found in late 2020 in Southern England and USA. These mutations make the virus 70% more transmissible. The mutation was on the spike protein and the COVID-19 targeted this spike protein mutation. Beta was found in South Africa and Nigeria. It spreads more easily but worsens the illness. Gamma, Founded in January 2021. It travelled from Brazil to Japan and by the end of the month reached the USA. It is more contagious than the earlier strains. Infected people who have already had COVID-19. Delta, It was spotted in India in December 2020. The surge in the second wave in mid April 2021 was caused because of this mutation. Currently found in 43 countries including the USA, UK, Singapore, Australia etc. Earlier mutations were mostly in aged people but this mutation was causing more in young people According to "Variants of Coronavirus"(2021).

Figure 1.

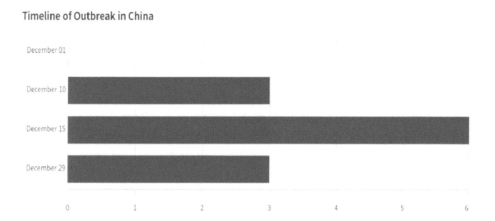

GROWTH OF COVID-19 FROM ORIGIN TO 1ST LOCKDOWN

Covid-19 originated from China and the first case of the Covid-19 in India was found on January 30, 2020. After that the cases increased day by day at a rapid speed. This increment has affected us so badly because there wasn't any remedy to stop it. Every sector was affected badly by it, the most affected were the lives of people who relied on daily wages. At the initial stages no one really thought it would be out of our hands to control that we will have to declare a nationwide lockdown.

Figure 2.

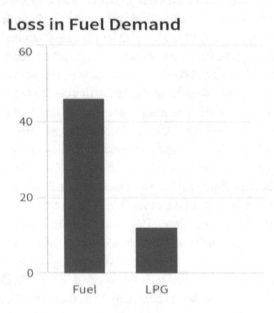

Loss in Fuel Demand

Lockdown was a very urgent requirement of that time but in order to do that on this large scale, there are many variables which need to be taken into account because the necessities like food, water etc. which are essential for survival are equally important as the lockdown was.

India has the second largest school system after China. Due to COVID-19 almost 90% of schools, colleges and universities were closed impacting a total of 320 million students in India (Pothula,2021). To cope up with this situation online learning came into the picture but this was challenging as most people live in areas without internet connectivity. A large population was untouched by online learning and most government-run schools were poor-equipped. There was a huge disparity between the urban and rural areas in terms of online learning. Only 4.4% households in rural areas had computers as compared to 23.4% in urban areas. And households with internet connectivity in rural and urban areas are 14.9% and 42% respectively(Modi & Postaria,2020). This was a huge disparity which needed to be dealt with. Moreover, due to the sudden switch towards online learning, it was not planned efficiently and the curriculum was not designed for such a format. Online learning is a passive learning process and as a result of this students were losing interest and there were low levels of attention span(Misra,2020). The difficulty was not only for the students but teachers also faced difficulty in switching to online learning as they were unprepared for online education. Due to changes in the examination and assessment format, changing the format of student recruitment for colleges and higher studies was also needed and those students planning to study abroad were stuck without any information due to restrictions on travelling (Gautam,2020). Education is the necessity for an individual and for the development of the society or any nation.

As mentioned earlier, there are so many variables and depending on them the resources need to be managed. But taking in account all the variables and making an insight from it is a very tedious job to do, but it needs to be done and with the time constraints it becomes more difficult to do this.

Figure 3. (COVID19-India API,2021)

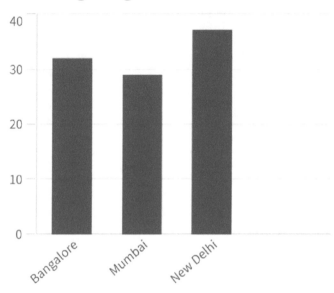

IMPACT ON ECONOMY

Covid-19 impacted us in many ways, one of them was on the Economy. Almost every economic sector was disruptively hit by Covid-19. Major parts which constitute the economy are agriculture, exports and imports, energy, stock market, etc. In April 2020, exports and imports both had a loss by 36.65% and 47.36% respectively.

Figure 4.

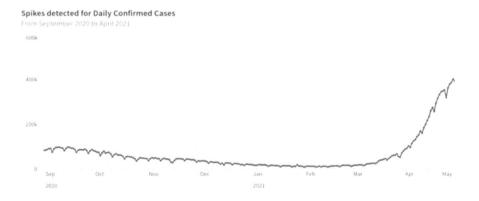

Figure 5.

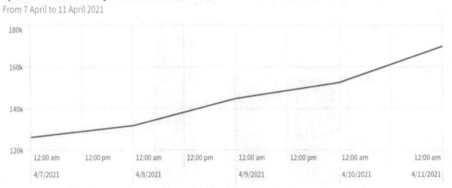

Figure 6.

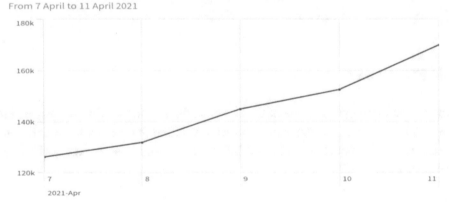

Most farmers were not even able to yield and those who did, 60% of them faced loss. The problem was not only restricted to this season but farmers also faced yielding for the next season. Tea industry faced a huge revenue loss. Tea exports fell from 8% to 33% in March 2020.

In the energy sector, night light radiance is well connected with the economy and there was a drastic decrease in it. New Delhi had the biggest loss by 37.2% followed by Bangalore and Mumbai by 32% and 29% respectively. Fuel demand in April 2020, fell by 46% as compared to the previous year. Cooking gas (LPG) also faced a loss by 12%.

On 23 March 2020, the stock market faced one of the worst losses in history. Sensex fell by 4000 points i.e., 13.15% and NSE NIFTY by 1150 points i.e., 12.98%. Overall, the markets faced a huge loss.

During lockdown the price of fuels were increasing continuously which impacted the citizens as well as the overall economy. The increase in the fuel price impacted people who own personal vehicles as their monthly budget was disturbed. High fuel prices also impacted the automobile sector which is one of the largest sources of employment in the country and there was observed a dip in sales of automobiles

Figure 7.

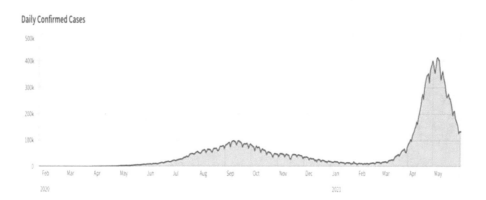

especially passenger and two-wheeler vehicles. Companies related to logistics and transportation were also suffering due to increase in the fuel price and they increased their service rate, transport and freight increased around 10-15% in their cost. Most products which are commonly used in any household are mostly transported from other states and as the transportation costs were higher it impacted in the increment of the price of the products. Overall, everything which involved transportation or travelling either directly or indirectly were impacted in some way.

The inflation rate was higher as compared to last year, whereas in most of the countries there was a dip in the inflation According to "Under the shadow of Covid-19 pandemic, inflation bites India the hardest" (2020).

The rise in the food prices was affected due to inflation. Main reason for the food inflation spike was due to the transportation disruption due to lockdown, goods and delivery services were also disrupted. In October 2020 the food inflation surged to 11% but came down to 9.43% in November 2020(Inani,2021). The reason for the increase in the price mainly of pulses was due to a 30% shortage of labourers because of reverse migration, this resulted in 10-15% increase in the price. The food inflation rose to 8.6% in April 2020 from 7.8% in the previous month. The poor section of the people were the most affected due to food inflation According to "As RBI Remains Worried over Food Inflation, How Prices of Daal and Milk Rose During Covid-19 Lockdown"(2020).

66% of jobs were affected due to COVID-19 and 28% faced deduction from salaries and many were not even getting salary. To this the government asked private establishments to pay full wages to workers during COVID-19 and the employers who were not able to do so were asked to furnish their audited balance sheets and accounts in the court According to "Private companies claiming incapacity in paying full wages must place balance sheets in court: Centre tells SC"(2020).

SECOND WAVE OF COVID-19

With the outbreak of Covid-19 in India, everything and everyone faced challenges. But with time the situation was getting better. As a result of this mask-wearing and social distancing was not obeyed as strictly as it needed to be. Since April 2021, there has been a surge in Covid-19 infections in India. On an average there were over 3 lakh new cases daily. On April 02,2021 we observed the greatest number of

Figure 8.

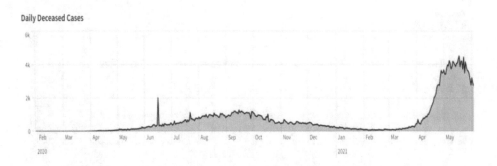

Figure 9.

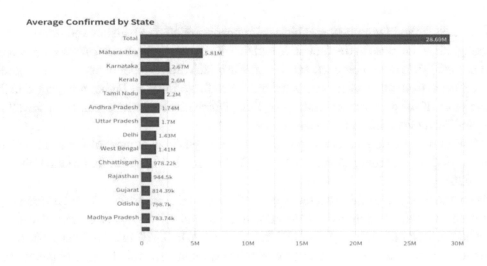

cases in the past 6 months. From April 7 to April 11 the number of cases grew very rapidly, the reason behind this rapid growth was because of large religious gathering and massive political rallies and as mentioned earlier no mask wearing and social distancing was taken seriously for this also. 80% - 85% of the positive cases in India were asymptomatic and they were not isolating themselves According to"What has changed in the second wave of Covid-19 in India?(2021). As a result, they were interacting freely with people and this also led to the surge in Covid-19 infections. During the first phase there was a large disparity between the cases in rural areas as compared to urban areas. When the second wave arrived, the disparity was almost negligible. The reason behind this was the travelling of people working in urban areas to the rural areas prior to the lockdown. The rapid growth in the rural areas was a serious point of concern because the houses were very close to each other and people there were not so aware. Maintaining social distance was very difficult under such circumstances. Also, medical facilities available in rural areas are not adequate. Providing medical supplies in rural areas from cities was inconvenient due to lockdown. Oxygen requirement during the second wave was more as compared to the first wave because during the second wave the virus mutated which made it stronger and it attacked directly on our lungs. As daily needs were stored during the first nationwide lockdown which resulted

Figure 10.

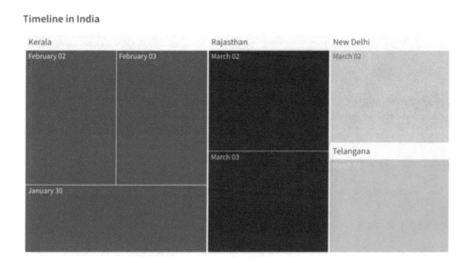

in its shortage for the first few weeks, the same thing happened with the oxygen cylinder. With time the need for oxygen cylinder was everywhere, even urban areas were suffering badly from the shortage of the oxygen cylinder and on top of that fulfilling the need of rural areas was out of question. Countries like USA, UK, Singapore, Australia, Saudi Arabia, UAE, France, Germany, Russia helped India in providing oxygen concentrators, generators and other medical supplies in fighting against the disease. Meanwhile the government took the initiative of laying down oxygen plants in 60 days.

The Indian Military helped in setting up Covid facilities and oxygen plants which were needed badly at that time. Not only the Indian Military but other industries also helped us in some ways. Ola provided the service of door-to-door delivery of oxygen tanks. The USA and other countries like the United Kingdom, European Union and Pakistan pledged to provide medical supplies to the country.

Figure 11.

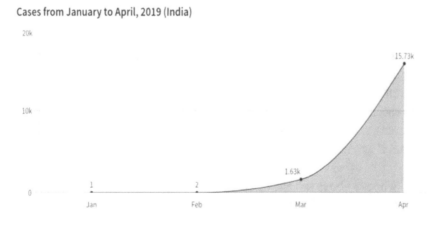

There was a significant fall in the number of cases for three consecutive days i.e., from 14 May to 17 May 2021. At present also the situation is better than the first few weeks of April but still the precautionary measures need to be followed strictly.

Figure 12.

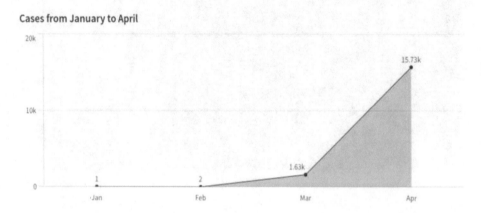

VACCINE AND ITS DISTRIBUTION

Vaccines are biologically prepared in order to fight against an infection. In India vaccines are provided free of cost and are supplied to neighbouring countries like Bangladesh, Myanmar, Nepal, Bhutan etc. to help them fight coronavirus According to "COVID-19 Updates"(2021). The coronavirus that causes COVID-19 has spikes of protein and these spikes allow the virus to attach to the cells and cause harm to it.The vaccine introduces the immune system to an inactive or weakened form of SARS-CoV-2 coronavirus or a part of it. This does not cause coronavirus and helps the body from future infection from the virus(Martin,2021). Vaccines recognise the spikes of protein as an enemy or foreigner and fight against it and lower the chances of getting COVID-19. In India two vaccines were authorized by the Central Drugs Standard Control Organization (CDSCO) According to "Frequently Asked Questions"(2021). First one is Covishield which is manufactured by Serum Institute of India (SII) and the other one manufactured by Bharat Biotech was named Covaxin According to "Can all adults get vaccinated in 2021" (2021). Both the vaccines completed their phase I and phase II trials. Covishield has completed its phase III trial in the United Kingdom.

India began the administration of the vaccines on January 16, 2021. According to "Timeline of the COVID-19 pandemic in India"(2021)

" First recipients were the health workers, working in direct contact of the Covid-19 patients.

In the First phase, vaccines were administered to only health workers and frontline workers such as police, paramilitary forces, sanitation workers and disaster management volunteers.

In the Second phase, it was administered to the following categories

1. All the residents who are above the age of 60 years.
2. All the residents whose age lies between 45 – 60 years with one or more qualifying health issues.

Figure 13.

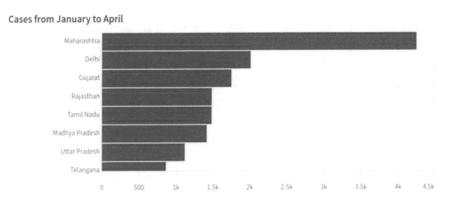

3.   Health care or frontline workers who were given the first dose in phase I.

In the Third phase Sputnik V was approved for distribution by the Drugs Controller General of India (DCGI) on April 12, 2021.
The next phase program will start from May 01, 2021 for all those who are above the age of 18 years.

Figure 14.

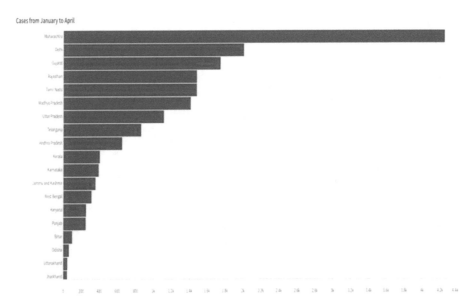

PRESENT SITUATION COMPARED TO COVID - 19 OUTBREAK

There is always a difference in the approach and damage when we encounter something for the first time as compared to the second time. This also happened when we were first hit by the first wave of Covid-19 as compared to when hit by the second wave. The first wave started around March 2020 and the nation-wide lockdown started from 25 March 2020 and the peak of the first wave was in the month of September 2020. The second wave started around the first week of March 2021.

During the first wave the cases were not so significant as compared to other countries like the United States, Brazil etc. and it was also less than the second wave. During the second wave India led the world in new and active cases. On 30 April 2021, India overtook Brazil and became the second country with most cases worldwide and was only behind the United States. The reason for this rapid growth is Holi on March 29, Kumbh mela in April, Sporting events such as IPL, State and Local elections.

When it comes to the economic impact in both waves, the market faced the greatest loss since 2007 during the first wave but it also strengthened the domestic resilience for the second wave. The domestic stock market has been in the positive rally since October 2020.

When the first nation-wide lockdown happened, people stocked food supplies and Retail and Consumer goods sales were doubled on 19 March 2020. This disrupted food supplies and led to a food crisis. But during the second wave no such thing happened.

Most of the situations were far better during the second wave as compared to the first wave except the number of new active cases and deceased rate.

Core areas like banking and payment are considered pillars of the economy. They were adopting digitalisation but due to pandemic it was accelerated in India by 3 to 5 years. There was an outbreak in digital payments, a surge was experienced in digital payments across online stores, small retail outlets, pharmacies, vegetables and other daily needs. Contactless payments such as QR code, wallets, UPI provide convenience, safety and security to consumers. By using these digital payment options maintaining social distance became manageable which was the need of the hour(Doshi,2020). There was a jump of 30% to digital transformation, 80% in cloud spending, 15% in customer experience. In short COVID -19 crisis accelerated our shift towards digitalisation According to "COVID-19 has accelerated digitisation process: study"(2020).

Many applications were developed to make our life easier during this pandemic. Coronavirus health monitoring app which makes us aware of the disease and its symptoms. Due to lockdown, work from home was made compulsory for some time and managing family with work was becoming very hectic on some days, food delivering apps and daily needs saved some time made the hectic routine manageable. Apart from daily needs there are several things any individual needs like clothes, electronics, stationery, etc. Mobile shopping apps were very useful with that According to "Top Mobile App Categories during COVID-19"(2021).

During the first lockdown phase a large population was untouched by online education but now the situation has reversed. Governments of respective states provided tablet or android phones to those who needed it, especially in rural areas. Online education has its own benefits like it is very affordable as compared to physical learning and can be studied anywhere at any time. Now the curriculum is also made according to that and study materials are provided online, again helping in social distancing.

Figure 15.

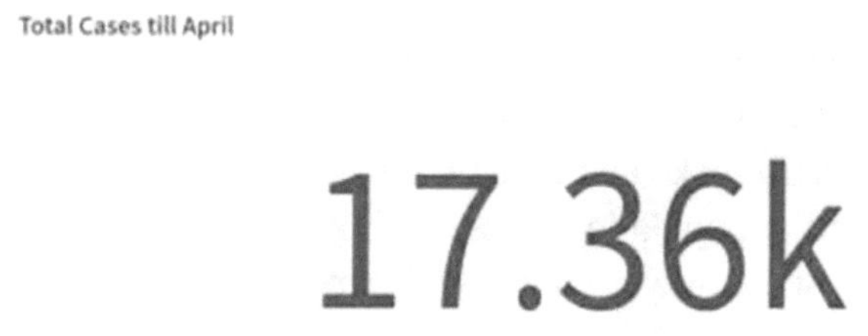

Total Cases till April
17.36k

Figure 16.

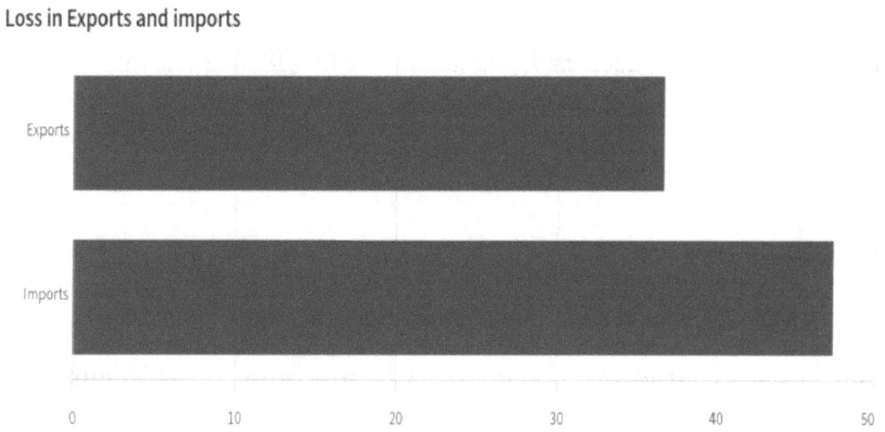

Loss in Exports and imports
Exports
Imports
0
10
20
30
40
50

Figure 17.

Loss in Stock Market
NIFTY
SENSEX
0
1
2
3
4
5
6
7
8
9
10
11
12
13
14

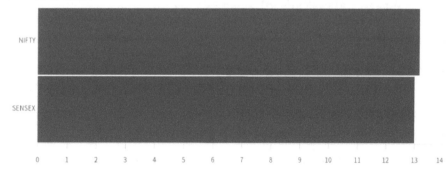

CONCLUSION

The pandemic affected the whole world and it not only affected any particular area or any particular section of people. It affected almost every sector and every section of people. This shows how deep were the roots of COVID-19. To make an impact there must be several factors considered to study the impact and to make most of the population aware of it in order to fight this pandemic. To display so many variables, one of the suitable ways is to show it through the dashboard as it makes understanding of the data in a simple and understandable way i.e. through graphs. Dashboard takes all the variables under one umbrella and shows the data in a way that it does not stress more on the cognitive load and eliminates the misunderstanding of the data. Real time dashboard saves time by highlighting the data which is relevant to us.

Qlik Sense is a data analytics application which allows users to create interactive dashboard, visualization and charts. Through Qlik Sense we can take dimensions and measures. By taking dimensions and measures we can create charts or visualizations which will represent our data in a visual form. Usually visualizing data makes it easy to understand. Another aspect of Qlik Sense is that it generates insights from the data provided to it and users can use these insights for their use. All the above visualizations were made using Qlik Sense.

REFERENCES

API. (2021, July 1). *COVID19-India API.* https://api.covid19india.org/

BBC. (2021, July 1). *India coronavirus: Can all adults get vaccinated in 2021?* https://www.bbc.com/news/world-asia-india-55571793

Digiteum. (2021, July 1). *Top Mobile App Categories during COVID-19.* https://www.digiteum.com/top-mobile-app-categories-covid/

e-Learning Industry. (2021, July 1). *Advantages And Disadvantages Of Online Learning.* https://el-earningindustry.com/advantages-and-disadvantages-online-learning

Express, F. (2021, July 1). *Private companies claiming incapacity in paying full wages must place balance sheets in court: Centre tells SC.* https://www.financialexpress.com/india-news/salary-cut-during-lockdown-supreme-court-home-ministry-order-private-companies-balance-sheet/1981053/

KPMG. (2021, July 1). *How COVID-19 is accelerating digitalisation for the….* https://home.kpmg/in/en/blogs/home/posts/2020/07/how-covid-19-accelerating-digitalisation-banking-payments-industry.html

Medical News Today. (2021, July 1). *How do COVID-19 vaccines work?* https://www.medicalnewstoday.com/articles/how-do-covid-19-vaccines-work

Ministry of External Affairs. (2021, July 1). *COVID-19 Updates.* https://www.mea.gov.in/vaccine-supply.htm

Ministry of Health and Family Welfare. (2021, July 1). *Frequently Asked Questions.* https://www.mohfw.gov.in/covid_vaccination/vaccination/faqs.html#about-the-vaccine

News 18. (2021, July 1). *As RBI Remains Worried over Food Inflation, How Prices of Daal and Milk Rose During Covid-19 Lockdown.* https://www.news18.com/news/india/as-rbi-remains-worried-over-food-inflation-how-prices-of-daal-milk-rose-during-lockdown-2662815.html

Report, G. S. (2021, July 1). *COVID-19's impact on education in India: It's not all bad news.* https://www.globalsistersreport.org/news/ministry/column/covid-19s-impact-education-india-its-not-all-bad-news

Sisense. (2021, July 1). *Real Time Dashboard.* https://www.sisense.com/glossary/real-time-dashboard/#:~:text=A%20real%2Dtime%20dashboard%20is,the%20most%20current%20data%20available.&text=Real%2Dtime%20dashboards%20can%20be,day%2Dto%2Dday%20basis

Standard, B. (2021, July 1). *Under the shadow of Covid-19 pandemic, inflation bites India the hardest.* https://www.business-standard.com/article/economy-policy/under-the-shadow-of-covid-19-pandemic-inflation-bites-india-the-hardest-120121600750_1.html

The Hindu. (2021, July 1). *COVID-19 has accelerated digitisation process: study.* https://www.thehindu.com/business/covid-19-has-accelerated-digitisation-process-study/article33243203.ece

The Indian Express. (2021, July 1). *Explained: What has changed in the second wave of Covid-19 in India?* https://indianexpress.com/article/explained/explained-whats-changed-in-second-wave-7289002/

The Quint. (2021, July 1). *India's Poor Are Eating Into Their Savings, Thanks To High Inflation And Covid-19.* https://www.bloombergquint.com/economy-finance/indias-poor-are-eating-into-their-savings-thanks-to-high-inflation-and-covid-19

Today, I. (2021, July 1). *Covid-19: 4 negative impacts and 4 opportunities created for education.* https://www.indiatoday.in/education-today/featurephilia/story/covid-19-4-negative-impacts-and-4-opportunities-created-for-education-1677206-2020-05-12

Web, M. D. (2021, July 1). *Variants of Coronavirus.* https://www.webmd.com/lung/coronavirus-strains#3

Wikipedia contributors. (2021a, July 1). COVID-19 pandemic in India. In *Wikipedia, The Free Encyclopedia.* Retrieved 18:55, July 1, 2021, from https://en.wikipedia.org/w/index.php?title=COVID-19_pandemic_in_India&oldid=1031367334

Wikipedia contributors. (2021b, June 29). Timeline of the COVID-19 pandemic in India (2021). In *Wikipedia, The Free Encyclopedia.* Retrieved 18:56, July 1, 2021, from https://en.wikipedia.org/w/index.php?title=Timeline_of_the_COVID-19_pandemic_in_India_(2021)&oldid=1030989391

Wikipedia contributors. (2021c, July 1). COVID-19 pandemic in India. In *Wikipedia, The Free Encyclopedia.* Retrieved 19:05, July 1, 2021, from https://en.wikipedia.org/w/index.php?title=COVID-19_pandemic_in_India&oldid=1031367334

World Economic Forum. (2021, July 1). *How COVID-19 deepens the digital education divide in India.* https://www.weforum.org/agenda/2020/10/how-covid-19-deepens-the-digital-education-divide-in-india/

Chapter 15
Corona:
The Development Invader

Mansha Sharma
Mithibai College, Mumbai University, India

Ajay Kumar Sharma
Human Resource Development Centre, Lovely Professional University, India

ABSTRACT

Coronavirus has come up as the worst nightmare in the form of a pandemic for progressive sapiens in terms of health, wealth, prosperity, and social wellbeing. To date, coronavirus has mutated to seven different shapes evolving into various variants. The main deliberation of catching the disease is carelessness and negligence of the citizens, and in developing countries like India, population and illiteracy makes it even more difficult to control the disease. However, immunity can be the superhero in fighting against the virus that invades the host. Although a strong immunity is important to fight the disease, the symptoms show at a later stage by the body of a human with a stronger immunity and cases are getting critical in this case. After a long struggle, scientists have come up with vaccines that are 90% efficient and show some side effects. The world is expected to function only if 'herd immunity' is achieved, but it is expected that wearing masks would be the new normal.

INTRODUCTION

The world has witnessed Pandemics and overcame the consequences successfully. With time, the technology gave an uplift to medical science, some unimaginable treatments, experiments came out to be successful. Although, this advancement in technology could not help the world in curing a virus like Corona virus which is responsible for global pandemic. Corona virus has come up as the worst nightmare in the form of a pandemic for progressive sapiens in terms of health, wealth, prosperity, and various social well beings.

DOI: 10.4018/978-1-7998-7188-0.ch015

BACKGROUND

Corona viruses are a family of viruses that causes infections like common cold. The strains of these viruses are often observed in animals like bats, camels, and this SARS- COV2 is expected to be determined from a bat while experimenting, in the virology labs of Wuhan, China.

When the virus started to spread in the 'Wet Market' of Wuhan, where animals were killed on the spot and sold to the consumers, it was thought that the strain affecting the humans came from the 'Pangolins' which are also noticed as scaly anteaters because bat was not sold in the market at that time. Later, the theories concluded, the variant was from the bat. On 11 February 2020, WHO named novel corona virus as COVID-19 where 'Co' stands for corona, 'Vi' stands for virus and 'D' stands for disease which emerged in 2019.

Since the Pandemic has started, the variant has mutated and evolved its shape seven times, making it difficult for the researchers to construct an effective vaccine or a medication to fight against the virus with minimum side effects.

HISTORY

Human corona virus, first portrayed during the 1960s, are liable for a considerable extent of upper respiratory lot diseases in kids. Since 2003, at any rate five new human Corona virus strains have been recognized. It is including the serious intense respiratory condition virus, which caused huge bleakness and mortality. The historical backdrop of human corona virus started in 1965 when Tyrrell and Bynoe found that they could entry an infection named B814. It was found in human undeveloped tracheal organ societies got from the respiratory plot of a child with a common virus.

The kid had regular indications and indications of the common cold and the washing was discovered to have the option to instigate common colds in volunteers tested intranasally. The infection, named B814, could be developed in human undeveloped organism tracheal organ tissue yet not in cell lines utilized around then for developing other known etiologic specialists of the common virus. (Parhlo, 30 March 2020)

EMERGENCE OF CORONA VIRUS

In 2019, China claimed that there was corona outbreak in the Wuhan City. The travel was held responsible for the spread of the virus outside the country. As the virus started to spread in the early 2020, the world went under lockdown and countries like Italy, America, India, Brazil and many more. The situation was out of control that the bodies were being dumped in big numbers in dump yards.

Every time a pandemic strike, it is expected to hit the population in four to five waves. The first was tackled with uttermost precautions and strictness. When things started to get normal countries unlocked the facilities that were under lockdown which emerged as the second wave of the corona virus, with variety of variants from different countries. The virus began to spread again and till date the world is cope up with the virus, although the vaccinations are in the market, citizens have become precautious, but it is observed that when a virus evolves, its transmissibility increases but the variant becomes less harmful, however, corona virus is becoming more transmissible and harmful with each evolution.

HOW HAS CORONA AFFECTED THE NATIONS?

As soon as the corona virus started to travel, it affected the country's GDP, especially developing countries like India which grows exponentially, dropped to 3.1%. Imagine a country like USA, which is considered as a leading nation, experienced a downgrade in its GDP during the global pandemic. Therefore, it was evident for developing countries to suffer. In addition to this, not just the GDP of the countries were infected from the virus, the aspects linked to it were tragically affected especially the businesses, crashed and companies had to sell out their shares, the industries had to turn down the outlets or franchise. The circumstances of most affected territories are discussed below:

1.   China:

On 31 December 2019, China reported 41 patients to WHO articulating that the patients were suffering from some mysterious kind of Pneumonia. The researchers concluded that the virus might have originated in the late November. After some speculation it was found that the virus was originated in the bats and later from scaly anteaters the virus spread to humans from the wet market of Wuhan City. After the conclusion to the origination, in January 2020 the market was shut. On 11 January 2020, China reported its first death from novel corona virus, since then, the globe is reporting deaths. Then, after this death, a Doctor, Li Wenliang from China insisted in a conference that the virus would lead to a pandemic and should be looked after but the doctor died himself due to corona virus as reported by the Chinese government who accused the doctor of spreading rumours about corona virus after more than 500 deaths were recorded. This gave a boom to a conspiracy theory that China could have used the variant of corona virus as a biological weapon against countries to become the leading nation of the world and overcome USA. WHO does not have proper statistics of China and the country is functioning very well in the pandemic and expected to surpass USA and become the succeeding country.

The first case that was reported outside China was in Thailand. 64-year-old women had a travel history from China. (Business insider, n.d.)

2.   United States of America:

On 21 January 2020, USA reported its first case of a Man in his 30's who had a travel history to Wuhan City. The Centre od Disease Control and Prevention (CDC) confirmed its first case in California which had no travel history and made no contact, this was the initiation of the local transmission in United States. On February 2020, USA reported its first death from covid and later, they were running out of space to bury the dead bodies. Th country was trying to control the situation on 25 May 2020 the death of George Floyd initiated the movement of 'Black lives Matter' and situation got worse in terms of peace and pandemic in USA under the Presidentship of Donald Trump.

This affected the country and there were certain movements initiated by the citizens of USA which made the situation worse like No mask movements which was very unnecessary!

It took corona virus two months to spread in all the 50 states of America, and an emergency was declared by Donald Trump where he sanctioned a 50 billion funding to fight against the disease. On 20 March 2020, an emergency was launched in New York and the situation has just gotten worse by then.

The pandemic affected the relations of USA with WHO and it has dropped out from the global health collective which would be implemented from July 2021. (ABC news, 22 September 2020)

3.   India:

India is the second most populated country after China. Landmass much lesser than United states or China. The nation recorded its first case on 30 January 2020, the similar day WHO declared COVID-19 as a global pandemic. A 20-year-old which came back from Wuhan was diagnosed positive in Kerala. When the first death was reported in India, the travel was suspended from 13 March to 15 April. These were the initiations of the pandemic affecting the economy of the country, and GDP started to downgrade and ended on to 3.1%.

India is a developing country, the sanitation, medical facilities to cover the whole population were quite mediocre and the virus all the businesses irrespective of its network. The country has the largest railway network which experienced immense loss at the time of pandemic. The Prime Minister of India, Narendra Modi did every bit to control the first wave and side by side banned the Chinese mobile phone applications that generated millions of revenues from the user consumption.

Gradually, the cases in India grew exponentially and India became the third most affected country after Brazil and Italy. The deaths increased; the below poverty line citizens walked thou-sands of kilometres to reach their home. The country saw its worst days, but the condition started to improve in September 2020. The government decided to unlock the country, which was the biggest mistake taken by the country according to WHO. While the country was resuming to recover, the corona virus was evolving itself to a variant which was deadlier than before, and India hit its second wave and went under lockdown again.

Several other countries were drastically affected like Italy, United Kingdom, where the death rates made records.

PENETRATION INSIDE THE HUMAN BODY

COVID-19 is a communicable disease that spreads through droplets in air and considered as an airborne disease. The virus has a high transmissibility rate and affects majorly the elderly age group and if proper care is not taken can be fatal. It affects the lungs and cause shortness of breath and ultimately the 02 level starts to decrease, and body fails to throw out Co2 and lungs get filled with Co2. This disease at its earliest was deadly for the people who were diabetic, had other health issues. Although, the younger generation could surpass the virus, the progress has made it transmissible to the youth. When an infectant sneezes without taking any precautions, considering the sickness is airborne, the virus accumulates on the surface and air and enters the nasal passage of the host who has not taken proper precautions gets infected and the respiratory system gets affected.

SYMPTOMS IN THE HUMAN BODY

Everybody reacts to an infection in a different way, the elementary indications are a sore throat, high fever, loss of smell and taste, shortness of breath in extreme condition, gastrointestinal complications, Fatigue. It is not compulsory that the infectant experiences all the symptoms. The immune system plays a vital role in regulating the antibodies and countering the virus to protect the host body initially. The body with a better immune system faces more complications in the treatment of disease as the immunity initially fights with the virus and shows negligible symptoms however when the body fails to respond the virus is established properly into the host and ready to act and infect the body and the treatment is delayed, whereas when a person with weak immunity comes across the virus the symptoms are reflected at an early stage and the treatment begins earlier and the infectant is cured before the situation gets critical.

TREATMENT OF THE DISEASE

As mentioned earlier, everybody reacts to the infection differently, similarly, every patient reacts to the medication differently. Some patients respond to the medicine progressively, while body of some patients might take time. The identification of the drug was a very complex task for the doctors because the researchers were failing to make a medicine and the medicines that were given to the public were causing serious stress and anxiety problems in patients.

When a patient is diagnosed with corona virus, the initiation of the treatment begins with isolation of the patient.

1.   In the hospital

The medication of corona virus that showed great results were of the drug 'Remdesivir'. This drug slows the replication of the virus and works as an antiviral medicine. The recovery time of the medicine was estimated to be 10 days. Although, this medicine was considered as a successful drug but later it started to show side effects including excessive anxiety in patients, which made the patients panicked and increased their heartbeat rates. So, later it was avoided in patients which suffered from anxiety.

Another medication that was given to control the inflammation is Dexamethasone which cured the inflammation to prevent the patients to maintain the medical condition. (Medical News Today, 25 January 2021)

2.   At home

80% of patients who are detected with corona virus do not need hospital treatment. There are various methods of taking care at home by taking proper sleep, keeping oneself hydrated by drinking plenty of water, taking the over counter pain relievers like acetaminophen, for body aches, drinking warm liquids to relax the sore throat, laying on either side of the body to make it easy for the body to cough.

At the early of pandemic, the medicine named hydroxychloroquine, which is generally used to treat malaria was used for the for the treatment of covid patients and later it was found out that the medicine could cause life threatening problems of heart, so it got discontinued. (Medical News Today, 25 January 2021)

PRECAUTIONS TO PREVENT THE SPREAD OF A DISEASE

It is believed that the precautions are always better than cure and this phrase should be a daily routine to fight the virus as a unit. It is the responsibility of the citizens of the globe to take uttermost precautions to avoid the spread of disease.

The elementary precautions could be:

1. A country could go under lockdown to break the chain of the infection, but this scenario affects the GDP of the countries and government has to unlock the country, here it is the responsibility of the residents of the nation to unite and fight against the virus to resume to a normal life. In that matter, wearing a proper mask, following social distancing, sanitizing the products around the environment etc. All these basic precautions should be taken.
2. Whenever a being experienced fever which lasts more than 3 days, the patient should consult the doctor and if the symptoms are similar to that of covid-19, isolate yourself as soon as you witness the signs and start with the medication.
3. It is believed that corona virus would stay in the environment as a guest forever and vaccinating oneself would be the wise decision to protect and take care of the self and family.
4. Leaving the house without a mask, sanitizer only if its necessary can only help to control when the waves strike the country.

CORONA VIRUS VARIANTS

The virus mutated a lot of times and with each mutation, it became more and more transmissible and harmful. WHO recorded various variants like alpha, beta, gamma, delta but the variant that was the most harmful was the delta variant.

The "delta variation" has come to rule features, having been found in India where it is anything but an outrageous flood in Covid-19 cases prior to spreading all throughout the planet. Yet presently a transformation of that variation has arisen, called "delta in addition to," which is beginning to stress worldwide specialists.

India has named delta in addition to a "variation of concern," and there are fears that it might be more contagious. In the U.K., Public Health England noted in its last outline that standard filtering of Covid cases in the nation (where the delta variation is currently liable for most new contaminations) has discovered just about 40 instances of the fresher variation, which has procured the spike protein change K417N, for example delta in addition to.

As of 16 June 2021, cases of the delta plus variant had also been identified in the U.S. (83 cases at the time the report was published last Friday) as well as Poland, Canada, turkey, India, Japan, Nepal, Portugal, Russia, and Switzerland. (CNBC, 24 June 2021)

FUTURE WITH CORONA VIRUS

It is not certain whether Coronavirus will turn into a persistent occasional illness. There is an excessive amount of vulnerability about the likelihood and recurrence of rise of new variations, the decrease in immunization viability for every variation, the basic inquiry of cross-variation invulnerability, and the consistency of safe human conduct. Be that as it may, the possibility of constant and occasional Coronavirus is genuine. If invulnerability from disease for a similar SARS-CoV-2 variation or antibody inferred insusceptibility winds down, the possibility would increment further. There is a lot to learn in the coming a long time about variations, antibodies, and insusceptibility. Repetitive occasional Coronavirus could require both wellbeing framework change and significant social change for the existence of high-hazard people in the cold weather months. There is a critical need to get ready for such a situation by adjusting reconnaissance, clinical reaction, general wellbeing reaction, and financial projects.

There is developing idealism and expectation that by uprightness of progressing inoculation endeavours, irregularity (declining contaminations through August), and normally procured insusceptibility, by spring and late-spring 2021 in the US there will be a considerable decrease in the quantity of passing's and hospitalizations identified with Coronavirus. Be that as it may, this idealism should be tempered by a few significant variables. The probability of accomplishing group invulnerability against SARS-CoV-2 is low essentially on the grounds that not all people in the US are qualified to be inoculated and a fourth of qualified people will probably decay to be vaccinated. Additionally, the antibodies do not give full resistance against disease, and the at present accessible immunizations are less compelling against variation B.1.351, and perhaps different variations. Appropriately, general society and wellbeing frameworks need to anticipate the likelihood that Coronavirus will persevere and turn into an intermittent occasional infection.

Three key contemplations will make accomplishing group insusceptibility against Coronavirus testing. To start with, antibodies will reduce affect keeping disease from the B.1.351 variation. Moderna and Pfizer immunizations have a general viability against suggestive illness of around 95% for wild-type variations, though adenovirus vector antibodies, like the Janssen/Johnson and Johnson immunization, have adequacy closer to 70%. Proof on antibody viability for forestalling contamination, notwithstanding, comes just from 1 gathering in the AstraZeneca preliminary that showed 55% assurance against disease as estimated through week-by-week nasal swabs versus 70% insurance for suggestive disease.2 Besides, for the 3 immunizations tried against the B.1.351 variation, Janssen, Novavax, and AstraZeneca announced adequacy gauges for indicative infection of 57%,3 49%,4 and a measurably nonsignificant rate, separately. On the off chance that the B.1.351 variation becomes predominant, a straightforward computation proposes that the total viability of antibodies for forestalling B.1.351 transmission in the US could be just half (ie, in light of flow adequacy of 90% to forestall suggestive sickness × 20% decrease of adequacy for forestalling contamination contrasted and indicative infection and expecting a normal decrease in adequacy for B.1.351 of 33% [excluding the measurably inconsequential assurance from the AstraZeneca vaccine]).

Second, insufficient people will get the antibody. Since the antibodies are right now not approved for use in youngsters, just roughly 75% of US people are qualified to be inoculated. Maybe more significant over the long haul, not all people are willing be vaccinated. Information gathered every day through Facebook's Information for Acceptable drive give ideal data on the extent of people who react yes or "indeed, presumably" to the inquiry, Will you take the immunization whenever offered it? These positive reactions in regards to probability of immunization receipt expanded in January 2021 and have reached 71%,5 like the 72% reaction in a broadly delegate sample.6 Even with a compelling supported antibody for youngsters, if B.1.351 or some other variation becomes prevailing, the US can expect antibody determined insusceptibility to reach just 37.5% (the assessed possible half total viability for transmission × 75% of people getting the immunization) in 2021 if all stock and organization challenges are survived.

Third, there is worry about the degree to which past diseases from one variation shield people from reinfection for certain new variations. Novavax detailed that in a stage 2b clinical preliminary in South Africa, the Coronavirus occurrence rate in the fake treatment bunch, dominatingly from variation B.1.351, was 3.9% both among people with Coronavirus seropositivity and the individuals who were Coronavirus seronegative.7 The understanding by Novavax of this finding has been that previous disease gives no invulnerability against new variations. If that is valid, group resistance can be accomplished distinctly through inoculation. However, on the off chance that B.1.351 spreads broadly, antibody determined resistance will probably be a lot of lower than the levels needed to arrive at crowd insusceptibility by the 2021-2022 northern side of the equator winter. (Health data organization, 3 March 2021)

REFERENCES

ABC News. (2020). *Timeline how corona virus started.* https://abcnews.go.com/Health/timeline-coronavirus-started/story?id=69435165

CNBC. (2021). *Delta covid variant has a new variant delta plus.* https://www.cnbc.com/2021/06/24/delta-plus-covid-variant-heres-what-you-need-to-know.html

IHME. (2021). *The potential future of covid pandemic.* http://www.healthdata.org/research-article/potential-future-covid-19-pandemic

Medical News Today. (2021). *Are treatments available for covid 19.* https://www.medicalnewstoday.com/articles/coronavirus-treatment#care-at-home

PARHLO. (n.d.). *COVID: A brief history of deadly corona virus.* https://www.parhlo.com/history-of-coronavirus

Compilation of References

Croft, P., Altman, D. G., Deeks, J. J., Dunn, K. M., Hay, A. D., Hemingway, H., LeResche, L., Peat, G., Perel, P., Petersen, S. E., Riley, R. D., Roberts, I., Sharpe, M., Stevens, R. J., Van Der Windt, D. A., Von Korff, M., & Timmis, A. (2015). The science of clinical practice: Disease diagnosis or patient prognosis? Evidence about "what is likely to happen" should shape clinical practice. *BMC Medicine*, *13*(1), 20. doi:10.118612916-014-0265-4 PMID:25637245

Kundu, A. K., Fattah, S. A., & Wahid, K. A. (2020). Least square saliency transformation of capsule endoscopy images for PDF model based multiple gastrointestinal disease classification. *IEEE Access: Practical Innovations, Open Solutions*, *8*, 58509–58521. doi:10.1109/ACCESS.2020.2982870

Reeves, J. J., Hollandsworth, H. M., Torriani, F. J., Taplitz, R., Abeles, S., Tai-Seale, M., Millen, M., Clay, B. J., & Longhurst, C. A. (2020). Rapid response to COVID-19: Health informatics support for outbreak management in an academic health system. *Journal of the American Medical Informatics Association: JAMIA*, *27*(6), 853–859. doi:10.1093/jamia/ocaa037 PMID:32208481

Singh, A. (2020). *Parallel 3-Parent Genetic Algorithm with Application to Routing in Wireless Mesh Networks, Implementations and Applications of Machine Learning*. Springer.

Sutton, R. S., & Barto, A. G. (2018). *Reinforcement learning: An introduction*. MIT Press.

Albawi, S., Mohammed, T. A., & Al-Zawi, S. (2017). Understanding of a convolutional neural network. In *2017 International Conference on Engineering and Technology (ICET)*. IEEE. 10.1109/ICEngTechnol.2017.8308186

Malmir, B., Amini, M., & Chang, S. I. (2017). A medical decision support system for dis- ease diagnosis under uncertainty. *Expert Systems with Applications*, *88*, 95–108. doi:10.1016/j.eswa.2017.06.031

Mantas, J. (2020). The Importance of Health Informatics in Public Health During the COVID-19 Pandemic. *Studies in Health Technology and Informatics*, *272*, 487–488. doi:10.3233/SHTI200602 PMID:32604709

Wei, W., Liu, Z., Huang, L., Nebout, A., Le Meur, O., Zhang, T., ... Xu, L. (2020). Predicting atypical visual saliency for autism spectrum disorder via scale-adaptive inception module and discriminative region enhancement loss. *Neurocomputing*. Advance online publication. doi:10.1016/j.neucom.2020.06.125

Benson, N. M., Edgcomb, J. B., Landman, A. B., & Zima, B. T. (2020). Leveraging Clinical Informatics to Improve Child Mental Health Care. *Journal of the American Academy of Child and Adolescent Psychiatry*, *59*(12), 1314–1317. doi:10.1016/j.jaac.2020.06.014 PMID:33248526

Mehran, M., & Saraf Esmaili, S. (2020). Optic Disc Detection in Retinal Fundus Images Based on Saliency Map. *Signal Processing and Renewable Energy*, *4*(4), 65–80.

Nilashi, M., Ibrahim, O., Ahmadi, H., & Shahmoradi, L. (2017). O. bin Ibrahim, H. Ahmadi, L. Shahmoradi, An analytical method for diseases prediction using machine learning techniques. *Computers & Chemical Engineering*, *106*(106), 212–223. doi:10.1016/j.compchemeng.2017.06.011

Vishwanathan, S. V. M., & Narasimha Murty, M. (2002). SSVM: a simple SVM algorithm. In *Proceedings of the 2002 International Joint Conference on Neural Networks. IJCNN'02* (Cat. No. 02CH37290). IEEE. 10.1109/IJCNN.2002.1007516

Brijain, M. (2014). *A survey on decision tree algorithm for classification*. Academic Press.

Ferreira, D. S., Ramalho, G. L., Medeiros, F. N., Bianchi, A. G., Carneiro, C. M., & Ushizima, D. M. (2019, April). Saliency-Driven System With Deep Learning for Cell Image Classification. In *2019 IEEE 16th International Symposium on Biomedical Imaging (ISBI 2019)* (pp. 1284-1287). IEEE. 10.1109/ISBI.2019.8759398

Flach, P. A. (2016). ROC analysis. In *Encyclopedia of Machine Learning and Data Mining* (pp. 1–8). Springer.

Lin, C. T., Bookman, K., Sieja, A., Markley, K., Altman, R. L., Sippel, J., Perica, K., Reece, L., Davis, C., Horowitz, E., Pisney, L., Sottile, P. D., Kao, D., Adrian, B., Szkil, M., Griffin, J., Youngwerth, J., Drew, B., & Pell, J. (2020). Clinical informatics accelerates health system adaptation to the COVID-19 pandemic: Examples from Colorado. *Journal of the American Medical Informatics Association: JAMIA*, *27*(12), 1955–1963. doi:10.1093/jamia/ocaa171 PMID:32687152

Nashi, M., Ibrahim, O., Ahmadi, H., Shahmoradi, L., & Farahmand, M. (2018). A hybrid intelligent system for the prediction of Parkinson's disease progression using machine learning techniques. *Biocybernetics and Biomedical Engineering*, *38*(1), 1–15. doi:10.1016/j.bbe.2017.09.002

Adeel, A., Khan, M. A., Sharif, M., Azam, F., Shah, J. H., Umer, T., & Wan, S. (2019). Diagnosis and recognition of grape leaf diseases: An automated system based on a novel saliency approach and canonical correlation analysis based multiple features fusion. *Sustainable Computing: Informatics and Systems*, *24*, 100349. doi:10.1016/j.suscom.2019.08.002

Belgiu, M., & Drăguţ, L. (2016). Random forest in remote sensing: A review of applications and future directions. *ISPRS Journal of Photogrammetry and Remote Sensing*, *114*, 24–31. doi:10.1016/j.isprsjprs.2016.01.011

Dagliati, A., Malovini, A., Tibollo, V., & Bellazzi, R. (2021). Health informatics and EHR to support clinical research in the COVID-19 pandemic: An overview. *Briefings in Bioinformatics*, *22*(2), 812–822. doi:10.1093/bib/bbaa418 PMID:33454728

Dhingra, G., Kumar, V., & Joshi, H. D. (2018). Study of digital image processing techniques for leaf disease detection and classification. *Multimedia Tools and Applications*, *77*(15), 19951–20000. doi:10.100711042-017-5445-8

Nashi, M., Ahmadi, H., Shahmoradi, L., Mardani, A., & Ibrahim, O. (2017). E. Yade- garidehkordi, Knowledge discovery and diseases prediction: A comparative study of machine learning techniques. *J. Soft Comput. Decis. Support Syst.*, *4*, 8–16.

Abu, M. A., Indra, N. H., Abd Rahman, A. H., Sapiee, N. A., & Ahmad, I. (2019). A study on Image Classification based on Deep Learning and Tensorflow. *International Journal of Engineering Research & Technology (Ahmedabad)*, *12*(4), 563–569.

Barakati, S. S., Topaz, M., Peltonen, L. M., Mitchell, J., Alhuwail, D., Risling, T., & Ronquillo, C. (2020). Health Informatics Solutions in Response to COVID-19: Preliminary Insights from an International Survey. *Studies in Health Technology and Informatics*, *275*, 222–223. doi:10.3233/SHTI200727 PMID:33227773

Hebert, L. E., Weuve, J., Scherr, P. A., & Evans, D. A. (2013). Alzheimer disease in the United States (2010-2050) estimated using the 2010 Census. *Neurology*, *80*(19), 1778–1783. doi:10.1212/WNL.0b013e31828726f5 PMID:23390181

Pesce, E., Withey, S. J., Ypsilantis, P. P., Bakewell, R., Goh, V., & Montana, G. (2019). Learning to detect chest radiographs containing pulmonary lesions using visual attention networks. *Medical Image Analysis*, *53*, 26–38. doi:10.1016/j.media.2018.12.007 PMID:30660946

Zhang, S. (2017). Learning k for knn classification. *ACM Transactions on Intelligent Systems and Technology*, *8*(3), 1–19.

Borji, A. (2018). *Saliency prediction in the deep learning era: Successes, limitations, and future challenges.* arXiv preprint arXiv:1810.03716.

Ruta, D., & Gabrys, B. (2005). Classifier selection for majority voting. *Information Fusion*, *6*(1), 63–81. doi:10.1016/j.inffus.2004.04.008

Sharma, R., & Singh, A. (2019). Overview of different machine learning techniques for plant disease detection. *Journal of the Gujarat Research Society*, *21*(6), 416–425.

Sylvestre, E., Thuny, R. M., Cecilia-Joseph, E., Gueye, P., Chabartier, C., Brouste, Y., Mehdaoui, H., Najioullah, F., Pierre-François, S., Abel, S., Cabié, A., & Dramé, M. (2020). Health informatics support for outbreak management: How to respond without an electronic health record? *Journal of the American Medical Informatics Association: JAMIA*, *27*(11), 1828–1829. doi:10.1093/jamia/ocaa183 PMID:32761100

Vinyals, O., Toshev, A., Bengio, S., & Erhan, D. (2015). Show and tell: a neural image caption generator. *Proceedings of the IEEE Conference on Computer Vision and Pattern Recognition, 3156*–3164. 10.1109/CVPR.2015.7298935

Balduzzi, D. (2017). The shattered gradients problem: If resnets are the answer, then what is the question? In *International Conference on Machine Learning*. PMLR.

Banerjee, S., Mitra, S., & Shankar, B. U. (2018). Automated 3D segmentation of brain tumor using visual saliency. *Information Sciences*, *424*, 337–353. doi:10.1016/j.ins.2017.10.011

Juhn, Y., & Liu, H. (2020). Artificial intelligence approaches using natural language processing to advance EHR-based clinical research. *The Journal of Allergy and Clinical Immunology*, *145*(2), 463–469. doi:10.1016/j.jaci.2019.12.897 PMID:31883846

Sharma, R., Singh, A., & Sharma, V. (2018). Potato Leaf Diseases Identification using CNN. *Journal of Emerging Technologies and Innovative Research*, *5*(12), 519–527.

Wu, Y. (2016). Google's neural machine translation system: bridging the gap between human and machine translation. Preprint at https://arxiv.org/ abs/1609.08144

Kannan, A. (2016). Smart reply: automated response suggestion for email. In *Proceedings of the 22nd ACM SIGKDD International Conference on Knowledge Discovery and Data Mining*. ACM. 10.1145/2939672.2939801

Mitra, S., Banerjee, S., & Hayashi, Y. (2017). Volumetric brain tumour detection from MRI using visual saliency. *PLoS One*, *12*(11), e0187209. doi:10.1371/journal.pone.0187209 PMID:29095877

Thanapol, P., Lavangnananda, K., Bouvry, P., Pinel, F., & Leprévost, F. (2020, October). Reducing Overfitting and Improving Generalization in Training Convolutional Neural Network (CNN) under Limited Sample Sizes in Image Recognition. In *2020-5th International Conference on Information Technology (InCIT)* (pp. 300-305). IEEE.

Wu, S., Roberts, K., Datta, S., Du, J., Ji, Z., Si, Y., Soni, S., Wang, Q., Wei, Q., Xiang, Y., Zhao, B., & Xu, H. (2020). Deep learning in clinical natural language processing: A methodical review. *Journal of the American Medical Informatics Association: JAMIA*, *27*(3), 457–470. doi:10.1093/jamia/ocz200 PMID:31794016

Zhu, Q. (2018). A deep-local-global feature fusion framework for high spatial resolution imagery scene classification. *Remote Sensing, 10*(4), 568.

He, K. (2016). Deep residual learning for image recognition. *Proceedings of the IEEE conference on computer vision and pattern recognition.*

Low, D. M., Rumker, L., Talkar, T., Torous, J., Cecchi, G., & Ghosh, S. S. (2020). Natural Language Processing Reveals Vulnerable Mental Health Support Groups and Heightened Health Anxiety on Reddit During COVID-19: Observational Study. *Journal of Medical Internet Research, 22*(10), e22635. doi:10.2196/22635 PMID:32936777

Park, S., & Kwak, N. (2016, November). Analysis on the dropout effect in convolutional neural networks. In *Asian conference on computer vision* (pp. 189-204). Springer.

The Office of the National Coordinator for Health Information Technology. (2017). *Quick stats: health IT dashboard.* https://dashboard.healthit.gov/quickstats/ quickstats.php

Zou, X., Zhao, X., Yang, Y., & Li, N. (2016). Learning-Based Visual Saliency Model for Detecting Diabetic Macular Edema in Retinal Image. *Computational Intelligence and Neuroscience, 2016*, 7496735. doi:10.1155/2016/7496735 PMID:26884750

Bali, B., & Garba, E. J. (2021). Neuro-fuzzy Approach for Prediction of Neurological Disorders: A Systematic Review. *SN. Computer Science, 2*(4), 307. doi:10.100742979-021-00710-9

Demner-Fushman, D., Elhadad, N., & Friedman, C. (2021). Natural language processing for health-related texts. In *Biomedical Informatics* (pp. 241–272). Springer. doi:10.1007/978-3-030-58721-5_8

LeCun, Y., Bengio, Y., & Hinton, G. (2015). Deep learning. *Nature, 521*(7553), 436–444. doi:10.1038/nature14539 PMID:26017442

Noh, H. (2017). Large-scale image retrieval with attentive deep local features. *Proceedings of the IEEE international conference on computer vision.* 10.1109/ICCV.2017.374

O'Mahony, N., Campbell, S., Carvalho, A., Harapanahalli, S., Hernandez, G. V., Krpalkova, L., ... Walsh, J. (2019, April). Deep learning vs. traditional computer vision. In *Science and Information Conference* (pp. 128-144). Springer.

Banerjee, S., Mitra, S., Shankar, B. U., & Hayashi, Y. (2016). A novel GBM saliency detection model using multi-channel MRI. *PLoS One, 11*(1), e0146388. doi:10.1371/journal.pone.0146388 PMID:26752735

Perez, L., & Wang, J. (2017). The effectiveness of data augmentation in image classification using deep learning. arXiv preprint arXiv:1712.04621.

Shickel, B., Tighe, P. J., Bihorac, A., & Rashidi, P. (2017). Deep EHR: A survey of recent advances in deep learning techniques for electronic health record (EHR) analysis. *IEEE Journal of Biomedical and Health Informatics, 22*(5), 1589–1604. doi:10.1109/JBHI.2017.2767063 PMID:29989977

Shoenbill, K., Song, Y., Gress, L., Johnson, H., Smith, M., & Mendonca, E. A. (2020). Natural language processing of lifestyle modification documentation. *Health Informatics Journal, 26*(1), 388–405. doi:10.1177/1460458218824742 PMID:30791802

Szegedy, C. (2016). Rethinking the inception architecture for computer vision. *Proceedings of the IEEE conference on computer vision and pattern recognition.* 10.1109/CVPR.2016.308

Bhatt & Patalia. (2017). Indian monuments classification using support vector machine. *International Journal of Electrical and Computer Engineering, 7*(4), 1952.

Dornauer, V., Jahn, F., Hoeffner, K., Winter, A., & Ammenwerth, E. (2020). Use of Natural Language Processing for Precise Retrieval of Key Elements of Health IT Evaluation Studies. *Studies in Health Technology and Informatics*, *272*, 95–98. doi:10.3233/SHTI200502 PMID:32604609

Mahapatra, D., Roy, P. K., Sedai, S., & Garnavi, R. (2016). Retinal image quality classification using saliency maps and CNNs. In *International Workshop on Machine Learning in Medical Imaging* (pp. 172-179). Springer. 10.1007/978-3-319-47157-0_21

Rajkomar, A., Oren, E., Chen, K., Dai, A. M., Hajaj, N., Hardt, M., Liu, P. J., Liu, X., Marcus, J., Sun, M., Sundberg, P., Yee, H., Zhang, K., Zhang, Y., Flores, G., Duggan, G. E., Irvine, J., Le, Q., Litsch, K., ... Dean, J. (2018). Scalable and accurate deep learning with electronic health records. *NPJ Digital Medicine*, *1*(1), 18. doi:10.103841746-018-0029-1 PMID:31304302

Alzheimer's Association. (2006). *Early-Onset Dementia: A National Challenge, a Future Crisis*. Alzheimer's Association.

Goodfellow, I. (2016). Deep learning: Vol. 1. *No. 2*. MIT Press.

Rueda, A., González, F., & Romero, E. (2013). Saliency-based characterization of group differences for magnetic resonance disease classification. *Dyna*, *80*(178), 21–28.

Vaci, N., Liu, Q., Kormilitzin, A., De Crescenzo, F., Kurtulmus, A., Harvey, J., O'Dell, B., Innocent, S., Tomlinson, A., Cipriani, A., & Nevado-Holgado, A. (2020). Natural language processing for structuring clinical text data on depression using UK-CRIS. *Evidence-Based Mental Health*, *23*(1), 21–26. doi:10.1136/ebmental-2019-300134 PMID:32046989

Abbood, A., Ullrich, A., Busche, R., & Ghozzi, S. (2020). EventEpi-A natural language processing framework for event-based surveillance. *PLoS Computational Biology*, *16*(11), e1008277. doi:10.1371/journal.pcbi.1008277 PMID:33216746

Erol, O. K., & Eksin, I. (2006). A new optimization method: Big Bang-Big Crunch. *Advances in Engineering Software*, *37*(2), 106–111. doi:10.1016/j.advengsoft.2005.04.005

Li, N., Bi, H., Zhang, Z., & Kong, X. (2018). Performance Comparison of Saliency Detection. Advances in Multimedia. doi:10.1155/2018/9497083

Richard. (2010). *Computer Vision: Algorithm and Application*. Academic Press.

Yang, X., Yang, H., Lyu, T., Yang, S., Guo, Y., Bian, J., Xu, H., & Wu, Y. (2020). A Natural Language Processing Tool to Extract Quantitative Smoking Status from Clinical Narratives. medRxiv. doi:10.1101/2020.10.30.20223511

Yang, X.-S. (2010). A new metaheuristic bat-inspired algorithm. Nature inspired cooperative strategies for optimization (NICSO 2010), 65–74. doi:10.1007/978-3-642-12538-6_6

Yosinski, J., Clune, J., Bengio, Y., & Lipson, L. (2014). How transferable are features in deep neural networks? Advances in Neural Information Processing Systems, 3320–3328.

He, S., Wu, Q. H., & Saunders, J. (2009). Group search optimizer: An optimization algorithm inspired by animal searching behavior. *IEEE Transactions on Evolutionary Computation*, *13*(5), 973–990. doi:10.1109/TEVC.2009.2011992

Lee, J., Yoon, W., Kim, S., Kim, D., Kim, S., So, C. H., & Kang, J. (2020). BioBERT: A pre-trained biomedical language representation model for biomedical text mining. *Bioinformatics (Oxford, England)*, *36*(4), 1234–1240. doi:10.1093/bioinformatics/btz682 PMID:31501885

Szegedy, C., Liu, W., Jia, Y., Sermanet, P., Reed, S., Anguelov, D., & Rabinovich, A. (2015). Going deeper with convolutions. In *Proceedings of the IEEE conference on computer vision and pattern recognition*. IEEE. 10.1109/CVPR.2015.7298594

Binitha, S., & Sathya, S. S. (2012). A survey of bio inspired optimization algorithms. *International Journal of Soft Computing and Engineering, 2*(2), 137–151.

Giummarra, M. J., Lau, G., & Gabbe, B. J. (2020). Evaluation of text mining to reduce screening workload for injury-focused systematic reviews. *Injury Prevention, 26*(1), 55–60. doi:10.1136/injuryprev-2019-043247

Szegedy, C., Ioffe, S., Vanhoucke, V., & Alemi, A. A. (2017). Inception-v4, inception-resnet and the impact of residual connections on learning. Association for the Advancement of Artificial Intelligence (AAAI), 4.

He, K., Zhang, X., Ren, S., & Sun, J. (2016a). Deep residual learning for image recognition. In *Proceedings of the IEEE conference on computer vision and pattern recognition*. IEEE. 10.1109/CVPR.2016.90

Rafiq, M. Y., Bugmann, G., & Easterbrook, D. J. (2001). Neural network design for engineering applications. *Computers & Structures, 79*(17), 1541–1552. doi:10.1016/S0045-7949(01)00039-6

Uronen, L., Moen, H., Teperi, S., Martimo, K. P., Hartiala, J., & Salanterä, S. (2020). Towards automated detection of psychosocial risk factors with text mining. *Occupational Medicine (Oxford, England), 70*(3), 203–206. doi:10.1093/occmed/kqaa022 PMID:32086511

Singh, Kumar, Walia, & Chakravorty. (2015). Face Recognition: A Combined Parallel BB-BC & PCA Approach to Feature Selection. *International Journal of Computer Science & Information Technology, 2*(2), 1-5.

Wu, C. S., Kuo, C. J., Su, C. H., Wang, S. H., & Dai, H. J. (2020). Using text mining to extract depressive symptoms and to validate the diagnosis of major depressive disorder from electronic health records. *Journal of Affective Disorders, 260*, 617–623. doi:10.1016/j.jad.2019.09.044 PMID:31541973

Khaleghi, T., Murat, A., Arslanturk, S., & Davies, E. (2020). Automated Surgical Term Clustering: A Text Mining Approach for Unstructured Textual Surgery Descriptions. *IEEE Journal of Biomedical and Health Informatics, 24*(7), 2107–2118. doi:10.1109/JBHI.2019.2956973 PMID:31796420

Krizhevsky, A., Sutskever, I., & Hinton, G. E. (2012). Imagenet classification with deep convolutional neural networks. Advances in neural information processing systems, 1097–1105.

Singh, A., Kumar, S., Singh, A., & Walia, S. S. (2019). Three-parent GA: A Global Optimization Algorithm. *Journal of Multiple-Valued Logic and Soft Computing, 32*, 407–423.

Cronin, R. M., Jimison, H., & Johnson, K. B. (2021). Personal Health Informatics. In E. H. Shortliffe & J. J. Cimino (Eds.), *Biomedical Informatics*. Springer. doi:10.1007/978-3-030-58721-5_11

Hinton, G., Deng, L., Yu, D., Dahl, G., Mohamed, A., Jaitly, N., Senior, A., Vanhoucke, V., Nguyen, P., Sainath, T., & Kingsbury, B. (2012). Deep neural networks for acoustic modeling in speech recognition: The shared views of four research groups. *IEEE Signal Processing Magazine, 29*(6), 82–97. doi:10.1109/MSP.2012.2205597

Magliani, F., Fontanini, T., & Prati, A. (2019). Landmark recognition: From small-scale to large-scale retrieval. Springer.

Roy, S., & Bhunia, G. S. (n.d.). Spatial prediction of COVID-19 epidemic using ARIMA techniques in India. *Data in Brief, 29*, 105340.

Sharma, P., Hans, P., & Gupta, S. C. (2020, January). Classification Of Plant Leaf Diseases Using Machine Learning And Image Preprocessing Techniques. In *2020 10th International Conference on Cloud Computing, Data Science & Engineering (Confluence)* (pp. 480-484). IEEE. 10.1109/Confluence47617.2020.9057889

Siuly, S., & Zhang, Y. (2016). Medical Big Data: Neurological Diseases Diagnosis Through Medical Data Analysis. *Data Sci. Eng., 1*(2), 54–64. doi:10.100741019-016-0011-3

Kumar, S., Singh, A., & Walia, S. S. (2018). Parallel Big Bang - Big Crunch Global Optimization Algorithm: Performance and its Applications to routing in WMNs. *Wireless Personal Communications, Springer, 100*(4), 1601–1618. doi:10.100711277-018-5656-y

Szegedy, C., Liu, W., Jia, Y., Sermanet, P., Reed, S., Anguelov, D., Erhan, D., Vanhoucke, V., & Rabinovich, A. (2015). Going deeper with convolutions. *Proceedings of the IEEE conference on computer vision and pattern recognition*, 1–9.

Wang, L. L., & Lo, K. (2021). Text mining approaches for dealing with the rapidly expanding literature on COVID-19. *Briefings in Bioinformatics, 22*(2), 781–799. doi:10.1093/bib/bbaa296 PMID:33279995

Glowacki, E. M., Wilcox, G. B., & Glowacki, J. B. (2021). Identifying #addiction concerns on twitter during the COVID-19 pandemic: A text mining analysis. *Substance abuse, 42*(1), 39–46. doi:10.1080/08897077.2020.1822489 PMID:32970973

Singh, A., Kumar, S., & Walia, S. S. (2020). Parallel 3-Parent Genetic Algorithm with Application to Routing in Wireless Mesh Networks. In *Implementations and Applications of Machine Learning* (pp. 1–28). Springer. doi:10.1007/978-3-030-37830-1_1

Simonyan, K., & Zisserman, A. (2014). Very deep convolutional networks for large-scale image recognition. arXiv Prepr. arXiv:1409.1556.

Hoo-Chang, S., Roth, H. R., Gao, M., Lu, L., Xu, Z., Nogues, I., Yao, J., Mollura, D., & Summers, R. M. (2016). Deep convolutional neural networks for computer-aided detection: CNN architectures, dataset characteristics and transfer learning. *IEEE Transactions on Medical Imaging, 35*(5), 1285–1298. doi:10.1109/TMI.2016.2528162 PMID:26886976

Chu, R., Sun, Y., Li, Y., Liu, Z., Zhang, C., & Wei, Y. (2019). Vehicle re-identification with viewpoint-aware metric learning. In *Proceedings of the IEEE/CVF International Conference on Computer Vision* (pp. 8282-8291). IEEE.

Daza, J. C., & Rueda, A. (2016, September). Classification of Alzheimer's disease in mri using visual saliency information. In *2016 IEEE 11th Colombian Computing Conference (CCC)* (pp. 1-7). IEEE. 10.1109/ColumbianCC.2016.7750796

Le Glaz, A., Haralambous, Y., Kim-Dufor, D. H., Lenca, P., Billot, R., Ryan, T. C., Marsh, J., DeVylder, J., Walter, M., Berrouiguet, S., & Lemey, C. (2021). Machine Learning and Natural Language Processing in Mental Health: Systematic Review. *Journal of Medical Internet Research, 23*(5), e15708. doi:10.2196/15708 PMID:33944788

Liu, Q., Liu, X., Jiang, B., & Yang, W. (2011). Forecasting incidence of hemorrhagic fever with renal syndrome in China using ARIMA model. *BMC Infectious Diseases, 11*(1), 218. doi:10.1186/1471-2334-11-218 PMID:21838933

Russakovsky, O., Deng, J., Su, H., Krause, J., Satheesh, S., Ma, S., Huang, Z., Karpathy, A., Khosla, A., Bernstein, M., Berg, A. C., & Fei-Fei, L. (2015). Imagenet large scale visual recognition challenge. *International Journal of Computer Vision, 115*(3), 211–252. doi:10.100711263-015-0816-y

Zheng, Y.-T. (2009). Tour the world: building a web-scale landmark recognition engine. In *2009 IEEE Conference on Computer Vision and Pattern Recognition*. IEEE. 10.1109/CVPR.2009.5206749

Ben-Ahmed, O., Lecellier, F., Paccalin, M., & Fernandez-Maloigne, C. (2017). Multi-view visual saliency-based MRI classification for Alzheimer's disease diagnosis. In *2017 Seventh International Conference on Image Processing Theory, Tools and Applications (IPTA)* (pp. 1-6). IEEE. 10.1109/IPTA.2017.8310118

Chen, T., Yap, K.-H., & Zhang, D. (2014). Discriminative soft bag-of-visual phrase for mobile landmark recognition. *IEEE Transactions on Multimedia, 16*(3), 612–622. doi:10.1109/TMM.2014.2301978

Elgendi, M., Nasir, M. U., Tang, Q., Smith, D., Grenier, J. P., Batte, C., ... Nicolaou, S. (2021). The effectiveness of image augmentation in deep learning networks for detecting COVID-19: A geometric transformation perspective. *Frontiers in Medicine*, 8. PMID:33732718

Hirschberg, J., & Manning, C. D. (2015). Advances in natural language processing. *Science*, *349*(6245), 261–266. doi:10.1126cience.aaa8685 PMID:26185244

Sharma, M., Mondal, S., Bhattacharjee, S., & Jabalia, N. (n.d.). Emerging Trends of Bioinformatics in Health Informatics. *Computational Intelligence in Healthcare, 343*.

Armstrong, N., & Hilton, P. (2014). doing diagnosis: Whether and how clinicians use a diagnostic tool of uncertain clinical utility. *Social Science & Medicine*, *120*, 208–214. doi:10.1016/j.socscimed.2014.09.032 PMID:25259659

Bhatnagar, S., Lal, V., Gupta, S. D., & Gupta, O. P. (2012). Forecasting incidence of dengue in Rajasthan, using time series analyses. *Indian Journal of Public Health*, *56*(4), 281. doi:10.4103/0019-557X.106415 PMID:23354138

Gadgil, S., Endo, M., Wen, E., Ng, A. Y., & Rajpurkar, P. (2021). *CheXseg: Combining Expert Annotations with DNN-generated Saliency Maps for X-ray Segmentation*. arXiv preprint arXiv:2102.10484.

Magge, A., Klein, A., Miranda-Escalada, A., Al-Garadi, M. A., Alimova, I., Miftahutdinov, Z., . . . Gonzalez, G. (2021, June). *Proceedings of the Sixth Social Media Mining for Health (# SMM4H) Workshop and Shared Task*. Academic Press.

Wang, E. K., Chen, C. M., Hassan, M. M., & Almogren, A. (2020). A deep learning based medical image segmentation technique in Internet-of-Medical-Things domain. *Future Generation Computer Systems*, *108*, 135–144. doi:10.1016/j.future.2020.02.054

Weyand, T. (2020). Google landmarks dataset v2-a large-scale benchmark for instance-level recognition and retrieval. *Proceedings of the IEEE/CVF Conference on Computer Vision and Pattern Recognition*.

Chen, D. (2011). Residual enhanced visual vectors for on-device image matching. In *2011 Conference Record of the Forty Fifth Asilomar Conference on Signals, Systems and Computers (ASILOMAR)*. IEEE. 10.1109/ACSSC.2011.6190128

Han, N., Srivastava, S., Xu, A., Klein, D., & Beyeler, M. (2021). *Deep Learning—Based Scene Simplification for Bionic Vision*. arXiv preprint arXiv:2102.00297.

Kaur, A., Kaur, L., & Singh, A. (2021). State-of-the-art segmentation techniques and future directions for multiple sclerosis brain lesions. *Archives of Computational Methods in Engineering*, *28*(3), 951–977. doi:10.100711831-020-09403-7

Manikandan, M., Velavan, A., & Singh, Z. (2016). Forecasting the trend in cases of Ebola virus disease in west African countries using auto regressive integrated moving average models Int. *Journal of Community Medicine & Public Health*, *3*, 615–618.

Scully, J. L. (2004). what is a disease? *EMBO Reports*, *5*(7), 650–653. doi:10.1038j.embor.7400195 PMID:15229637

Walsh, J., Cave, J., & Griffiths, F. (2021). Spontaneously Generated Online Patient Experience of Modafinil: A Qualitative and NLP Analysis. *Frontiers in Digital Health*, *3*, 10. doi:10.3389/fdgth.2021.598431

Digan, W., Névéol, A., Neuraz, A., Wack, M., Baudoin, D., Burgun, A., & Rance, B. (2021). Can reproducibility be improved in clinical natural language processing? A study of 7 clinical NLP suites. *Journal of the American Medical Informatics Association: JAMIA*, *28*(3), 504–515. doi:10.1093/jamia/ocaa261 PMID:33319904

Jordan, M. I., & Mitchell, T. M. (2015). Machine learning: Trends, perspectives, and prospects. *Science*, *349*(6245), 255–260. doi:10.1126cience.aaa8415 PMID:26185243

Leaman, R., Islamaj Do ̆gan, R., & Lu, Z. (2013). DNorm: Disease name normalization with pairwise learning to rank. *Bioinformatics (Oxford, England)*, *29*(22), 2909–2917. doi:10.1093/bioinformatics/btt474 PMID:23969135

Patel, A., Swaminarayan, P., & Patel, M. (2021). Identification of Nutrition's Deficiency in Plant and Prediction of Nutrition Requirement Using Image Processing. In *Proceedings of the Second International Conference on Information Management and Machine Intelligence* (pp. 463-469). Springer. 10.1007/978-981-15-9689-6_50

Serte, S., & Serener, A. (2021). Graph-based saliency and ensembles of convolutional neural networks for glaucoma detection. *IET Image Processing*, *15*(3), 797–804. doi:10.1049/ipr2.12063

Zhang, X., Zhang, T., Young, A. A., & Li, X. (2014). Applications and comparisons of four time series models in epidemiological surveillance data. *PLoS One*, *9*(2), e88075. doi:10.1371/journal.pone.0088075 PMID:24505382

Caruana, R., & Niculescu-Mizil, A. (2006). An empirical comparison of supervised learning algorithms. *Proceedings of the 23rd international conference on Machine learning*. 10.1145/1143844.1143865

Committee on Diagnostic Error in Health Care. (2015). *Board on Health Care Services, Institute of Medicine, T.N.A.o, Sciences, Improving Diagnosis in Health Care*. The National Academies Press.

Sran, P. K., Gupta, S., & Singh, S. (2020). Segmentation based image compression of brain magnetic resonance images using visual saliency. *Biomedical Signal Processing and Control*, *62*, 102089. doi:10.1016/j.bspc.2020.102089

Tayefi, M., Ngo, P., Chomutare, T., Dalianis, H., Salvi, E., Budrionis, A., & Godtliebsen, F. (2021). Challenges and opportunities beyond structured data in analysis of electronic health records. *Wiley Interdisciplinary Reviews: Computational Statistics*, 1549.

Toennies, K. D. (2017). Feature Detection. In *Guide to Medical Image Analysis* (pp. 173–207). Springer. doi:10.1007/978-1-4471-7320-5_5

Must-Know Data Breach Statistics for 2021. (n.d.). *IBM*. https://www.varonis.com/blog/data-breach-statistics/

Barlow, H. B. (1989). Unsupervised learning. *Neural Computation*, *1*(3), 295–311. doi:10.1162/neco.1989.1.3.295

Jagadeesh, K., & Rajendran, A. (n.d.). Machine Learning Approaches for Analysis in Healthcare Informatics. In Machine Learning and Analytics in Healthcare Systems (pp. 105-122). CRC Press.

Scheuermann, R. H., Ceusters, W., & Smith, B. (2009). Toward an ontological treatment of disease and diagnosis. *Summit on Translational Bioinformatics*, *2009*, 116–120. PMID:21347182

Singh, Kumar, Walia, & Chakravorty. (2015). Face Recognition: A Combined Parallel BB-BC & PCA Approach to Feature Selection. *International Journal of Computer Science & Information Technology, 2*(2), 1-5.

Verma, P., Negi, C. S., Pant, M., & Saxena, A. (2020). *Deep Saliency: A Deep Learning based Saliency Approach to detect Covid-19 through x-ray images*. Academic Press.

ABC News. (2020). *Timeline how corona virus started*. https://abcnews.go.com/Health/timeline-coronavirus-started/story?id=69435165

Abolmaali, S. (2021). A comparative study of SIR Model, Linear Regression, Logistic Function and ARIMA Model for forecasting COVID-19 cases. doi:10.1101/2021.05.24.21257594

Aguiar, M., Stollenwerk, N., Kooi, B. W., Simos, T. E., Psihoyios, G., Tsitouras, C., & Anastassi, Z. (2011). *The Stochastic Multi-strain Dengue Model: Analysis of the Dynamics*. Academic Press.

Ai, T., Yang, Z., Hou, H., Zhan, C., Chen, C., Wenzhi, L., Tao, Q., & Sun, Z. (2020). Correlation of chest ct and rt-pcr testing in coronavirus disease 2019 (covid-19) in China: A report. *Radiology*, *296*(2), E32–E40. Advance online publication. doi:10.1148/radiol.2020200642 PMID:32101510

Al-Antari, Al-Masni, Choi, Han, & Kim. (2018). (2018). A fully integrated computer-aided diagnosis system for digital x-ray mammograms via deep learning detection, segmentation, and classification. *International Journal of Medical Informatics, 117*, 44-54.

Al-Hiary, Bani-Ahmad, Reyalat, Braik, & Al-Rahamneh. (2011). Fast and Accurate Detection and Classification of Plant Diseases. *International Journal of Computer Applications, 17*(1).

Ali, I. (2016). AI4COVID-19: AI-Enabled Preliminary Diagnosis for COVID-19 from Cough Samples via an App. *IEEE Access, 4*, 1–12.

Allahi, F., Fateh, A., Revetria, R., & Cianci, R. (2021). The COVID-19 epidemic and evaluating the corresponding responses to crisis management in refugees: A system dynamic approach. *Journal of Humanitarian Logistics and Supply Chain Management, 11*(2), 347–366. doi:10.1108/JHLSCM-09-2020-0077

Allam, Z., & Jones, D. S. (2020). On the Coronavirus (COVID-19) Outbreak and the Smart City Network: Universal Data Sharing Standards Coupled with Artificial Intelligence (AI) to Benefit Urban Health Monitoring and Management. *Healthcare MDPI, 8*(1), 46. doi:10.3390/healthcare8010046

Alloghani, M. (2020). A Systematic Review on Supervised and Unsupervised Machine Learning Algorithms for Data Science. In *Unsupervised and Semi-Supervised Learning.* Springer Nature Switzerland AG 2020.

Almeshal, A. M., Almazrouee, A. I., Alenizi, M. R., & Alhajeri, S. N. (2020). Forecasting the Spread of COVID-19 in Kuwait Using Compartmental and Logistic Regression Models. *Applied Sciences (Basel, Switzerland), 10*(10), 3402. doi:10.3390/app10103402

Al-Raeei, M., El-Daher, M., & Solieva, O. (2021). Applying SEIR model without vaccination for COVID-19 in case of the United States, Russia, the United Kingdom, Brazil, France, and India. *Epidemiologic Methods, 10*(s1), 20200036. doi:10.1515/em-2020-0036

Alvarez, F. E., Argente, D., & Lippi, F. (2020). *A simple planning problem for COVID-19 lockdown. Tech. Rep.* National Bureau of Economic Research. doi:10.3386/w26981

Amayomordecai. (2020, April 26). *Heart disease risk prediction machine learning.* Kaggle. https://www.kaggle.com/amayomordecai/heart-disease-risk-prediction-machine-learning

Amundsen, E. J., Stigum, H., Rottingen, J. A., & Aalen, O. O. (2004). Definition and estimation of an actual reproduction number describing past infectious disease transmission: application to HIV epidemics among homosexual men in Denmark, Norway and Sweden. *Epidemiology and Infection.*

API. (2021, July 1). *COVID19-India API.* https://api.covid19india.org/

appsstore.ai. (2020). *Intelligent apps for any IP Cameras.* appsstore.ai.

Arkin, R. C., Fujita, M., Takagi, T., & Hasegawa, R. (2001), Ethological modeling and architecture for an entertainment robot. *IEEE Int. Conf. Robotics & Automation.*

Atkeson, A., Kopecky, K., & Zha, T. (2020). *Estimating and Forecasting Disease Scenarios for COVID-19 with an SIR Model.* doi:10.3386/w27335

Badnakhe, M. R., & Deshmukh, P. R. (2012, March). Infected Leaf Analysis and Comparison by Otsu Threshold and k-Means Clustering. *International Journal of Advanced Research in Computer Science and Software Engineering, 2*(3).

Baldé, M. A. (2020). Fitting SIR model to COVID-19 pandemic data and comparative forecasting with machine learning. doi:10.1101/2020.04.26.20081042

Bandyopadhyay, S. K., & Dutta, S. (2020). Machine learning approach for confirmation of COVID-19 cases: positive, negative, death and release. doi:10.1101/2020.03.25.20043505

Bangert. (2018). *Smart Condition Monitoring Using Machine Learning.* Algorithmica technologies GmbH.

Basu & Campbell. (2020). Going by the numbers: Learning and modeling COVID-19 disease dynamics. 0960-0779/ doi:10.1016/j.chaos.2020.110140

Basu, M. (2020, 7 July). India's R value increases for the first time in 3 months – at 1.19 from 1.11 a week ago. *The Print India.* https://www.theprint.in/

BBC. (2021, July 1). *India coronavirus: Can all adults get vaccinated in 2021?* https://www.bbc.com/news/world-asia-india-55571793

Behnood, G. (2018). *North American.* https://spectrum.ieee.org/biomedical/devices/ai-could-provide-momentbymoment-nursing-for-a-hospitals-sickest-patients

Belfiore, Urraro, Grassi, Giacobbe, Patelli, Cappabianca, & Reginelli. (2020). *Artificial intelligence to codify lung CT in Covid-19 patients.*(doi:10.100711547-020-01195-x

Berkane, S., Harizi, I., & Tayebi, A. (2021). Modeling the Effect of Population-Wide Vaccination on the Evolution of COVID-19 Epidemic in Canada. doi:10.1101/2021.02.05.21250572

Best, J., & the ZDNet News Website. (2020). *AI and the coronavirus fight: How artificial intelligence is taking on CO-VID-19.* https://www.zdnet.com/article/ai-and-the-coronavirus-fight-how-artificial-intelligence-is-taking-on-covid-19/

Bhange, M., & Hingoliwala, H. A. (2015). Smart Farming: Pomegranate Disease Detection Using Image Processing. *Second International Symposium on Computer Vision and the Internet,* 58, 280-288. 10.1016/j.procs.2015.08.022

Boudrioua, M. S., & Boudrioua, A. (2020). Predicting the COVID-19 epidemic in Algeria using the SIR model. doi:10.1101/2020.04.25.20079467

Broga, D. (2020). *How Taiwan used tech to fight COVID-19.* https://www.techuk.org/insights/news/item/17187-how-taiwan-used-techto-

Brune, R. (2008). *A Stochastic Model for Panic Behaviour in Disease Dynamics.* Academic Press.

Busso, C., Deng, Z., Yildirim, S., Bulut, M., Lee, C. M., Kazem Zadeh, A., Lee, S. B., Neumann, U., & Narayanan, S. (2004). *Analysis of Emotion Recognition using Facial Expression, Speech and Multimodal Information.* ICMI.

Butt, C., Gill, J., Chun, D., & Babu, B. A. (2020). Deep learning system to screen coronavirus disease 2019 pneumonia. *Applied Intelligence, Springer,* 2020, 1–7.

Caccavo, D. (2020). Chinese and Italian COVID-19 outbreaks can be correctly described by a modified SIRD model. doi:10.1101/2020.03.19.20039388

Calafiore, G. C., Novara, C., & Possieri, C. (2020). A time-varying SIRD model for the COVID-19 contagion in Italy. *Annual Reviews in Control,* 50, 361–372. doi:10.1016/j.arcontrol.2020.10.005 PMID:33132739

Celesti, F., Celesti, A., Carnevale, L., Galletta, A., Campo, S., Romano, A., Bramanti, P., & Villari, M. (2017). *Big data analytics in genomics: the point on deep learning solutions. IEEE symposium on computers and communications (ISCC).* IEEE.

Chahal, A., & Gulia, P. (2019). Machine Learning and Deep Learning. *International Journal of Innovative Technology and Exploring Engineering,* 8(12), 4910-4914.

Chahal, A., & Gulia, P. (2019). Machine Learning and Deep Learning. *International Journal of Innovative Technology and Exploring Engineering*, *8*(12).

Char, D.S. (2018). Implementing Machine Learning in Health Care — Addressing Ethical Challenges. *N Engl J Med*, *378*(11), 981–983.

Chatterjee, S., Sarkar, A., Chatterjee, S., Karmakar, M., & Paul, R. (2020). Studying the progress of COVID-19 outbreak in India using SIRD model. doi:10.1101/2020.05.11.20098681

Chattopadhyay, A. K., Choudhury, D., Ghosh, G., Kundu, B., & Nath, S. K. (2021). Infection kinetics of Covid-19 and containment strategy. *Scientific Reports*, *11*(1), 11606. doi:10.103841598-021-90698-2 PMID:34078929

Chen & Guestrin. (2016). *XGBoost: A Scalable Tree Boosting System KDD.* . doi:10.1145/2939672.2939785

Chen, M., Kuo, C., & Chan, W. K. (2021). Control of COVID-19 Pandemic: Vaccination Strategies Simulation under Probabilistic Node-Level Model. *2021 6th International Conference on Intelligent Computing and Signal Processing (ICSP)*.

Chen, X., Li, J., Xiao, C., & Yang, P. (2020). Numerical solution and parameter estimation for uncertain SIR model with application to COVID-19. *Fuzzy Optimization and Decision Making*, *20*(2), 189–208. doi:10.100710700-020-09342-9

Chowell, G., Castillo-Chavez, C., Fenimore, P. W., Kribs-Zaleta, C. M., Arriola, L., & Hyman, J. M. (2004). Model parameters and outbreak control for SARS. *Emerging Infectious Diseases*, *10*(7), 1258–1263. doi:10.3201/eid1007.030647 PMID:15324546

Chuo, F., Tiing, S., & Labadin, J. (2008). A Simple Deterministic Model for the Spread of Hand, Foot and Mouth Disease (HFMD) in Sarawak. *2008 Second Asia International Conference on Modelling & Simulation (AMS)*.

CNBC. (2021). *Delta covid variant has a new variant delta plus.* https://www.cnbc.com/2021/06/24/delta-plus-covid-variant-heres-what-you-need-to-know.html

Copeland, B. J., & Proudfoot, D. (2007). Artificial Intelligence: History, Foundations, And Philosophical Issues. Handbook of the Philosophy of Science. Philosophy of Psychology and Cognitive Science, 429-485.

Corbett. (2017, April 25). The Real-World Benefits of Machine Learning in Healthcare. *The Medical Officer*.

Cordelli, E., Tortora, M., Sicilia, R., & Soda, P. (2020). Time-Window SIQR Analysis of COVID-19 Outbreak and Containment Measures in Italy. *2020 IEEE 33rd International Symposium on Computer-Based Medical Systems (CBMS)*.

COVID-19 Pandemic Sparks 72% Ransomware Growth, Mobile Vulnerabilities Grow 50%, Skybox Security. (2021). https://www.prnewswire.com/in/news-releases/covid-19-pandemic-sparks-72-ransomware-growth-mobile-vulnerabilities-grow-50--817268901.html

COVID-19 Projections. (2020). https://covid19.healthdata.org/united-states-of-america

Covid19India. (2020). Available from https://www.covid19india.org/

Crokidakis, N. (2020). COVID-19 spreading in Rio de Janeiro, Brazil: Do the policies of social isolation really work? doi:10.1101/2020.04.27.20081737

Cun, Y.L., Bengio, Y., & Hinton, G. (2015). Deep Learning. *Nature*, *521*, 438-444.

Dalvi Rd, F., Zago, G. T., & Andreão, R. V. (2016). Heartbeat classification system based on neural networks and dimensionality reduction. *Research on Biomedical Engineering*, *32*(4), 318–326. doi:10.1590/2446-4740.05815

Das, S., Ghosh, P., Sen, B., & Mukhopadhyay, I. (2020). *Critical community size for COVID- 19–a model based approach to provide a rationale behind the lockdown.* arXiv preprint arXiv: 200403126.

datarobot.com. (2020). *Enabling the AI-Driven Enterprise.* http://www.datarobot.com

Davenport, T., & Kalakota, R. (2019). The potential for artificial intelligence in healthcare. *Future Healthcare Journal,* 6(2), 94–98. doi:10.7861/futurehosp.6-2-94 PMID:31363513

Devi, M. N., Balamurugan, A., & Kris, M. R. (2016). Developing a Modified Logistic Regression Model for Diabetes Mellitus and Identifying the Important Factors of Type II Dm. *Indian Journal of Science and Technology.*

Devlin, J., Chang, M.-W., Lee, K., & Toutanova, K. (2018). *BERT: Pre-training of Deep Bidirectional Transformers for Language Understanding.* arXiv:1810.04805v2

Devlin, J., & Chang, M.-W. (2019). *Open Sourcing BERT: State-of-the-Art Pre-training for Natural Language Processing.* Google AI Blog.

Dey, A. K., Sharma, M., & Meshram, M. R. (2016). Image Processing Based Leaf Rot Disease, Detection of Betel Vine (Piper BetleL.). *International Conference on Computational Modeling and Security,* 85, 748-754.

Digiteum. (2021, July 1). *Top Mobile App Categories during COVID-19.* https://www.digiteum.com/top-mobile-app-categories-covid/

Domingos, P. (2012). A Few Useful Things to Know About Machine Learning. *Communications of the ACM,* 55(10), 1–10. doi:10.1145/2347736.2347755

Domino's India data hacked? 1 million credit card details, phone numbers allegedly leaked. (2021). *Business Today.* https://www.businesstoday.in/latest/corporate/story/omg-dominos-india-hacked-1-million-credit-card-details-names-phone-numbers-leaked-293943-2021-04-20

During, R. (2020). *COVID-19.* https://www.govtech.com/blogs/lohrmann-on-cybersecurity/ransomware-during-covid-19.html

e-Learning Industry. (2021, July 1). *Advantages And Disadvantages Of Online Learning.* https://elearningindustry.com/advantages-and-disadvantages-online-learning

Engels, E. A., Pfeiffer, R. M., Goedert, J. J., Virgo, P., McNeel, T. S., Scoppa, S. M., & Biggar, R. J. (2006). Trends in cancer risk among people with AIDS in the United States 1980–2002. *AIDS (London, England),* 20(12), 1645–1654. doi:10.1097/01.aids.0000238411.75324.59 PMID:16868446

Epidemics, COVID-19 Hospital Impact Model for. (2020). https://penn-chime.phl.io

EstradaM. A. R. (2020). *The Uses of Drones in Case of Massive Epidemics.* doi:10.2139srn.3546547

Express, F. (2021, July 1). *Private companies claiming incapacity in paying full wages must place balance sheets in court: Centre tells SC.* https://www.financialexpress.com/india-news/salary-cut-during-lockdown-supreme-court-home-ministry-order-private-companies-balance-sheet/1981053/

Fang, T. (2006). A kind of epidemic model with infectious force in both latent period and infected period and nonlinear infection rate. *J. Biomath.,* 21(3), 345–350.

Fatima & Pasha. (2014). Survey of Machine Learning Algorithms for Disease Diagnostic. *JILSA,* 9(1).

Ferretti, L., Wymant, C., Kendall, M., Zhao, L., Nurtay, A., Abeler-Dörner, L., Parker, M., Bonsall, D., & Fraser, C. (2020). *Quantifying SARS-CoV-2 transmission suggests epidemic control with digital contact tracing.* doi:10.1126cience.abb6936

Franco, L., & Treves, A. (2001). A neural network facial expression recognition system using unsupervised local processing. In *Proceedings of the 2nd International Symposium on Image and Signal Processing and Analysis*. IEEE. 10.1109/ISPA.2001.938703

Gao, Yang, Lin, & Park. (2018). *Computer vision in healthcare applications.* doi:10.1155/2018/5157020

Garcia & Barbedo. (2016). *A review on the main challenges in automatic plant disease identification based on visible range images.* Science Direct, Biosystems Engineering.

Gavhale, K. R., & Gawande, U. (2014). An Overview of the Research on Plant Leaves Disease Detection using Image Processing Techniques. *IOSR Journal of Computer Engineering*, *16*(1), 10–16.

Gay, C. (2003). Dye and N., 2003. "Modeling the SARS epidemic. *Science*, *300*(5627), 1884–1885. PMID:12766208

Ghahraman, Z. (2004). Unsupervised Learning. *Machine Learning, LNAI, 3176*, 72–112.

GholamiB.HaddadW. M.BaileyJ. M. (2018). https://spectrum.ieee.org/biomedical/devices/ai-could-provide-momentby-moment-nursing-for-a-hospitals-sickest-patients

Ghosh, S., & Singh, A. (2020). The scope of Artificial Intelligence in mankind: A detailed review. *Journal of Physics: Conference Series*, *1531*, 012045.

Gibbons, J.A. (2019). Machine learning in medicine: a practical introduction. *BMC Medical Research Methodology,* 19-64.

Global News. (2020). *Global news.* http://globalnews.ca

Gris, K. V., Coutu, J. P., & Gris, D. (2017). Supervised and Unsupervised Learning Technology in the Study of Rodent Behavior. *Frontiers in Behavioral Neuroscience, Vol, 11*, 141–143. doi:10.3389/fnbeh.2017.00141 PMID:28804452

Gulshan, Peng, & Coram. (2016). *Development and Validation of a Deep Learning Algorithm for Detection of Diabetic Retinopathy in Retinal Fundus Photographs.* doi:10.1001/jama.2016.17216 PMID:27898976

Gutierrez, G. (2020). *Artificial Intelligence in the Intensive Care Unit.* doi:10.118613054-020-2785-y

Hafeez, M. F. A. (2020). *Covid-resnet: A deep learning framework for screening of covid19 from radiographs.* arXiv preprint arXiv:2003.14395

Haleem, Ibrahim, & Abid. (2020). *Artificial Intelligence (AI) applications for COVID-19 pandemic.* doi:10.1016/j.dsx.2020.04.012

Hara, N. (2007). Global stability of a delayed SIR epidemic model with density dependent birth and death rates. *Journal of Computational and Applied Mathematics*, *201*(2), 339–347. doi:10.1016/j.cam.2005.12.034

Hattori, A., & Sturm, R. (2013). The obesity epidemic and changes in self-report biases in BMI. *Obesity (Silver Spring, Md.)*, *21*(4), 856–860. doi:10.1002/oby.20313 PMID:23712990

Hertz, L. (2020). *Face Mask Detection System using Artificial Intelligence.* https://www.leewayhertz.com/face-mask-detection-system/

Hochreiter, S., & Schmidhuber, J. (1997). Long short-term memory. *Neural Comput.*

Hosmer, D. W., Lemeshow, S., & Sturdivant, R. X. (2013). *Applied Logistic Regression.* Wiley Series in Probability and Statistics. doi:10.1002/9781118548387

Hota, A. (2014). *Development and Validation of Statistical and Deterministic Models Used to Predict Dengue Fever in Mexico* [Bachelors Dissertation]. Harvard University.

Houthooft, R., Ruyssinck, J., van der Herten, J., Stijven, S., Couckuyt, I., Gadeyne, B., Ongenae, F., Colpaert, K., Decruyenaere, J., Dhaene, T., & De Turck, F. (2015). Predictive modelling of survival and length of stay in critically ill patients using sequential organ failure scores. *Artificial Intelligence in Medicine, 63*(3), 191–207. doi:10.1016/j.artmed.2014.12.009 PMID:25579436

Hu, Z., Ge, Q., Jin, L., & Xiong, M. (2020). *Artificial intelligence forecasting of COVID-19 in China.* arXiv preprint: 200207112.

Huang, Y., Sun, M., & Sui, Y. (2020). *How Digital Contact Tracing Slowed Covid-19 in East Asia.* https://hbr.org/2020/04/how-digital-contact-tracing-slowed-covid-19-in-east-asia

ICMR COVID Study Group, COVID Epidemiology & Data Management Team, COVID Laboratory Team, & VRDLN Team. (2020). Laboratory surveillance for SARS-CoV-2 in India: Performance of testing & descriptive epidemiology of detected COVID-19. *The Indian Journal of Medical Research, 151*, 424–437. doi:10.4103/ijmr.IJMR_1896_20

Ideris, S. H. B. (2016). *The development of stochastic SIR and S(I^m I^f) R models for heterosexual HIV and AIDS disease mapping in Malaysia* [Masters Dissertation, Universiti Pendidikan Sultan Idris]. UPSI Digital Repository.

Ideris, S. H., Malim, M. R., & Shaadan, N. (2021). Relative Risk Estimation for Human Leptospirosis Disease in Malaysia Based on Existing Models and Discrete Space-Time Stochastic Sir Model. *Pertanika Journal of Science & Technology, 29*(2). Advance online publication. doi:10.47836/pjst.29.2.20

IHME. (2021). *The potential future of covid pandemic.* http://www.healthdata.org/research-article/potential-future-covid-19-pandemic

Imai, N. (2020). *Transmissibility of 2019-nCoV, WHO Collaborating Centre Infect. Dis. Model. MRC Centre Global Infect.Dis. Anal. J-IDEA, Imperial Coll.* doi:10.25561/77148

Impact of digital surge during Covid-19 pandemic: A viewpoint on research and practice. (2020). https://www.ncbi.nlm.nih.gov/pmc/articles/PMC7280123/

Ince, T., Kiranyaz, S., & Gabbouj, M. A. (2009). generic and robust system for automated patient-specific classification of ECG signals. *IEEE Transactions on Biomedical Engineering, 56*(5), 1415–1426. doi:10.1109/TBME.2009.2013934 PMID:19203885

Infographics. (2020). *Machine Learning in Healthcare: Examples, Tips & Resources for Implementing into Your Care Practice.* Author.

International Business, Times. (2020). *Scientists develop new AI model that can predict coronavirus without testing.* https://www.ibtimes.sg/scientists-develop-new-ai-model-that-can-predict-coronavirus-without-testing-44889

IoT Privacy and Security. Challenges and Solutions. (2020). https://www.mdpi.com/2076-3417/10/12/4102/pdf

Jacimovski, S., & Kekić, D. (2010). A mathematical SIR model for epidemic emergency. *NBP - Journal of Criminalistics and Law, 15*, 65-76.

Jahanshahi, H., Munoz-Pacheco, J. M., Bekiros, S., & Alotaibi, N. D. (2021). A fractional-order SIRD model with time-dependent memory indexes for encompassing the multi-fractional characteristics of the COVID-19. *Chaos, Solitons, and Fractals, 143*, 110632. doi:10.1016/j.chaos.2020.110632 PMID:33519121

Jhuria, M., Kumar, A., & Borse, R. (2013). Image Processing For Smart Farming: Detection Of Disease And Fruit Grading. *Proceedings of the 2013 IEEE Second International Conference on Image Information Processing (ICIIP-2013).* 10.1109/ICIIP.2013.6707647

Jiang, F. (2017). Artificial intelligence in healthcare: past, present, and future. *Stroke and Vascular Neurology*, *2*, 230-243.

Jiang, F. (2017). Artificial intelligence in healthcare: Past, present and future. Stroke and Vascular Neurology. *BMJ (Clinical Research Ed.)*, *2017*, 230–243.

Jin, C., Chen, W., Cao, Y., Xu, Z., Zhang, X., Deng, L., Zheng, C., Zhou, J., Shi, H., & Feng, J. (2020). Development and evaluation of an ai system for covid-19 diagnosis. doi:10.1101/2020.03.20.20039834

Jo, H., Son, H., Hwang, H. J., & Jung, S. Y. (2020). *Analysis of COVID-19 spread in South Korea using the SIR model with time-dependent parameters and deep learning*. Academic Press.

Jong, M.C.M., & de., Diekmann, O., & Heesterbeek, H. (1995). How Does Transmission of Infection Depend on Transmission Size*? Publications of the Newton Institute*, *5*, 84–94.

Journal, R. (2020). *Radiology Journal.* https://pubs.rsna.org/journal/radiology

Kapoor, A., Guha, S., Kanti Das, M., Goswami, K. C., & Yadav, R. (2020). Digital healthcare: The only solution for better healthcare during COVID-19 pandemic? *Indian Heart Journal*, *72*(2), 61–64. doi:10.1016/j.ihj.2020.04.001 PMID:32534691

Katal, S., Pouraryan, A., & Gholamrezanezhad, A. (2021). COVID-19 vaccine is here: Practical considerations for clinical imaging applications. *Clinical Imaging*, *76*, 38–41. doi:10.1016/j.clinimag.2021.01.023 PMID:33548891

Kato, F., Tainaka, K., Sone, S., Morita, S., Iida, H., & Yoshimura, J. (2011). Combined effects of prevention and quarantine on a breakout in SIR model. *Scientific Reports*, *1*(1), 10. doi:10.1038rep00010 PMID:22355529

Katsis, C. D., Katertsidis, N., Ganiatsas, G., & Fotiadis, D. I. (2008). Toward Emotion Recognition in Car Racing Drivers: A Bio signal Processing Approach. *IEEE Transactions on Systems, Man, and Cybernetics.*

Kaur, N., & Goyal, K. (2021). Uncertainty Quantification of Stochastic Epidemic SIR Models Using B-spline Polynomial Chaos. *Regular and Chaotic Dynamics*, *26*(1), 22–38. doi:10.1134/S1560354721010020

Kelly, C. (2019). Key challenges for delivering clinical impact with artificial intelligence. *BMC Medicine*, *17*(195), 1–9.

Kermack, W.O., & McKendrick, A.G. (1991). *Contributions to the mathematical theory of epidemics–I*. Academic Press.

Kermack, W. O., & McKendrick, A. G. (1927). A contribution to the mathematical theory of epidemics. *Proceedings of the Royal Society of London. Series B, Containing Papers of a Biological Character*, *115*, 700–721.

Ketchell, M. (2020). *Why Singapore's coronavirus response worked – and what we can all learn.* https://theconversation.com/why-singapores-coronavirus-response-worked-and-what-we-can-all-learn-134024

Khalid, M., & Khan, F. (2016). Stability Analysis of Deterministic Mathematical Model for Zika Virus. *British Journal of Mathematics & Computer Science*, *19*(4), 1–10. doi:10.9734/BJMCS/2016/29834

Kleinbaum, D. G., & Klein, M. (2010a). Introduction to Logistic Regression. *Logistic Regression,* 1–39.

Kleinbaum, D. G., & Klein, M. (2010b). Important Special Cases of the Logistic Model. Logistic Regression. *Logistic Regression,* 41–71.

Kotsia, I., & Pitas, I. (2007, January). Facial Expression Recognition in Image Sequences Using Geometric Deformation Features and Support Vector Machines. *IEEE Transactions on Image Processing*, *16*(1), 172–187.

KPMG. (2021, July 1). *How COVID-19 is accelerating digitalisation for the....* https://home.kpmg/in/en/blogs/home/posts/2020/07/how-covid-19-accelerating-digitalisation-banking-payments-industry.html

Krieger. (2017). *Google computers trained to detect cancer*. Bay Area News Group.

Kubota. (2017). *Stanford researchers have trained an algorithm to diagnose skin cancer*. Academic Press.

Kumar, Gupta, & Srivastava. (2020). *A review of modern technologies for tackling COVID-19 pandemic*. doi:10.1016/j.dsx.2020.05.008

Kumar, V. (2020). *Tackling COVID-19: The Technology behind Contact Tracing*. https://www.mygreatlearning.com/blog/covid-contact-tracing/

Kuniya, T. (2020). Evaluation of the effect of the state of emergency for the first wave of COVID-19 in Japan. *Infectious Disease Modelling*, *5*, 580–587. doi:10.1016/j.idm.2020.08.004 PMID:32844135

Kushta, E., & Prenga, D. (2021). Extended log periodic approach in analysing local critical behaviour–case study for Covid-19 spread in Albania. *Journal of Physics: Conference Series*, *1730*(1), 012056. doi:10.1088/1742-6596/1730/1/012056

Lalwani, S., Sahni, G., Mewara, B., & Kumar, R. (2020). Predicting optimal lockdown period with parametric approach using three-phase maturation SIRD model for COVID-19 pandemic. *Chaos, Solitons, and Fractals*, 138. PMID:32834574

Le, J. (2019). *The 5 Trends Dominating Computer Vision*. https://heartbeat.fritz.ai/the-5-trends-that-dominated-computer-vision-in-2018-de38fbb9bd86

Ledzewicz, U., & Schattler, H. (2011). On optimal singular controls for a general SIR-model with vaccination and treatment. *Conference Publications 2011*.

Letko, M., Marzi, A., & Munster, V. (2020). Functional assessment of cell entry and receptor usage for SARS-CoV-2 and other lineage B beta coronaviruses. *Nature, 5*, 562–569. PMID:32094589

Li, J., Wang, Y., Wu, J., Ai, J., Zhang, H., Gamber, M., Li, W., Zhang, W.-H., & Sun, W. (2020). Do Stay at Home Orders and Cloth Face Coverings Control COVID-19 in New York City? Results From a SIER Model Based on Real-world Data. *Open Forum Infectious Diseases*, *8*(2), ofaa442. doi:10.1093/ofid/ofaa442 PMID:33553466

Li, L. (2020). Artificial Intelligence Distinguishes COVID-19 from Community-Acquired Pneumonia on Chest CT. *Radiology*. Advance online publication. doi:10.1148/radiol.2020200905

Lin, Zhou, Faghri, Shaw, & Campbell. (2019). *Analysis and prediction of unplanned intensive care unit readmission using recurrent neural networks with long short term memory*. Academic Press.

Li, S., Lin, Y., Zhu, T., Fan, M., Xu, S., Qiu, W., Chen, C., Li, L., Wang, Y., Yan, J., Wong, J., Naing, L., & Xu, S. (2021). Development and external evaluation of predictions models for mortality of COVID-19 patients using machine learning method. *Neural Computing & Applications*. PMID:33424133

Liyana, Ibeni, Salikon, & Salleh. (2019). Comparative analysis on bayesian classification for breast cancer problem. *Computer Science, Bulletin of Electrical Engineering and Informatics*.

Lounis, M. (2021). Estimation of epidemiological indicators of COVID-19 in Algeria with an SIRD model. *Eurasian Journal of Medicine and Oncology*.

Ma'sum, M. A., Jatmiko, W., & Suhartanto, H. (2016). Enhanced tele ECG system using hadoop framework to deal with big data processing. In *International workshop on Big Data and information security (IWBIS)*. New York: IEEE. 10.1109/IWBIS.2016.7872900

Maetschke, S. R., Madhamshettiwa, P. B., Davis, M. J., & Ragan, M. A. (2013). Supervised, semi-supervised and unsupervised inference of gene regulatory networks. *Briefing in Bioinformatics, Vol, 15*(2), 195–211. doi:10.1093/bib/bbt034 PMID:23698722

Maghdid, H. S., Ghafoor, K. Z., Sadiq, A. S., Curran, K., & Rabie, K. (2020). A novel AI-enabled framework to diagnose coronavirus COVID 19 using smartphone embedded sensors: design study. doi:10.1109/IRI49571.2020.00033

Mahrouf, M., Boukhouima, A., Zine, H., Lotfi, E. M., Torres, D. F., & Yousfi, N. (2021). Modeling and Forecasting of COVID-19 Spreading by Delayed Stochastic Differential Equations. *Axioms*, *10*(1), 18. doi:10.3390/axioms10010018

Maki, K. (2020). A delayed SEIQR epidemic model of COVID-19 in Tokyo. doi:10.1101/2020.08.18.20177709

Malhotra, B., & Kashyap, V. (2020). Progression of COVID-19 in Indian States - Forecasting Endpoints Using SIR and Logistic Growth Models. doi:10.1101/2020.05.15.20103028

Malik, A., Kumar, N., & Alam, K. (2021). Estimation of parameter of fractional order COVID-19 SIQR epidemic model. *Materials Today: Proceedings*.

Maruthappu, M. (2018). Debate & Analysis Artificial intelligence in medicine: Current trends and future possibilities. *The British Journal of General Practice*, 143–144.

Medical News Today. (2021). *Are treatments available for covid 19.* https://www.medicalnewstoday.com/articles/coronavirus-treatment#care-at-home

Medical News Today. (2021, July 1). *How do COVID-19 vaccines work?* https://www.medicalnewstoday.com/articles/how-do-covid-19-vaccines-work

Mila, A. L., Carriquiry, A. L., & Yang, X. B. (2004). Logistic Regression Modeling of Prevalence of Soybean Sclerotinia Stem Rot in the North-Central Region of the United States. *Phytopathology*, *94*(1), 102–110. doi:10.1094/PHYTO.2004.94.1.102 PMID:18943826

Ming-Yen, N., & Elaine, Y. P. (2020). Imaging profile of the covid-19 infection: Radiologic findings and literature review. *Radiology. Cardiothoracic Imaging*, *2*(1), e200034. doi:10.1148/ryct.2020200034 PMID:33778547

Ministry of External Affairs. (2021, July 1). *COVID-19 Updates.* https://www.mea.gov.in/vaccine-supply.htm

Ministry of Health and Family Welfare. (2021, July 1). *Frequently Asked Questions.* https://www.mohfw.gov.in/covid_vaccination/vaccination/faqs.html#about-the-vaccine

Mitra, G. (2020). *Vehant Technologies' Uses AI For Social Distancing, Face Mask And Vehicle Detection.* https://www.expresscomputer.in/indiaincfightscovid19/vehant-technologies-uses-ai-for-social-distancing-face-mask-and-vehicle-detection/55421/

Mohamed, I. A., Aissa, A. B., Hussein, L. F., Taloba, A. I., & Kallel, T. (2021). A new model for epidemic prediction: COVID-19 in kingdom Saudi Arabia case study. *Materials Today: Proceedings*. Advance online publication. doi:10.1016/j.matpr.2021.01.088 PMID:33520671

Mooney, P. (2018). *Chest X-Ray.* https://www.kaggle.com/paultimothymooney/chest-xray-pneumonia

Muhammad, I., & Ya, Z. (2015). *Supervised machine learning approaches A survey.* State Journal on Soft Computing. doi:10.21917/ijsc.2015.0133

Mwanga, E. P., Minja, E. G., Mrimi, E., Jiménez, M. G., Swai, J. K., Abbasi, S., . . . Okumu, F. O. (2019). Detection of malaria parasites in dried human blood spots using mid-infrared spectroscopy and logistic regression analysis. doi:10.1101/19001206

Nain, M., Sharma, S., & Chaurasia, S. (2021). Safety and Compliance Management System Using Computer Vision and Deep Learning. *IOP Conference Series: Materials Science and Engineering*.

Narin, A., Kaya, C., & Pamuk, Z. (2020). *Automatic detection of coronavirus disease (covid-19) using x-ray images and deep convolutional neural networks.* arXiv preprint arXiv:2003.10849

Nashif, S., Raihan, M. R., & Imam, M. H. (2019). *Heart Disease Detection by Using Machine Learning Algorithms and a Real-Time Cardiovascular Health Monitoring System. World Journal of Engineering and Technology.*

Nassar, A.P., Jr., & Caruso, P. (2016). *ICU physicians are unable to accurately predict length of stay at admission: a prospective study.* doi:10.1093/intqhc/mzv112

Ndiaye, B., & Tendeng, L., & Seck, D. (2020). *Analysis of the COVID-19 pandemic by SIR model and machine learning technics for forecasting.* ResearchGate database.

Neher, R. A., Dyrdak, R., Druelle, V., Hodcroft, E. B., & Albert, J. (2020). Potential impact of seasonal forcing on a SARS-CoV-2 pandemic. *Swiss Medical Weekly.* PMID:32176808

Nesteruk, I., & Benlagha, N. (2021). Predictions of COVID-19 Pandemic Dynamics in Ukraine and Qatar Based on Generalized SIR Model. *Innovative Biosystems and Bioengineering, 5*(1), 37–46. doi:10.20535/ibb.2021.5.1.228605

News 18. (2021, July 1). *As RBI Remains Worried over Food Inflation, How Prices of Daal and Milk Rose During Covid-19 Lockdown.* https://www.news18.com/news/india/as-rbi-remains-worried-over-food-inflation-how-prices-of-daal-milk-rose-during-lockdown-2662815.html

Nguyen, T.T., Waurn, G., & Campus, P. (2020). *Artificial intelligence in the battle against coronavirus (COVID-19): A survey and future research directions.* doi:10.13140/RG.2.2.36491.23846

O'Brien, J. (2014). *Using hidden Markov models and spark to mine ECG data.* Academic Press.

Odagaki, T. (2021). Exact properties of SIQR model for COVID-19. *Physica A, 564,* 125564. doi:10.1016/j.physa.2020.125564 PMID:33250562

Omar, A. H., & Hasan, Y. A. (2013). Numerical simulations of an SIR epidemic model with random initial states. *ScienceAsia, 39S*(1), 42. doi:10.2306cienceasia1513-1874.2013.39S.042

Omrani, E., Khoshnevisan, B., Shamshirband, S., Saboohi, H., Anuar, N.B., & Nasir, M.H.N. (2014). Potential of radial basis function-based support vector regression for apple disease detection. *Journal of Measurement,* 233-252.

Ou. (2020). Characterization of spike glycoprotein of SARS-CoV-2 on virus entry and its immune cross-reactivity with SARS-CoV. *Nature Communications, 2,*16-20.

PARHLO. (n.d.). *COVID: A brief history of deadly corona virus.* https://www.parhlo.com/history-of-coronavirus

Pedersen, M. G., & Meneghini, M. (2020b). Data-driven estimation of change points reveals correlation between face mask use and accelerated curtailing of the COVID-19 epidemic in Italy. doi:10.1101/2020.06.29.20141523

Pedersen, M. G., & Meneghini, M. (2020c). A simple method to quantify country-specific effects of COVID-19 containment measures. doi:10.1101/2020.04.07.20057075

Pedersen, M., & Meneghini, M. (2020a). *Quantifying undetected COVID-19 cases and effects of containment measures in Italy: Predicting phase 2 dynamics.* . doi:10.13140/RG.2.2.11753.85600

Peng, M. (2020). Artificial intelligence application in COVID-19 diagnosis and prediction. SSRN *Electronic Journal,* 1-17. doi:10.2139srn.3541119

Pérez, Aguilar, & Dapena. (2020). MIHR: A Human-Robot Interaction Model. *IEEE Latin America Transactions, 18*(9), 1521-1529.

Perra, N., Balcan, D., Gonçalves, B., & Vespignani, A. (2011). Towards a Characterization of Behavior-Disease Models. *PLoS One*, 6(8), e23084. Advance online publication. doi:10.1371/journal.pone.0023084 PMID:21826228

Phadikar, S., & Sil, J. (2008). Rice Disease Identification using Pattern Recognition. *Proceedings of 11th International Conference on Computer and Information Technology (ICCIT 2008)*.

Pirouz, B. (2020). Investigating a serious challenge in the sustainable development process: Analysis of confirmed cases of COVID-19 (New Type of Coronavirus) Through a Binary Classification Using Artificial Intelligence and Regression Analysis. *Sustainability*.

Pisani, P., Renna, M. D., Conversano, F., Casciaro, E., Muratore, M., Quarta, E., Di Paola, M., & Casciaro, S. (2013). Screening and early diagnosis of osteoporosis through x-ray and ultrasound based techniques. *World Journal of Radiology*, 5(11), 398. doi:10.4329/wjr.v5.i11.398 PMID:24349644

ProtocolB. T. (2020). https://bluetrace.io/

Pujari, J. D., Yakkundimath, R., & Byadgi, A. S. (2015). Image Processing Based Detection of Fungal Diseases In Plants. *International Conference on Information and Communication Technologies*, 46, 1802-1808. 10.1016/j.procs.2015.02.137

Qi, X., Jiang, Z., & Yu, Q. (2016). *Machine Learning based CT radiomics model for predicting hospital stay in patients with pneumonia associated with SARSCoV-2 infection: A multicentre study.*. doi:10.1016/S0031-3955(16)31867-3

Rahardiantoro, S., & Sakamoto, W. (2021). Clustering Regions Based on Socio-Economic Factors Which Affected the Number of COVID-19 Cases in Java Island. *Journal of Physics: Conference Series*, 1863(1), 012014. doi:10.1088/1742-6596/1863/1/012014

Rao, A. S. R. (2020). Identification of COVID-19 Can be Quicker through Artificial Intelligence framework using a Mobile Phone-Based Survey in the Populations when Cities/Towns Are Under Quarantine. *Infection Control and Hospital Epidemiology*, 1–18.

RenZ. (2013). *A Case Study of Using Refined Epidemic SIR Model to Analyse Bad Takeover and the Distributions of Well-Performed, Bad-Performed and Bankrupt Companies*. Available at https://ssrn.com/abstract=2513691

Report, G. S. (2021, July 1). *COVID-19's impact on education in India: It's not all bad news*. https://www.globalsistersreport.org/news/ministry/column/covid-19s-impact-education-india-its-not-all-bad-news

Rodas, F., Paredes, M., Celis, G., & Pullas-Tapia, G. (2020). *Use of mathematical models for epidemiological simulation of Covid-19 in Ecuador*. Academic Press.

Rosebrock, A. (2018). *OpenCV Face Recognition, PyImageSearch*. https://www.pyimagesearch.com/2018/09/24/opencv-face-recognition/

Saaidia, M., Zermi, N., & Ramdani, M. (2014). Facial Expression Recognition Using Neural Network Trained with Zernike Moments. *2014 4th International Conference on Artificial Intelligence with Applications in Engineering and Technology*, 187-192. 10.1109/ICAIET.2014.39

Saito, M. M., Imoto, S., Yamaguchi, R., Miyano, S., & Higuchi, T. (2014). Parameter estimation in multi-compartment SIR model. *17th International Conference on Information Fusion (FUSION)*, 1-5.

Salman, F. M. (2020). COVID-19 Detection using Artificial Intelligence. *International Journal of Academic Engineering Research*, 4(3), 18–25.

Sathya, R., & Abraham, A. (2013). Comparison of Supervised and Unsupervised Learning Algorithms for Pattern Classification. *International Journal of Advanced Research in Artificial Intelligence, Vol, 2*(2), 34–38. doi:10.14569/IJARAI.2013.020206

Sato, A., Ito, I., Sawai, H., & Iwata, K. (2015). An epidemic simulation with a delayed stochastic SIR model based on international socioeconomic-technological databases. *2015 IEEE International Conference on Big Data (Big Data).* 10.1109/BigData.2015.7364074

Scenarios, COVID-19. (2020). *COVID-19 Scenarios.* https://neherlab.org/covid19/

Schmidhuber, J. (2015). Deep learning in neural networks: An overview. *Neural Networks, 61*, 85–117.

Sedaghat, A., Alkhatib, F., Mostafaeipour, N., & Oloomi, S. A. (2020). Prediction of COVID-19 Dynamics in Kuwait using SIRD Model. *International Journal of Medical Sciences, 7*. Advance online publication. doi:10.15342/ijms.7.170

Sen, M. D., & Ibeas, A. (2021). On an SE(Is)(Ih)AR epidemic model with combined vaccination and antiviral controls for COVID-19 pandemic. *Advances in Difference Equations, 2021*(1). doi:10.118613662-021-03248-5

Sethy, P. K., & Behera, S. K. (2020). Detection of coronavirus disease (COVID-19) based on deep features. doi:10.20944/preprints202003.0300.v1

Setzer, E. (2020). *Contact-Tracing Apps in the United States.* https://www.lawfareblog.com/contact-tracing-apps-united-states

Shastri, S., Singh, K., Kumar, S., Kour, P., & Mansotra, V. (2020). Time series forecasting of Covid-19 using deep learning models: India-USA comparative case study. *Chaos, Solitons, and Fractals, 140*, 110227. doi:10.1016/j.chaos.2020.110227 PMID:32843824

Shi, H., Lee, K., Lee, H., Ho, W., Sun, D., Wang, J., & Chiu, C. (2012). Comparison of Artificial Neural Network and Logistic Regression Models for Predicting In-Hospital Mortality after Primary Liver Cancer Surgery. *PLoS One, 7*(4), e35781. doi:10.1371/journal.pone.0035781 PMID:22563399

Sisense. (2021, July 1). *Real Time Dashboard.* https://www.sisense.com/glossary/real-time-dashboard/#:~:text=A%20real%2Dtime%20dashboard%20is,the%20most%20current%20data%20available.&text=Real%2Dtime%20dashboards%20can%20be,day%2Dto%2Dday%20basis

Sommer. (2019). *Israel Unveils Open Source App to Warn Users of Coronavirus Cases.* https://www.haaretz.com/israel-news/israel-unveils-app-that-uses-tracking-to-tell-users-if-they-were-near-virus-cases-1.8702055

Song, Y., Zheng, S., Li, L., Zhang, X., Zhang, X., & Huang, Z. (2020). Deep learning enables accurate diagnosis of novel coronavirus (COVID-19) with CT images. medRxiv.

Sotoodeh & Ho. (2019). *Improving length of stay prediction using a hidden Markov model.* Academic Press.

Speidel, Wilfley, Star-Lack, Heanue, & Van Lysel. (2006). Scanning-beam digital x-ray (sbdx) technology for interventional and diagnostic cardiac angiography. *Medical Physics, 33*(8), 2714-2727.

Standard, B. (2021, July 1). *Under the shadow of Covid-19 pandemic, inflation bites India the hardest.* https://www.business-standard.com/article/economy-policy/under-the-shadow-of-covid-19-pandemic-inflation-bites-india-the-hardest-120121600750_1.html

Sugiyanto, S., & Abrori, M. (2020). A Mathematical Model of the Covid-19 Cases in Indonesia (Under and Without Lockdown Enforcement). *Biology, Medicine, & Natural Product Chemistry, 9*(1), 15–19. doi:10.14421/biomedich.2020.91.15-19

Sun, H., Qiu, Y., Yan, H., Huang, Y., Zhu, Y., Gu, J., & Chen, S. (2021). Tracking Reproductivity of COVID-19 Epidemic in China with Varying Coefficient SIR Model. *Journal of Data Science: JDS*, 455–472. doi:10.6339/JDS.202007_18(3).0010

Supervised Machine Learning. (n.d.). *What is, Algorithms with Examples.* Guru99. https://www.guru99.com/supervised-machine-learning.html

Thangadurai & Padmavathi. (2014). Computer Visionimage Enhancement For Plant Leaves Disease Detection. *World Congress on Computing and Communication Technologies.*

The Hindu. (2021, July 1). *COVID-19 has accelerated digitisation process: study.* https://www.thehindu.com/business/covid-19-has-accelerated-digitisation-process-study/article33243203.ece

The Indian Express. (2020). *Mumbai hospitals run out of beds for critical Covid patients.* https://indianexpress.com/article/cities/mumbai/mumbai-hospitals-run-out-of-beds-for-critical-covid-patients-6407221/

The Indian Express. (2021, July 1). *Explained: What has changed in the second wave of Covid-19 in India?* https://indianexpress.com/article/explained/explained-whats-changed-in-second-wave-7289002/

The Quint. (2021, July 1). *India's Poor Are Eating Into Their Savings, Thanks To High Inflation And Covid-19.* https://www.bloombergquint.com/economy-finance/indias-poor-are-eating-into-their-savings-thanks-to-high-inflation-and-covid-19

Thomas. (2020). *15 examples of machine learning in healthcare that are revolutionizing medicine.* Academic Press.

Today, I. (2021, July 1). *Covid-19: 4 negative impacts and 4 opportunities created for education.* https://www.indiatoday.in/education-today/featurephilia/story/covid-19-4-negative-impacts-and-4-opportunities-created-for-education-1677206-2020-05-12

Tovissodé, C. F., Doumatè, J. T., & Kakaï, R. G. (2021). A Hybrid Modeling Technique of Epidemic Outbreaks with Application to COVID-19 Dynamics in West Africa. *Biology (Basel)*, *10*(5), 365. doi:10.3390/biology10050365 PMID:33922834

Tsang, S. (2020). *Contact tracing apps being deployed around the world.* https://iapp.org/news/a/here-are-the-contact-tracing-apps-being-employed-around-the-world/

Ulhaq, A., Khan, A., Gomes, D., & Paul, M. (2020). Computer vision for COVID-19 control. *Survey.* arXiv2004.09420

Valenzuela, T. D., Roe, D. J., Cretin, S., Spaite, D. W., & Larsen, M. P. (1997). Estimating Effectiveness of Cardiac Arrest Interventions. *Circulation*, *96*(10), 3308–3313. doi:10.1161/01.CIR.96.10.3308 PMID:9396421

Vembandasamy, K., Sasipriya, R., & Deepa, E. (2015). Heart Diseases Detection Using Naive Bayes Algorithm. IJISET-International Journal of Innovative Science. *Engineering & Technology*, *2*, 441–444.

Verma, V., & Priyanka. (2020). *Study of lockdown/testing mitigation strategies on stochastic sir model and its comparison with South Korea, Germany and New York data.* arXiv preprint arXiv:2006.14373.

Wang, H., Li, G., Ma, Z., & Li, X. (2012). Image Recognition of Plant Diseases Based on Principal Component Analysis and Neural Networks. In *8th International Conference on Natural Computation (ICNC 2012)* (pp. 246-251). IEEE.

Wang, New, & Sun. (2020). *Response to COVID-19 in Taiwan big data analytics, new technology, and proactive testing.* doi:10.1001/jama.2020.3151

Wang, P. (2019). On Defining Artificial Intelligence. *Journal of Artificial General Intelligence, 10*(2), 1-37.

Wang, S., Kang, B., Ma, J., Zeng, X., Xiao, M., & Guo, J. (2020). A deep learning algorithm using CT images to screen for Corona Virus Disease (COVID-19). medRxiv. doi:10.1101/2020.02.14.20023028

Waringa, Lindvallc, & Umeton. (2020). *Automated machine learning*. Academic Press.

Web, M. D. (2021, July 1). *Variants of Coronavirus.* https://www.webmd.com/lung/coronavirus-strains#3

Website. (2020). *Computed Tomography (CT) - Chest.* https://www.radiologyinfo.org/en/info

WHO reports fivefold increase in cyber attacks, urges vigilance. (2020). *WHO.* https://www.who.int/news/item/23-04-2020-who-reports-fivefold-increase-in-cyber-attacks-urges-vigilance

Wickramaarachchi, W. P. T. M., & Perera, S. S. (2021). An SIER model to estimate optimal transmission rate and initial parameters of COVD-19 dynamic in Sri Lanka. *Alexandria Engineering Journal, 60*(1), 1557–1563. doi:10.1016/j.aej.2020.11.010

Wikipedia contributors. (2021a, July 1). COVID-19 pandemic in India. In *Wikipedia, The Free Encyclopedia*. Retrieved 18:55, July 1, 2021, from https://en.wikipedia.org/w/index.php?title=COVID-19_pandemic_in_India&oldid=1031367334

Wikipedia contributors. (2021b, June 29). Timeline of the COVID-19 pandemic in India (2021). In *Wikipedia, The Free Encyclopedia*. Retrieved 18:56, July 1, 2021, from https://en.wikipedia.org/w/index.php?title=Timeline_of_the_CO-VID-19_pandemic_in_India_(2021)&oldid=1030989391

Wikipedia contributors. (2021c, July 1). COVID-19 pandemic in India. In *Wikipedia, The Free Encyclopedia*. Retrieved 19:05, July 1, 2021, from https://en.wikipedia.org/w/index.php?title=COVID-19_pandemic_in_India&oldid=1031367334

Wong & Wang. (2020). *Covid-net: A tailored deep convolutional neural network design for detection of covid-19 cases from chest radiography images.* arXiv preprint arXiv:2003.09871.

World Economic Forum. (2021, July 1). *How COVID-19 deepens the digital education divide in India.* https://www.weforum.org/agenda/2020/10/how-covid-19-deepens-the-digital-education-divide-in-india/

World Health Organization. (2020). *WHO Coronavirus Disease (COVID-19) Dashboard.* https://covid19.who.int/

World Health. (2020). *Contact tracing apps: Which countries are doing what.* https://health.economictimes.indiatimes.com/news/diagnostics/contact-tracing-apps-which-countries-are-doing-what/75440095

Wu, F., Zhao, S., Yu, B., Chen, Y.-M., Wang, W., Song, Z.-G., Hu, Y., Tao, Z.-W., Tian, J.-H., Pei, Y.-Y., Yuan, M.-L., Zhang, Y.-L., Dai, F.-H., Liu, Y., Wang, Q.-M., Zheng, J.-J., Xu, L., Holmes, E. C., & Zhang, Y.-Z. (2020). 'A new coronavirus associated with human respiratory disease in china'. *Nature, 579*(7798), 265–284. doi:10.103841586-020-2008-3 PMID:32015508

Wu, J. T., Leung, K., Bushman, M., Kishore, N., Niehus, R., de Salazar, P. M., Cowling, B. J., Lipsitch, M., & Leung, G. M. (2020). Estimating the clinical severity of COVID-19 from the transmission dynamics in Wuhan, China. *Nature Medicine, Vol, 26*(4), 506–510. doi:10.103841591-020-0822-7 PMID:32284616

Wynants, L. (2020). Prediction models for diagnosis and prognosis of covid-19 infection: a systematic review and critical appraisal. *BMJ Open, 369*, 1-11.

Xu, B. (2020). Epidemiological data from the COVID-19 outbreak, real-time case information. Nature, 7(106), 1-6.

Xu, B. (2020). Epidemiological data from the COVID-19 outbreak, real-time case information. *Scientific Data, 7*,106.

Xu, X., Jiang, X., & Ma, C. (2020). *Deep learning system to screen coronavirus disease 2019 pneumonia.* https://arxiv.org/abs/2002.09334

Xu, Y., Li, X., Zhu, B., Liang, H., Fang, C., Gong, Y., Guo, Q., Sun, X., Zhao, D., Shen, J., Zhang, H., Liu, H., Xia, H., Tang, J., Zhang, K., & Gong, S. (2020). Characteristics of pediatric SARS-CoV-2 infection and potential evidence for persistent fecal viral shedding. *Nature Medicine, Vol, 26*(4), 502–505. doi:10.103841591-020-0817-4 PMID:32284613

Yan, L., & Zhang, H.-T. (2020). A machine learning-based model for survival prediction in patients with severe CO-VID-19 infection. doi:10.1101/2020.02.27.20028027

Yang, Z. (2020). Modified SEIR and AI prediction of the trend of the epidemic of COVID-19 in China under public health interventions. *Journal of Thoracic Disease,* 1-18.

Yang, Zeng, Wang, Wong, Liang, & Zanin. (2020). Modified SEIR and AI prediction of the epidemics trend of COVID-19 in China under public health interventions. *J Thorac Dis 2020, 12*(3), 165.

Yang, B., Cao, J., Ni, R., & Zhang, Y. (2018). Facial Expression Recognition Using Weighted Mixture Deep Neural Network Based on Double-Channel Facial Images. *IEEE Access: Practical Innovations, Open Solutions, 6,* 4630–4640.

Yan, Y., Huang, Y., Chen, S., Shen, C., & Wang, H. (2020). Joint Deep Learning of Facial Expression Synthesis and Recognition. *IEEE Transactions on Multimedia, 22*(11), 2792–2807.

Yao & Leng. (2020). *Introduction to Computer Vision with Watson and OpenCV.* https://www.coursera.org/learn/introduction-computer-vision-watson-opencv/

Yu & Koltun. (2016). *Multi-scale context aggregation by dilated convolutions.* Academic Press.

Yuang, S.-L., Han, L. T., & Ma, Z. E. (2001). A kind of epidemic model having infectious force in both latent period and infected period. *J. Biomath., 16*(4), 392–398.

Zhang, G., & Liu, X. (2020). Prediction and control of COVID-19 infection based on a hybrid intelligent model. doi:10.1101/2020.10.22.20218032

Zhang, C., Wang, X., & Li, X. (2010). Design of Monitoring and Control Plant Disease System Based on DSP&FPGA. *Second International Conference on Networks Security, Wireless Communications and Trusted Computing.*

Zhang, K., Huang, Y., Du, Y., & Wang, L. (2017). Facial Expression Recognition Based on Deep Evolutional Spatial-Temporal Networks. *IEEE Transactions on Image Processing, 26*(9), 4193–4203.

Zhang, S., Tjortjis, C., Zeng, X., Qiao, H., Buchan, I., & Keane, J. (2009). Comparing data mining methods with logistic regression in childhood obesity prediction. *Information Systems Frontiers, 11*(4), 449–460. doi:10.100710796-009-9157-0

Zhang, Z., Sheng, C., Ma, Z., & Li, D. (2004). The outbreak pattern of the SARS cases in Asia. *Chinese Science Bulletin, 49*(17), 1819–1823. doi:10.1007/BF03183407 PMID:32214712

Zheng, Du, Wang, Zhang, Cui, Kang, Yang, Lou, Chi, Long, Ma, Yuan, Zhang, Zhang, Ye, & Xin. (2020). *Predicting COVID-19 in China Using Hybrid AI Model.* IEEE.). doi:10.1109/TCYB.2020.2990162

Zhou, P., Yang, X.-L., Wang, X.-G., Hu, B., Zhang, L., Zhang, W., Si, H.-R., Zhu, Y., Li, B., Huang, C.-L., Chen, H.-D., Chen, J., Luo, Y., Guo, H., Jiang, R.-D., Liu, M.-Q., Chen, Y., Shen, X.-R., Wang, X., ... Shi, Z.-L. (2020). A pneumonia outbreak associated with a new coronavirus of probable bat origin. *Nature, 579*(7798), 270–289. doi:10.103841586-020-2012-7 PMID:32015507

About the Contributors

Kanishk Bansal is a Research Scholar pursuing Ph.D. in computer applications with AI as the area of research.

Snigdha Behara is an electronics engineer turned user experience designer who advocates for social causes through her innovation and design. She is an advocate for mental health and hopes to destigmatize it by initiating important conversations.

Sandeep Chaurasia is working in the department of CSE, School of Computing & I.T. in Manipal University Jaipur since November 2020. He completed his PhD (Engineering) in 2014 in the area of Supervised Machine Learning and M. Tech in Computer Science in the year 2009. He has done his B.E. in Computer Engineering in the year 2006. He has around 13 years of rich experience in academics and one year in industry. He has more than more than 30 publications in International / national journals/ conference proceedings. He has 4 software copyright in his account. He is a SMIEEE, LMCSI, MACM and member of Machine Intelligence Research labs - USA. He is also member of reviewer board of various journals and technical program committee of several reputed conferences. His research interests include Machine Learning and Soft Computing and other areas of interest are Algorithms, Artificial Intelligence. He is associated with Machine Learning for more than 9 years. Currently working in the area of application of machine / Deep learning in natural language processing like semantic analysis & lexical analysis. He has guided 1 PhD and guiding 4 PhD students in the area of NLP, Intrusion detection, food adulteration using AI techniques. He is also active member of special interest group and initiative by MIR labs to connect the researchers & professional across the globe. He is active cooperate relation and faculty placement coordinator in department of computer science & engineering, He has conducted various campus drives and assist students to achieve quality placements.

Gowhar Dar has a master's in computer applications (MCA) from the University of Kashmir. Gowhar Mohiuddin is a research scholar at Lovely Professional University Punjab and is currently working on diagnosis and detection of Alzheimer's diseases using deep learning.

Megha Nain is currently working as an Assistant Professor in the Department of Computer Science and Engineering at Poornima University Jaipur since July 2021. She is pursuing her PhD degree in the domain of Computer Vision and Deep Learning at Manipal University Jaipur since January 2020. She completed her master's, MSc. Tech in Industrial Mathematics and Computer Applications from Jamia Millia Islamia University, Delhi, in the year 2015 and B.Sc. Mathematics (honours) from Delhi University, in the year 2011. Previously she worked as an Assistant Professor in the department of CSE at NIMS University, Jaipur for a year and worked in the IT sector for more than 3 years. Along with her PhD work, she also reviews various scientific journals such as IEEE Access and the International Journal of Intelligent Systems. Her research interests include Computer Vision and Deep Learning.

Sonia Rani is PhD Scholar at Lovely Professional University Punjab India. Her Research interest is applied machine learning data analytics and natural language processing.

Gaurav K. Roy received his Master's degree from Lovely Professional University, India & Application Security Engineering from EC Council University, USA. He is a data privacy and security researcher by hobby, Sr. Content Developer by profession, and an international trainer by passion. This gold-medalist has a deep interest in the security and data analysis domain for the past six years. He has provided freelance security to government and private organizations of his country. His Hall of Fames, Acknowledgement emails, and Bug bounties are proof of that. He has also reviewed many online courses and tutorials on cybersecurity, game development, programming and authored many e-learning tutorials on top platforms as well. He has more than 3.5 lacs students worldwide, and his online courses and study materials on different platforms are some of the most viewed courses in the e-learning industry. He has recently got the record holder title in the India Book of Records. He is also a published author of the Book named: Cybersecurity and Digital Privacy – A Universal Approach. Last, but not least, he has published more than 14 research papers in national &international journals.

Sreelakshmi S. has completed her Master of Philosophy (M.Phil.) in Computer Science with a specialization in Medical Image Processing, from the Indian Institute of Information Technology and Management - Kerala (IIITM-K) under Cochin University of Science and Technology (CUSAT). She has also completed her Masters and Bachelors in Computer Science from Kannur University. Sreelakshmi has also obtained her Master of Arts Degree in Psychology from Indira Gandhi National Open University (IGNOU), New Delhi, India. Her research interests include Cognitive computing, Computational Psychology, and Medical Image Processing.

Shilpa Sharma is presently working as Associate Professor in the department of Computer Applications at Manipal University Jaipur. She has completed her PhD (Computer Science) in 2013 in Software Engineering. She has done her MCA in the year 2006. She has around 15 years of rich experience in academics and 8 years of post-PhD experience. She has more than more than 20 publications in International / national journals/conference proceedings. Her research interests include Software Engineering, AI and its applications and Image Processing. She has guided 3 PhD and guiding 3 PhD students in Deep Learning and Cyber Security. She is also member of reviewer board of various journals and technical program committee of several reputed conferences.

Ashok Sharma, MS (Computer Science), Ph.D. (Machine Learning and Cloud Computing), has 18 Years of Teaching Experiences in Higher Education and He has worked in Various Reputed Institution of Higher Learning in India in different capacity. His area of Interest is Machine Learning, Cloud Computing and Data Science. He is certified in Beidou Technology from Shanghai Jio Tong University ,Shanghai, Leveraging Technology for Effective Teaching in the Classroom and Beyond from International Institute of Information Technology, Bangalore, Internet of Things and Introduction to Big Data from

University of California San Diego. He has attended 30+ DST/AICTE sponsored Training in different Technologies and He is presently holding position of Associate Professor in School of Computer Science and Engineering, Lovely Professional University, Phagwara, India and 8 PhD Scholars are working under his guidance in the area of Cloud Computing, Data Science and Cognitive Behaviour Analysis.

Rahul Sharma with 9 years of teaching experience and is working as Assistant Professor, Department of Computer Applications, Govt. Degree College Kathua, J&K, India. Mr. Rahul Sharma is doing his research work from School of Computer Applications, Lovely Professional University Jalandhar, Punjab, India under the guidence of Dr. Amar Singh.

Amar Singh is working as Associate Professor at School of Computer Applications, Lovely Professional University Jalandhar, Punjab, India. He has published international research papers in reputed international journals. Proposed new efficent algorithms and apporaches in fields like Artificial Intelligence, Wireless Mesh Networks, Soft Computing etc. Dr. Amar Singh has been involved in imparting hands-on training in different workshops on different topics of Machine Learning and Soft Computing.

Sudip Singh is working as UP Government officer in Power Sector on SAP Project. Have about 15 years of work experience in IT and power. Worked with Accenture on Microsoft Business Intelligence Technologies. Holds various technology certifications MCTS (Microsoft Certified Technology Specialist), MCPDEA etc. Passionate about Data Science and Machine Learning. Holds B.Tech Degree in Computer Science.

Chandan Tanvi Mandapati is pursuing her MS in Statistics and Data Analytics from Lovely Professional University (2020-2022). She is a certified data analyst from IABAC and is a member of various data science associations. She writes mainly on the use of machine learning models for medical concerns and promotes the usage of Artificially Intelligent methodologies paired with Visual Analytics.

Anoop V. S. has completed his Doctor of Philosophy (Ph.D.) and Master of Philosophy (M.Phil.) from the Indian Institute of Information Technology and Management - Kerala (IIITM-K) under Cochin University of Science and Technology (CUSAT). Anoop is currently working as a Senior Scientist (Research & Training) at Kerala Blockchain Academy under Kerala University of Digital Sciences, Innovation and Technology. In his previous role, he worked as an Assistant Professor in Computer Science at Rajagiri College of Social Sciences, Kochi. He has also worked as a Senior Data Scientist with CogTalk at Dubai Future Accelerator for implementing Artificial Intelligence solutions for Etisalat Digital and Etihad Airways. Anoop is an experienced Software Engineer with more than five years of experience working with US-based MNCs in Technopark, Thiruvananthapuram. He has completed many industry internships on Artificial Intelligence and implemented text mining algorithms to solve complex business problems. Anoop's research interests are primarily in Applied Text Mining, Information Retrieval, and Blockchain. He has several publications in his credit that include edited books, book chapters, articles in international journals, and conference proceedings.

Index

U

V

W

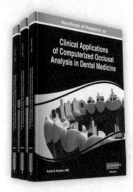
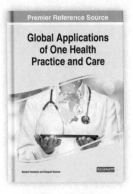
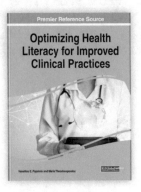
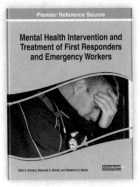
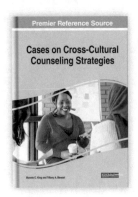
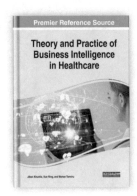
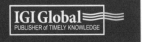

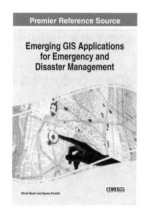
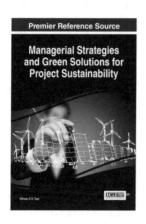
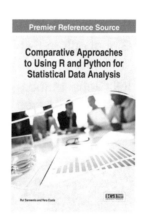
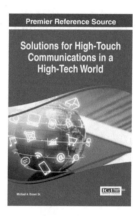